THE GREAT BOOK OF BUSINESS SECRETS

10 9 8 7 6 5 4 3 2 1

Boardroom® Classics publishes the advice of expert authorities in
many fields. But the use of this material is not a substitute for
legal, accounting, or other professional services. Consult a
competent professional for answers to your specific questions.

Library of Congress Cataloging-in-Publication Data
The Great Book of Business Secrets
    p.cm.
    Includes index.
    ISBN 0-88723-050-4

Boardroom® Classics is a registered trademark of
Boardroom® Reports, Inc.
330 W. 42nd Street, New York, NY 10036

Printed in the United States of America

THE GREAT BOOK OF BUSINESS SECRETS

Contents

Contents v

vi Contents

Contents vii

viii Contents

x Contents

Contents xiii

xiv Contents

6 • EXECUTIVE LIFE

Part I

**THE GREAT BOOK
OF BUSINESS SECRETS**

Effective Management Techniques

Chapter 1
Managing People

What Makes An Effective Manager?

There is no such thing as one single effective executive personality. Those effective executives vary widely in temperament, operating style, abilities, knowledge, and interests. What they do have in common are certain practices. The key ones:

1. Know where their time goes. In any organization, executives have little control over their time. The trick is to systematically manage whatever time can be brought under their own control.

2. Focus on results.

3. Build on strengths. Capitalize on their own and those of their superiors, colleagues and subordinates.

4. Concentrate on the few major areas where superior performance will produce outstanding results. They set priorities, follow them.

5. Make decisions based on dissenting opinions. To judge, alternatives from which to choose are important. Dissent brings these out.

Source: Peter F. Drucker, *The Effective Executive*, Harper & Row, New York.

Leadership Skills

Management-training courses help executives sharpen existing skills and may encourage them to acquire others. But training rarely gives them the type of inherent interpersonal skills needed to manage a dynamic company successfully.

Some of the most critical managerial talents:

■Ability to use their power and personality to change their own style when necessary and to influence others.

■Courage to make a decision when risk is present.

■Capability to motivate others by knowing when to exert their power and when to avoid the use of it.

■Endurance. Training courses can teach executives time-management techniques, but the techniques can't keep them alert during a 12-hour day.

■Objectivity. It's virtually impossible to teach managers to avoid their own biases when evaluating others.

■Optimism.

Source: George E. Manners, Jr., of Rensselaer Polytechnic Institute, and Joseph A. Steger, director of human resources, Colt Industries, Inc., quoted in *Inside R&D*, Fort Lee, NJ.

Improving Leadership Abilities

■Make decisions that support independent employee behavior within organizational limits.

■Take time each day to think about general business and social trends. Then look for ways the company can benefit from them.

■Learn more about individual subordinates to better match their jobs to their goals and abilities.

■Review your most recent decisions. If too many were risk-free, it could be a danger sign.

■Note the dimensions of recent changes. If all were minor, it might be a sign of reluctance to change.

■Evaluate all your current duties to see whether delegating some of them to subordinates might help develop their abilities.

Source: Donald B. Miller, *Working with People*, CBI Publishing, Boston.

Leadership And Outstanding Leadership

Most people have the ability to lead others, but won't do it unless they find themselves in a situation that gets them excited enough to take the reins. Finding the ideal opportunity for leadership skills to flourish is tough enough. But it's only half the battle. Once you're in the right spot, you must pay attention to five basic rules of outstanding leadership...

1. Challenge the ways things are done. Maintaining the status quo breeds mediocre performance. At its best, it's management—keeping things operating smoothly, efficiently and under control—not leadership. Leaders look for ways to radically improve the way the organization works. That doesn't mean 5%–20% improvements—it means hundreds of percent gains.

The first step is to search for opportunities for significant change. A leader won't necessarily have to come up with the idea and the solution, however. Challenges seek out leaders as well as the other way around. Many of the best leaders are thrust into the situation in which they wind up performing at their best.

The Patricia M. Carrigan story: She became the first woman assembly plant manager in the history of General Motors in 1982. She was initially puzzled and worried about the assignment. As a trained clinical psychologist, she had spent more time in education than in the auto industry at the time she took charge of the Lakewood plant with a troubled labor history. Within two years, Lakewood was transformed. Absenteeism was down from 25% to 9% (saving more than $8 million annually). Sickness and accident costs were cut by two-thirds. Grievances, which had once totaled more than 5,500 cases, were down to nearly zero.

Carrigan involved the workers in making changes and spent time explaining why new performance standards were necessary, asking for workers' ideas, and training them to meet the new requirements. When Carrigan was eventually reassigned to another plant, the union local gave her a plaque that said, in part: "...we, the members of Local 34, honor Pat M. Carrigan for her leadership, courage, risk-taking and honesty...we will always warmly remember Pat M. Carrigan as one of us."

Critical to fomenting change: Experimenting and taking risks. That means keeping communication channels open for new products, processes and services to flow into the organization. Keep up contact with people actually doing the work to uncover better ideas on improving the process.

Successful leaders are quick to point to past mistakes as essential to their ultimate success. Ski instructors say, "If you're not falling, you're not learning."

Essential: Endurance in the face of stress. Leaders take stress in stride. When they encounter a stressful event, they consider it interesting...feel they can influence its outcome...and see it as an opportunity for development.

2. Create a vision that others can identify with. Vision can be called a personal agenda, purpose, legacy, dream or goal—but leaders know it as a clear sense of direction. Vince Lombardi said of good coaching: "If you don't know what the end result is supposed to look like, you can't get there."

For leaders, end results begin as impressions, but become more concrete as they have to explain them to those they are working with. The head of Diamond Shamrock described what a leader needed in a rapidly changing environment as "a simple compass—which indicates the general direction to be taken and allows you to use your own ingenuity in overcoming various difficulties."

The next step is being able to communicate that vision so that others can be excited about working toward it. That happens, however, only if followers find the purpose appealing.

Trap: Trying to make visions out of mundane matters such as job descriptions or product specifications. To find the broadest common ground in an organization, the vision must transcend day-to-day work and uplift—even ennoble—human aspirations.

3. Enable others to act. Leaders make the people they work with feel like owners—not hired hands. They know that relationships are the keys to maximizing support for their projects—and they make sure that when they win, everyone wins.

Example: As executive vice president of Springfield Remanufacturing Center Corporation, Mike Carrigan first worked up his own budget projections. But he then involved everyone down the line in the company's planning by asking each manager and supervisor to be personally responsible for verifying the accuracy of one of his projections.

For several weeks, the managers went around the plant asking employees about their needs, testing assumptions, double-checking with suppliers and buyers. Then, when they came back with their findings, Carrigan told them that their findings would be accepted as the budget figures for the coming fiscal year. They had to set their own budgets and they had to live with them. If they wanted to complain, they had to complain to themselves.

People will work wholeheartedly only with a leader they trust—so a leader must be the first to demonstrate commitment and trustworthiness. When a would-be leader doesn't fulfill a promise, it is virtually impossible to rebuild relationships with others. There is always a nagging feeling of doubt about credibility.

Executives who have a hard time trusting others often fail as leaders because they view the world around them as filled with competitors—people whose interests are opposed to their own. That makes them unwilling (or unable) to build strong teams. As a result, their missions often fail.

4. Show others the way by setting an example. If leaders ask followers to observe certain standards, they have to live by the same rules.

Example: Betsy Sanders, an executive at the Nordstrom retailing firm, remembers when the owner, Bruce Nordstrom, walked through her department one day, overheard a conversation between two customers and then came to her and said "See those two ladies over there? They say they're unhappy about something in the store. Find out what it is and see if we can fix it!"

Sanders found out that the women liked two dresses in an expensive department of the store but couldn't afford them. She brought the women down to the moderate-price dress department and helped them make a selection.

Hours later, Nordstrom took a break from a major negotiation meeting to stop by Sanders' department and check with her about what the customers wanted and what she had done about it. This display of concern for the customer by the owner impressed Sanders enormously.

The incident was over ten years ago, but Sanders still remembers it in her day-to-day work at the firm.

5. Recognize and reward accomplishments. Leaders bring out the best in people—getting them to achieve more than they themselves believed they could accomplish. They don't give up on people because doing so means to them that they're giving up on themselves. To get people to persist and to achieve extraordinary results, they provide clear directions, substantial encouragement, personal attention and constant feedback.

It's important to give rewards not only when the job is completed, but to punctuate the experience with small wins to provide momentum, and to reinforce people's understanding of the company's definition of high standards and outstanding achievement.

Source: Barry Posner, Ph.D., associate professor of management and director of graduate education, Leavey School of Business and Administration, Santa Clara University, Santa Clara, CA 95053 and coauthor, with James M. Kouzes, of *The Leadership Challenge,* Jossey-Bass, 350 Sansome St., San Francisco 94104.

Manager? Leader? There Is A Big Difference

Nineteenth-century America was notable for its adventurers and its writers—the titans who made the industrial revolution, the explorers who opened up the West, the writers who defined us as a nation and a people.

Twentieth-century America started to build on the promise of their accomplishments, but something went wrong. Since World War II, the U.S. has been notable chiefly for its bureaucrats and managers, its organization men, its wheeler-dealers who have remade, and in some cases, unmade, the institutions of America. But...where are the leaders who will build America's future greatness?

How Businesses Buried Leadership

■By emphasizing management instead of pioneering. Many U.S. companies are well-managed but poorly led. Managers may be handling each day's routine tasks well, but no one asks...should "this" be done at all?

Problem: Routine work smothers creative planning and change. Also, because a routine is the easiest to deal with, there's an unconscious conspiracy to immerse ourselves in routine and avoid the tough questions, or to leave them to someone else. That's not leadership. Part of the fault lies with our schools of management. We teach people how to be good technicians or staff people. We don't train them for leadership.

■By insisting on harmony. Most organizations, by their very nature, strive too much for harmony. Their cohesiveness depends on a commonly held set of values, beliefs, norms and attitudes. Anyone who does not share the common culture is considered an outsider, a deviant.

Problem: Unanimity leads to stagnation. It's the deviant, the individual who sees things differently, who is the company's vital link to change and adaptation. Every leader, like King Lear, needs at least one Fool to challenge what is sacred and to herald the advent of cosmic shifts. But too many companies would rather risk obsolescence than make room for the nonconformists in their midst.

Breeding Leadership

To break through the barriers to strong leadership, companies must look for top executives with rare qualities…

■Talent for managing the dream. Leaders can create a compelling vision that takes people to a new place…and then translate that vision into reality. Managing the dream can be broken down into five parts…communicating the vision (Johnson & Johnson's James Burke spent 40% of his time communicating the company founder General Johnson's credo to 800 managers who debated every line), recruiting meticulously, rewarding, retraining and reorganizing.

Example: SAS Airline's CEO, Jan Carlzon, has a vision to make SAS one of the few air carriers to still be in existence in the year 2000. To accomplish this vision, he developed two goals…

1. To make SAS 1% better than its competitors in a hundred different ways.

2. To create a market niche.

He chose the business travelers. To attract them, he broke away from the traditional pyramid-shaped organization chart and created small, autonomous work groups. He put in profit-sharing plans and charged the groups with making every single interaction with customers into a meaningful "moment of truth."

■Ability to manage risk. Good leaders create an atmosphere where risk-taking is encouraged. As successful film producer Sydney Pollack tells his people, the only mistake is to do nothing.

■Ability to encourage reflective backtalk. Real leaders know the importance of having someone around who will tell them the truth. Almost all of the CEOs I've interviewed were still married to their first wives or husbands. I think the reason may be that the spouse is the one person a leader can really trust. The backtalk is reflective because it allows the leader to learn, to find out more about himself or herself.

■Intense curiosity. That growth is partly fueled by boundless curiosity. They read, look, explore, wonder, make connections. They know that the world is not static and they like to get out and talk to people who speak with different voices. In their jobs, they spend time in the field, looking at their own operations, talking with workers and customers. They want honest, valid feedback. That keeps them fresh, and gives the company new energy.

■Intense optimism. All successful leaders possess optimism, faith and hope. Ronald Reagan was a good example. When pollster Richard Wirthlin had to break it to the President that his approval rating, which hit record highs at the time of his assassination attempt, had fallen to an all-time low for any President in his second year of office, Reagan, with his eternal optimism, quipped: "Don't worry. I'll just go out there and try to get assassinated again."

Optimism and hope provide choices. Jimmy Carter was done in by his despairing "malaise" speech. He depressed us. Reagan, whatever his other flaws, gave us hope. Another example is comedian George Burns who said, "I can't die…I'm booked."

■Maintain high standards for subordinates. Leaders expect the best of the people around them. Most subordinates do what they believe they are expected to do. Jaime Escalante, a Los Angeles teacher, believed that students in a Los Angeles inner-city school could learn calculus…and they did.

■The Gretzky factor. Wayne Gretzky, the best hockey player of his generation, said that it's not as important to know where the puck is now as to know where it will be. Leaders know where markets and societies are going next, and where the organization must be if it is to grow.

■Take the long view. Good leaders have patience. Armand Hammer, at 89, set his long-range plans for only 10 years in advance because he wanted to be around to see them happen. One Japanese company has a 250-year plan. Michael Eisner of Disney has long been preparing for the 1992 European market.

■Create strategic alliances and partnerships—especially international ones. The shrewd leaders of the future will recognize the importance of creating alliances with other organizations whose fates are correlated with their own. Thus, the Norwegian counterpart of Federal Express is setting up a partnership with Federal Express. We're seeing many new joint ventures between U.S. companies and foreign partners.

Source: Warren Bennis, distinguished professor of business administration at the University of Southern California, and consultant to many large companies. He is the author of *Why Leaders Can't Lead,* Jossey-Bass Publishers, 350 Sansome St., San Francisco 94104, and *On Becoming a Leader,* Addison-Wesley Publishing, Reading, MA 01867.

Key Skills For Managers

■Interest in improving the way things are done.
■Continuing desire to initiate.
■Confidence in abilities and goals.
■Ability to develop, counsel and help others improve.
■Concern with the impact managerial actions have on the activities of others.
■Capacity to get others to follow the manager's lead.
■Knowledge of how to inspire teamwork.
■Capability of influencing others to form alliances or teams.
■Faith in others.
■Skill in oral and written communication.
■Tendency to put business needs before personal needs.
■Spontaneity of expression.
■Objectivity in a dispute.
■Knowledge of own strengths and weaknesses.
■Adaptability to change.
■Mental stamina to put in long hours.
■Logical thought.
■Ability to use information to create new, meaningful concepts.

Source: *International Management,* New York.

How Successful Managers Use Power

They share power with less-powerful employees. Aim: To extend decision-making to the individuals most affected by decisions.

...They downplay thier own power. Aim: To foster collaboration with co-workers who have less power. To do that, they must not only share power with co-workers, but they must de-emphasize their own superiority. This promotes equality, which in turn allows for constructive pooling of talents and resources between managers and subordinates.

...They use power for collective benefit. Instead of abusing power for personal gain, successful managers use power to make decisions that benefit the company as a whole.

...They practice restraint. Instead of reminding people at every opportunity about how much power they possess, successful managers give others the opportunity to influence events and take credit. Aim: To enhance morale by encouraging initiative and avoiding excessive control.

Source: Jay Hall, business psychologist, and president of management education consultants, Telemetrics International, Woodlands, TX, writing in *Management World,* 2360 Maryland Rd., Willow Grove, PA 19090.

Best Ways To Earn Respect And Trust

Managers' effectiveness depends heavily on the opinions of others about them.

Challenge: Making a good impression requires knowledge about how people form judgments about you.

Key Factors

Making a positive impression depends upon your ability to demonstrate...

■Credibility. You must deliver on promises and give accurate information about resources you need, completion dates, quality of the service you render, etc. Credibility also stems from technical skill and knowledge and who endorses you.

When, for example, a respected member of the organization says you are outstanding, that helps establish your credibility.

■Respect for other people's status. Most people are as sensitive to their status as they are to their economic interests. They need respect and recognition. In business, that means they seek deference...

1. They want to learn important information earlier rather than later.

2. They expect behavior from others that underscores their worth in the organization. Simply stopping by to chat informally with subordinates or peers indicates that you consider the relationships important. When you also share a new (and not publicly available) piece of information, you demonstrate respect for their status.

Relationships of mutual respect are almost always characterized by reciprocity—you give as much as you get. You don't keep telling other people what to do. You ask them for their opinions and ideas. You don't keep asking for things. You give as well. You place other people's goals on a par with your own. People who master these techniques earn enormous respect from important people in the company.

■Mastery of important social norms and symbols. People and groups differ in preferred styles of speaking (how formal, how much or little jargon, references to sports or families, etc.). To be effective, you must understand these norms and integrate them into your everyday interactions.

Example of how one executive earned respect and acclaim by his carefully crafted presentation...Directors still remember a talk given by a senior Kellogg executive several years ago. With colorful slides and other graphics, Horst Schroeder gave them a glimpse of his comprehensive grasp of the business. They gave him an ovation. He knew Kellogg so well...he could even remember some piece of equipment located in Sydney, Australia—and the cost of it. According to one insider: "You came away from meeting Horst feeling, 'This guy is going to take the company to new heights.'" (*Wall Street Journal,* 11/28/89.)

That's an example of an executive who knew what language to speak—how to impress the people whose respect he wanted to earn.

■Sensitivity to personality nuances. Individuals differ in how long they speak, the duration of comfortable pauses, how willing they are to listen to comments from others and even how frequently they wish to speak. To impress another person, you must be able to synchronize your speech pattern with that of the other person.

Also important is the ability to observe when the other person is disturbed by the interaction and shows stress (longer silences, unresponsiveness, looking away or becoming agitated). When you synchronize your own communication with that of others, you prevent them from becoming stressed.

■Persistence. Building favorable impressions requires reasonably frequent contacts with the people you're trying to impress. What is reasonable depends on the situation and how close the relationship is presumed to be. With a colleague, it might be daily, with a peer, every week or two, with an important outsider, it might be once or twice a month or just once a year.

What's important is that the contact not be solely dependent on the literal meaning of what you say. You must demonstrate all the components that go into making a favorable impression.

Source: Dr. Leonard R. Sayles, professor of management, Columbia University Graduate School of Business, New York and director, executive leadership research, Center for Creative Leadership, Greensboro, NC 27407.

Daily Coaching

Effective coaching is a day-to-day, not a once-a-year activity. The more time managers spend in a supportive role with subordinates, rather than doing work or telling them how to do it, the better the results will be. Important: The subordinate's role must be participative, not passive. A successful program requires involvement and commitment from the employee. The manager should tell the employee what's expected...provide assistance and support...offer feedback on performance...and reward on the basis of results.

Source: *Managerial Leadership in Perspective: Getting Back to Basics* by Burt K. Scanlan, professor of management, University of Oklahoma, Norman, OK 73069.

Six Keys To Effective Management/ Six Keys To Ineffective Management ...Your Choice

■When forced into an argument, ask an irrelevant question and lean back with a smug grin while your opponent tries to figure out what's going on. Then quickly change the subject.

■Listen intently while others are arguing a problem. Then pounce on a trite statement and bury them with it.

■Hire a brilliant assistant but keep him out of sight and out of the limelight.

■Walk briskly. That keeps questions from subordinates and superiors at a minimum.

■Keep your office door closed. That puts visitors on the defensive and gives the appearance that you're always in an important meeting.

■Always give orders verbally. That reduces the opportunity for potential rivals to accumulate a "Pearl Harbor" file.

Source: IBM Systems Science Institute, 11601 Wilshire Blvd., Los Angeles 90025.

Hard-Driving Managers

Hard-driving managers are valuable, but only to a point. They get maximum productivity from subordinates because their striving for perfection forces them to settle for nothing less than top performance. Trap: Driven managers are often plagued by a subconscious sense of inadequacy. They therefore drive harder to compensate for the inadequacies. Result: They expect too much of themselves and their subordinates. They ultimately exhaust themselves and force subordinates to quit in frustration. When that starts happening to a manager, it's time to talk to him about easing up. If that doesn't work, your choices may be limited.

Source: *The Levinson Letter,* 375 Concord Ave., Belmont, MA 02178.

An Open Door Isn't Enough

A manager who thinks he keeps an open door for workers should ask how often subordinates really walk in with problems. If the answer is "not often," the manager must do more to overcome workers' reluctance to bring bad news to the boss. Example: Schedule regular meetings with worker representatives from various departments to hear worker concerns. Make sure workers understand they are free to speak without fear of retribution. Then set a date by which management will answer all comments. Payoff: The most highly motivated workers are those who believe management does things for them as well as to them.

Source: Joyce S. Anderson, Anderson Associates, Margate, NJ, quoted in *Personnel Journal,* 245 Fischer Ave., Costa Mesa, CA 92626.

A Successful Manager

The ability to criticize constructively without destroying the recipient's morale is a key to management success. Important: Criticize the individual's behavior, not the individual, personally...Base criticism on specific criteria...Decide what improvement is realistic, and in what time frame...Choose the right time and the right place to deliver criticism...Involve the individual in a discussion, rather than deliver a lecture...State the solution you expect and how that solution will benefit the person.

Source: Hendrie Weisinger, Ph.D., author of *The Critical Edge,* Little, Brown & Co., 34 Beacon St., Boston, MA 02108.

Good Managers Get More Done

The word "manager" is widely misunderstood and frequently misused in the business world. A manager is not the same as an executive, though "manager" is used to refer to both. Problem: This clouds many would-be top executives' understanding of the tough process of growing from a manager into an executive.

Managers get things done. Executives decide what is worth doing. Many young managers think of themselves as executives, when in fact, their job is to get things done.

At The Beginning

Most important for new managers: Knowledge about the business of their company. As non-managerial professionals, they focus on a trade—engineering, accounting, etc. Professionals read trade journals and academic documents to learn more about their profession. However, when they become managers, their focus shifts to the company they work for. Their first job is learning everything there is to know about the company.

Preeminent on-the-job lesson for managers, on the way to becoming executives: Leadership. Good leadership isn't hereditary. Leadership is learned. It consists of...

■Communication. In any company, there are differences in people's skills, knowledge and values. The leader's job is to capitalize on differences and maximize each individual's contribution to the corporate purpose.

Example: A subordinate with no experience in an assignment given to him by a manager requires complete, understandable instruction to successfully finish the project. The manager who fails to provide such instruction will invariably blame the subordinate when the project fails, when in fact only the manager is to blame.

■Motivation. Leaders can't actually motivate subordinates, because only individuals can motivate themselves. The good leader, however, molds the workplace to allow motivated individuals to achieve more. He creates challenge, promotes growth, fosters accomplishment.

■Commitment. Commitment from subordinates comes from agreement. Agreement occurs when workers identify their own goals and values with those of the company and its managers. They are committed when they all agree on common goals.

Creating Systems

In order to grow from a manager to an executive, the manager must master the skill of creating systems. Systems are the tools of efficiency that enable a boss at any level to achieve results. The creation and management of systems grows increasingly complex and far-reaching as the learning curve from manger to executive is traveled.

Example: A new manager may have 10 people with basic assembly jobs he must coordinate. An executive may have many times that both inside the company and outside—bankers, accountants, vendors, key customers, etc.

Creating systems to run such increasingly complex business variables requires creativity, experimentation and vision. As individuals progress along the learning curve, they capitalize on systems to enhance their ability to manage more diversity.

Diversity Is Opportunity

An essential component of effective executive performance is the ability to handle and take advantage of diversity. Lower-level managers have minimal diversity—their job is to make the corporate machinery run. Their choices in doing so are few—and are usually relatively simple.

Executive decisions are more complex. Executive vision starts with creative thinking. Perhaps more than any single trait, respect for differences characterizes executives. Executives are constantly scanning their company and their environment for creative options, for new opportunities to make their company unique, and more distinctive.

Source: Kate McKeown, co-author with Lou Mobley, former director of IBM's Executive School, of *Beyond IBM: Leadership, Marketing and Finance for the 1990s,* Enter Publishing, 4201 Massachusetts Ave. NW, Washington, DC 20016. Ms. McKeown is president of McKeown & Company, Inc., a Washington, D.C. executive strategy consulting firm.

People Skills Versus People Management

Common management trap: Confusing people skills with people management. People skills involve being nice…getting along with people, avoiding conflict, making people feel good, having people like you.

But managers run into big trouble if they use only these skills, without the important people-management skills that involve confronting tough problems that sometimes cause bad feelings.

Example: A boss has a very competent employee, and is constantly praising him and encouraging him to keep up the good work. Trap: The employee stops advancing in the company because the manager, completely overlooking the importance of growth and challenge to the employee, fails to give him new, stimulating work. The boss is interested only in making the employee feel good, but in the process fails at his job of managing. The employee ultimately leaves the company.

To balance people skills and people management…

■Maintain high standards without being excessively empathetic. "People-skill" managers who are always nice to employees think they're doing a good job because they're understanding and empathetic. Trap: Being always understanding means excusing employees from meeting the company's standards. Best: Be understanding, while clearly telling employees what they must do to maintain good standing in the company.

■Instill pride in employees instead of lavishing affection. "People-skill" managers have the constant urge to tell employees how much they like them. They think this motivates. Reality: It demoralizes, because it removes the employees' sense of challenge. Better: Recognition of top performance. Recognizing genuine accomplishment instills pride in the employee and spurs him to greater achievement.

■Be prepared to confront tough realities even if morale must suffer. "People-skill" managers are afraid to tell employees that they must change the way they do their jobs if they want to remain valuable assets to the company. In tough times, this is unavoidable and the best managers are able to confront employees by telling them that, for example, they must do more work, or take a pay cut, or team up with others, if things are to improve—even if this creates a temporary morale problem.

■Manage conflict, instead of avoiding it. "People-skill" managers try desperately to avoid conflict. Better managers try to avoid conflict between employees, but accept that they can't always succeed and are prepared to confront conflict when it arises. They do use people skills to talk the conflict out with their people, but then they confront the problem, and make the changes necessary to resolve the conflict, even if it means one or both employees are temporarily unhappy because they must make adjustments.

Source: Harry Levinson, Ph.D., *The Levinson Letter,* 375 Concord Ave., Belmont, MA 02178.

Keys To Better Delegation

Most managers are reluctant to delegate because they are afraid that it will cause their department's performance to deteriorate. To lessen the fear:

■Train subordinates. Set aside time each week to groom staffers so they'll be able to handle new responsibilities well enough to make you feel confident about delegating new work.

■Be open with information. If workers feel that they're being kept in the dark about the company's operations and goals, they are likely to worry about making decisions and will do nothing because they won't feel they have the facts to make decisions. It's much better to run the small risk that proprietary information will leak out from the company than to make it impossible for subordinates to make informed decisions that can improve company productivity.

■Avoid oversupervising. When a manager is away from the office, calling constantly to check on what's being done will only impede subordinates' willingness to take the initiative to get a job done.

Source: Robert Half, Robert Half International, Box 3000, Menlo Pk, CA 94026.

The Executive's Spy Network

Apart from conventional sources of information, effective managers should consider tapping employees in the company who are naturally good sources.

Develop sources of information below the executive ranks. Well-placed secretaries and maintenance personnel have access to inside information. High-level employees may have too much at stake in their jobs to be unbiased sources.

Never pay information sources with money. Instead, compensate them with friendship, a well-timed family gift, personal concern.

Use multiple sources. By using employees with overlapping knowledge, a manager can double-check the information and reliability of sources.

Stress the need for early information. Give large rewards for it.

Encourage subordinates to air their grievances directly to you. Listen to what one manager has to say about others.

When evaluating information, look for the worst possible news. Listening to gossip and office informants can help the company anticipate a problem, but not if the executives are only looking for a rosy view to confirm their own actions.

When It's Wrong To Be Right

Manager's obsession with being right brings about rigidity of thinking. That stifles creativity, discourages risk taking, polarizes people over issues, and leads to the recycling of old ideas.

Highly intelligent executives with large egos and top positions to protect are usually the most effective at stifling the new ideas of others. The more intelligent the executive, the more capable the person is of defending a position, regardless of its merits.

Criticism is another way of bolstering the need to be right and screening out new ideas. Workers quickly decide that silence is the safest position when the boss aggressively pushes an idea. And the most timid workers even allow critical (and threatening) managers to preempt ideas and solutions that they actually originate.

Top management must support the right to be wrong to encourage the flow of fresh ideas and new approaches to the business. Some techniques that work at meetings:

■A rule that two positive points must be presented about an idea before one negative comment is made should be implemented. This puts the focus on positive aspects of an idea, promoting open-mindedness.

■Once an idea is presented, others at the meeting must make a positive comment, a negative comment, and add an interesting point to the idea. The goal is to provide creative spark to the discussion.

■Everyone at the meeting agrees to spend a few minutes considering another participant's idea, regardless of how radical or far-out it may seem.

Remember that thinking ability is not an inherited trait. Thinking is as much a learned skill as riding a bicycle. And the best thinkers are not always the most intelligent. Intelligent people are often caught between their need to be right and their egos.

Source: Eric M. Bienstock, Ph.D., managing director, The Edward de Bono School of Thinking, New York.

Giving And Taking Orders

Good managers expect subordinates to disagree sometimes. They don't want a yes response to every instruction. The best managers provide more ideas and projects than their subordinates can possibly accomplish. They want their staff members to use their knowledge and judgment in deciding priorities. Effective managers expect to be told when an instruction is faulty or can't be followed. They should be told by the employee who is closest to the situation when the realities contradict the boss' assumptions.

Well-managed companies encourage managers and subordinates to balance out these initiatives.

Managers should want to know about legitimate objections and barriers. They should provide a responsive ear to ideas and warnings the subordinates feel are important. But when time is critical, or when a broad view should prevail, the manager still can insist on going ahead.

Sensible subordinates must be able to blend the desire to be heard with the willingness to defer. Managers evaluate their employees on their ability to stand up and disagree. Also important is the employees' willingness to accept orders after their objections have been heard.

When order-giving generates a power struggle, the relationship has broken down badly and needs attention.

Criticism: How To Give It/How To Take It

The ability to give—and to accept—criticism productively is clearly important to success at all levels—individual, departmental, corporate.

Alarming: American business is handicapped by a negative approach to giving and receiving criticism. Examples:

■One of the top causes of job stress is lack of feedback, especially criticism.

■The two major reasons executives lose their jobs...insensitivity to others and an inability to allow for the views of others...are key traits of destructive critics.

Clearly, the need to improve our "critical skills" has become—critical.

The Problem With Criticism

Most people define criticism negatively—a way to find fault or to point out what's wrong or bad about someone. And we associate criticism with negative emotions. Criticism hurts, and, because it threatens our self-esteem, our reactions are usually defensive...anger and excuse-making.

Of course, criticism is destructive if it's used to insult or to embarrass someone, or to make oneself look good or feel powerful at another's expense.

Problem: People who are well-meaning in their criticism often hurt others.

By contrast, people with what I term "The Critical Edge" have learned to give (and accept) criticism in a way that motivates, influences or improves behavior in the context of work.

Helpful model: *TASK*, or *Teach Appropriate Skills and Knowledge*. By consciously shifting our minds to the TASK at hand, we can reverse our negative habits regarding criticism and begin to engender positive growth.

How To Criticize Productively

■Strategize. Plan your criticism in advance. Avoid spontaneous sarcasm or accusation. Think through exactly what you want to teach...and why. How can you best say this so the person will be receptive? What is a realistic time frame in which to expect improvement or change?

Example: A co-worker's first proposal was too long, detailed and dry. As she leaves the meeting, exhilarated that it is over, you say, "I thought you'd never finish! I almost fell asleep!" She is hurt, and resents your lack of support. Better: Say, "Nice job. I've been thinking—your research was so exhaustive, you may have lost a few of us. Next time, you might find it more effective to come right to the point, and then summarize the data."

■Protect self-esteem. Don't attack the person you're criticizing ("Your proposal was boring.")

Better: Help him/her to feel valuable. ("It's hard to cover such thorough research in a staff meeting. Would it be possible to provide the details in a handout? That way, we can study the numbers later.")

■Focus on improvement. People feel secure and motivated if it is clear they will have a chance to improve.

Example: "Your research gives us a firm base to build on. Let's develop a strategy from here."

■Time criticism carefully. Pay attention to the setting, the emotional state of the person you criticize, your own emotional state and whether others are present. Criticizing when you're angry, for example, is almost always counterproductive. Criticizing in front of others must be done carefully. If you have to criticize someone in front of peers, be sure to recognize the person first for his efforts, so the whole group hears that as well as the criticism.

Example: "I see you've done excellent research, Smith. Would you mind summarizing your findings for those of us with limited time? Then get a detailed report to the marketing people."

■Avoid criticizing when it is too late for the recipient to do anything about it. Example: "That report you sent out last week was terrible."

■Be interactive. Allow the person you are criticizing to respond.

Example: "Next time, I'd like you to focus more on the big picture. How do you think you can use your time more effectively? What can you do to tighten up your presentation and make it more lively? Think about it for a week and let me know."

■Be flexible. Be sure to communicate with an instructive approach rather than an authoritative one, which provokes resistance. Avoid rigid "should" statements that imply your way is the only way.

Example: Instead of saying, "You should never bore people with the details," try, "I know I appreciate it when meetings move along quickly. You could try summarizing your research. But maybe you feel it's important to back up your suggestions in detail? If so, let's find some alternatives to the two-hour meeting."

■Communicate concern. Criticism is much easier to accept if the recipient feels the critic is concerned with his welfare and growth.

Example: "I'll ask the Graphics Department to design an attractive cover for your report, and you can distribute it before our next meeting. Can you have it ready in two weeks?"

■State the incentive for the recipient. Example: "Your peers will appreciate your efforts to be more concise...You'll be more likely to achieve your objectives if you improve your meeting skills."

■Include the positives. Example: "Your attention to detail has always been one of your great strengths. We know we can trust your data."

Taking Criticism

When you can take the point of criticism and use its sharpness to work for you, you have the other side of The Critical Edge.

Best: Ask how you can improve. Then listen. If you skip into self-deprecation ("I'm a failure, he hates my proposal"), breathe slowly and remember you can learn from your critic. Then, follow up. ("Thanks for your help. Do you have any further suggestions?")

If You Are The Boss

Executives become more isolated the further they rise.

Drawback: They're robbed of feedback about their performance.

Essential: Ask for criticism from your peers and subordinates...and be sure to thank them for offering it.

Source: Hendrie Weisinger, Ph.D., psychologist specializing in anger and criticism. Dr. Weisinger teaches at UCLA's Anderson Graduate School of Management and conducts criticism seminars for corporate and government clients. His book is *The Critical Edge*, Harper & Row, 10 E. 53 St., New York 10022.

How To Reprimand Employees Without Humiliating Them

Effective ways to turn negative, humiliating employee reprimands into tactful, constructive criticism:

■Give employee an alibi for a mistake. Use the "I know, but..." approach. Example: "I know you've had a lot of paperwork lately, but these forms...."

■Take the blame for not preventing the mistake from happening. Example: "It's my fault for not mentioning this problem sooner, but...."

■Place the blame on conditions beyond his control. Example: "I know these federal regulations seem to complicate things, but...."

■Point out the benefits that come from the mistake. Example: "The way those reports were lost makes me think we should do something about our delivery system."

■Best time to dispense employee criticism: Early in the day and early in the week. Day-end fatigue can exaggerate criticism. The employee who is reprimanded just before his weekend begins goes home in a bad state of mind and blows discussion out of proportion by stewing about it all during the weekend.

For best results, time remarks so there's another chance to talk with the employee before the end of the day. A casual conversation—even a few words—after several hours will assure him that feelings toward him haven't changed, that his job isn't in jeopardy, and that there is confidence in his ability to resolve the problem.

Source: Herman Harrow, Envirotech Corp., in *Sales & Marketing Management*.

Employee Loyalty

It's no secret that employee loyalty isn't what it used to be...or that it's tougher today to maintain enthusiasm and integrity...but companies that work at it are succeeding. The best of them are building a stronger, more solidly based loyalty than ever before.

In the past, employee loyalty, although common, was really a blind, almost automatic loyalty. It came as much from employees' inertia as from anything the company did. Employees stayed with the companies they started at without asking why.

But today, employee values are different. A very large portion of employees simply don't care at all who they work for, as long as the paycheck is adequate. Beyond that, issues of career advancement, perks and other personal ambitions dictate where people work. The company's interests come last.

But companies that are working hard to break this mold have been able to build a deeper and stronger kind of loyalty. It's a "considered loyalty"—an "earned loyalty." This type of employee loyalty is one that management has taken an active role in cultivating and maintaining.

What can we learn from these companies?

Keys To Building Loyalty

Companies that have achieved the highest degree of loyalty are...

■Committed to open communication between management and workers. An environment of openness is as important to building loyalty as any specific program the company might adopt. But a policy of openness won't be effective if employees don't know about it. The openness must be communicated. Successful companies are actively marketing themselves to their employees as being committed to openness. They're creating an image of the company as an open place.

The specifics of open communications differ from company to company. In some companies, the approach is to "empower" employees, that is, to bring decision-making down to the level where it has the most impact. This makes employees feel better about the company—as well as making the company run better. Such a program says a lot about the company to prospective employees. It attracts and holds workers who find it important to have a degree of responsibility and autonomy.

Other companies take a paternalistic approach. Their brand of open communication is to keep employees informed about everything the company is doing. They assure employees that their interests won't be omitted in the decision-making process. They use research techniques to gather input from employees. It's the company, though, not the employees, that makes the decisions.

A company going through difficult times will acknowledge that fact to its employees. It will let them know that it recognizes that the steps it is taking are as traumatic and troublesome for the employees as they are for the company. It will tell employees that it is committed to keeping them informed. It will tell them, honestly, what the implications of the changes are. It will let them know as quickly as possible how the changes are going to affect them.

■Aware of family issues. These companies are setting up benefits programs that help employees deal with pressing family needs. Child care is an obvious example. Larger companies are offering employees more help in relocation.

Elder-care programs are being introduced in some companies. These companies have policies and referral programs to help employees who are caring for dependent elderly relatives. Some companies have a person on staff, called a family-resource consultant, to whom employees can turn for help.

Benefits programs such as these have a dual impact. They alleviate stress and thereby improve the employee's productivity. And they boost loyalty by showing that the company understands and is willing to accommodate the employee's family problems.

■Focusing on performance—as a way to recognize and reward outstanding workers. More companies are using incentive pay for star performers. And they are developing more detailed evaluations of individual performance.

Rather than having performance appraisals take place long after the fact, at the end of the year, managers are sitting down with employees on January 1 and looking ahead to the coming year. They're setting very specific individual goals for the employees.

This gives the individual a clear road map for the year ahead, showing how he/she is going to be evaluated. Employees who accomplish their goals see their rewards are tied closely to performance, and this is a strong motivator.

This type of evaluation system helps reinforce loyalty where the company wants to reinforce it—with outstanding performers. Their frustration, typically, is that they're neither recognized nor rewarded for what they perceive to be extra efforts. But this kind of system very closely ties their rewards to recognition of their effort. They see this as a preferable work environment.

One of the toughest issues facing business today is runaway health-care costs.

Companies are naturally concerned that cost-containment measures will erode employee loyalty.

Challenge: To gain employee acceptance for the changes the company must make. Employees must be made to see that their needs will be taken into account in dealing with this tough problem. Before making changes, the company should explain the magnitude of the problem, outline the alternatives it's considering, ask for employee input, and get employees to participate in devising a solution.

By acknowledging that employees are concerned with this issue too, and not simply making unilateral decisions, the company will be seen as a concerned employer. Loyalty will be enhanced, rather than deflated.

Source: Suzanne M. Kenney, national practice leader, listening services, Hewitt Associates, 100 Half Day Road, Lincolnshire, IL 60069.

Fear Versus Honesty

When fear pervades the workplace, productivity suffers, turnover soars and profitability usually drops. Major types of fear in the workplace...

■Fear of reprisal: Includes fear of termination, disciplining, transfer to undesirable position, etc. Fear is instilled through intimidation. When employees fear reprisal, witch hunts to fix blame become common.

■Fear of communicating: When employees fear being punished, they're reluctant to convey bad news to management.

■Fear of not knowing: This fear exists in companies where back-stabbing is a way of life. Managers must be informed about important activities in the company if they are to defend themselves against calculating co-workers.

■Fear of change: Managers with the most to lose are the most fearful of change. Managers who are protective of their turf resist change because they fear the unknown.

To Break Down Fears

■Emphasize teamwork, teaching, listening and leading. Replace management paranoia with basic beliefs of "honesty without fear." These include the belief that people want to contribute...people should be trusted...change is good...problems are opportunities.

■Change management policies. Meet often with employees, instead of defending barriers between management and lower levels. Encourage mistakes and use them as lessons, instead of punishing people for making them.

■Focus on fortifying employee confidence. Offer plenty of training, aimed at qualifying people for acceptance of greater responsibility. Then give them responsibility, reinforcing their sense of self-esteem.

Source: Gerald M. McBean and Ted A. Lowe, American Society of Quality Control, quoted in *Productivity*, 101 Merritt 7, Norwalk, CT 06851.

The Secrets Of Flexible People Management

Companies have restructured so thoroughly that they can no longer improve productivity by cutting staff.

Today's new challenge: Making sure that everyone on the leaner staff is top-notch...with fewer people doing more work, the company has even less tolerance for substandard performance.

Problem: The tight labor market is making this increasingly difficult. And—offering huge salary increases to keep especially valuable employees has its limits.

Today, management must be exceptionally innovative in managing the staff for maximum competitiveness...

The New Perk: Flexibility

The need to be more flexible in personnel management is particularly acute for companies that have a young workforce or a high proportion of female workers. But the issue isn't just parental leave when a new baby comes. It's equally important to parents of teenagers and to those whose aging parents are dependent on them.

Reason: The increased demands of a leaner organization, combined with the complex demands of personal life, force employees to seek out the least rigid work conditions possible. Successful companies are responding to these compelling social trends by:

■Offering more flexible work schedules. According to our annual survey of companies, 19% now have some system of flextime that applies to the whole organization. Another 22% offer flexible hours in some departments. Most companies that use flextime establish a core period, say, from 10 a.m. to 3 p.m., which is fully staffed and is when most of the work gets done. But workers are given the option of coming in early or staying late to round out their eight hours.

Companies that have substantial international business are using flextime to make sure the phones are covered to accommodate different time zones.

■Restructuring job descriptions to remove boundaries of responsibility, and cross-training workers so that they can substitute for one another during peak periods. As workers become more versatile and valuable contributors, many companies are rewarding them with more pay. Successful cross-training makes loss of one key employee much easier to adjust to.

■Introducing flexible benefit plans and child-care assistance. In addition, about 56% of the companies we survey are now offering wellness programs, on-site health clubs or financial assistance for those who join outside health clubs.

Help From Human Resources

To find the right strategy for your company, challenge all the old assumptions about hiring and managing people. Forget the personnel department mentality. Today's recruiting and training needs demand a sensitive human resources staff that can analyze the company's long-term people requirements and fill them with innovative staffing and training.

Key: The old personnel department must progress from the role of administration and legal compliance to an important agent of change and a program implementor. In companies where human resources people have proven their ability and won credibility with line managers, they are becoming full partners in accomplishing the company's strategic goals. These are the companies that are attracting the best workers.

Though flextime has proven valuable in attracting valued employees, it has hit a snag in the era of downsizing where smaller staffs are called upon to work longer, more intense hours to get the job done. In many companies, people are stressed, trying to accomplish the same amount of work with many fewer bodies. Managers fear that if workers are allowed to keep odd hours, the work may not get done.

Solution: Create rewards for getting the work done with incentive pay. Group-based incentive programs, such as gainsharing, reward workers with additional compensation when their unit achieves objectives valuable to the company.

Key: Management first defines with employees what is critical performance for their department. Then employees are paid for exceeding those goals. More and more companies are reducing the traditional merit pay budget, which essentially gives everybody the same raise, and instead putting those funds into pools to reward productive employees.

Powerful Results

Companies are quickly finding that trying these ideas has a powerful influence on the organization. People become more committed to their work and their teammates. They show up on time for work and even come in early and stay late.

What motivates them: The feeling that they can have an effect on the company's results. There's a sense of participation that they just don't get from rigid hours, rigid job descriptions, rigid hierarchies. These team goals even work better than profit sharing as an incentive because most employees are never able to see their own relationship to profits that often originate in parts of the company over which they have no control.

Source: Thomas B. Wilson, vice president and general manager, New England region, Hay Group, 5 Faneuil Hall Marketplace, Boston, MA 02109.

Managing Secrets

Dynamic management of employees is most effective if you concentrate on three groups of people: 1. The youngest workers, who represent tomorrow's potential. 2.

The most senior workers, whose experience can be invaluable. 3. The future managers, the special people who will have long-term careers at the company if properly identified and handled early on.

Source: *The Type 3 Company* by Georges Archier, chairman of the French Association of Quality Circles, Nichols Publishing, Box 96, New York 10024.

Good Bosses Give
Immediate Gratification

The subordinates that count most in any business are those who thrive on accomplishment, who are challenged by barriers and who enjoy showing what they can do in a tough situation. To these people, there's nothing more satisfying than the combination of accomplishment and recognition.

Real Achievement

Effective managers have learned to watch for subordinate "victories" and then to reward them. A victory is simply an accomplishment with two unique components:

■An unusual effort, initiative and/or creativity.

■Successfully attaining a tough goal.

Example: An employee who deals with a vendor to whom the company has been continuously paying a specified price, negotiates a 10% discount by combining the needs of several divisions. That's a clear case of individual initiative, coupled with concentrated effort that achieves a meaningful end. Such accomplishment should be immediately recognized and quickly rewarded. It's that kind of behavior that makes good companies better.

The reward does not have to be something major. The important thing is that it be spontaneous and genuine. It must reflect the fact that the boss really knows when employees have extended themselves and appreciates what they've done to improve the operations of the company.

Pressure To Conform

Unfortunately, many organizations punish achievement-oriented, high-energy employees. They are "joshed," even ridiculed for their hard work.

Many things conspire to discourage exceptional work when that is just what management is supposed to encourage. One often even hears managers talking about colleagues who are workaholics. They're accused of being insecure, lacking a good family life or being too self-centered as they try to demonstrate excellence.

Managers who recognize and applaud high performance not only counterbalance these negative social pressures, but can help to reverse them.

It's common to doubt whether employees really take seriously such gestures and to assume they appear trite. Reality: The people the company values most—those who thrive on achievement and recognition—do take such gestures eagerly.

When a generous reward follows a victory resulting from unusual effort, the recipient's sense of having "made it" is sparked. That spark is magical for motivated employees and they'll be spurred on to further accomplishments in the future.

Source: Dr. Leonard R. Sayles, professor of management, Columbia University Graduate School of Business, New York 10027.

The Most Powerful Motivator Of All, Personal Pride

Businesses have experimented with a host of strategies for making employees more productive—profit sharing, stock options, bonus plans, etc.

Many of these strategies work, but none spur employees to operate at maximum potential. Reason: Responsibility for one's own actions is more powerful than money as a motivator. To many companies, the concept of "participative management," which is based on decentralizing responsibility, is nothing new. But it has become such a buzzword that many companies believe they can raise productivity and morale by simply letting workers make more decisions. Reality: It's not that easy—more often it is a challenge.

The Challenge

The only way to ensure that employees push themselves to perform and to improve is to create a working environment that cultivates, rather than stifles, the most powerful motivator there is...personal pride. The pride in turning out quality products more efficiently comes only from giving individuals responsibility for their actions, thereby motivating them to demonstrate their proficiency. Other benefits:

■Fewer costly disputes.

■More ideas from workers on how to boost productivity.

■Strong teams of workers.

Example: W.L. Gore & Associates, the company that makes Gore-Tex and other synthetic materials. Employees don't have titles and are empowered to make decisions usually reserved for only high-level executives. At the end of the year, they even decide on the size of bonuses for themselves and their teammates. And, even in today's tight labor market, Gore has a backlog of applicants. Some recent hirees waited six years to join the company.

Getting Started

To give employees more control over their work...

■Bring decision-making down to an appropriate level. Twenty-five years ago, only a plant manager could stop the assembly line in a U.S. auto factory. In many plants today, people working on the assembly line can stop the line when they see something wrong. This way, many problems are solved before faulty units are moved down the line...and workers develop a sense of responsibility for the product. Quality and morale improve.

The optimum level of decision-making varies from industry to industry. To reach it, companies must be willing to experiment and then fine-tune.

Quality circles are often a good way to begin bringing decision-making to the shop floor, but circles alone aren't enough to motivate workers in the long term. Reasons: They don't include enough employees. Too often, those who do participate start to take on an elitist role.

■Listening to employees. It helps for managers to talk to the workers who report to them for at least five minutes each day. To some old-line managers, that might sound simplistic, but the fact is, the technique works. By knowing their workers, managers can:

■Spot problems at an early stage.

■Gain the confidence of the work force. This point can be vital when the company needs to make big changes in procedures.

Example: When a Japanese firm recently bought a financially troubled U.S. manufacturing company, it made virtually no changes in the product or production system. But it did reduce the number of managers. Then it asked the remaining supervisors to spend at least 15 minutes a day with each employee they manage. Managers argued that in view of their reduced number, they had no time to spend with each worker. The Japanese insisted, and the supervisors complied. Result: Supervisors discovered that it took them less time to manage when they spent a regular amount of time with each employee. Reason: Workers knew exactly what was expected of them, and they had ample opportunity each day to work out problems with the boss. Operational efficiency rose dramatically.

Essentials Of Listening

■Focus on solutions. When listening to employees, don't ask just about problems…ask also about how they would solve them. More often than not, workers know the solution.

■Follow up on suggestions. When an idea is good, reward it with an invitation to lunch, recognition or even a promotion or merit raise. If a worker's idea is impractical, daily talks give managers an opportunity to explain the difficulties.

■Reward workers for the company's productivity gains. Though bonuses may be small, they're powerful in creating peer pressure that steers employees toward higher productivity.

■Require managers to spend time periodically in low-level positions. Avis's legendary Bob Townsend, for example, temporarily worked on the switchboard. Results: He got a feel for what his employees did and problems they dealt with. Meanwhile, he gained trust and promoted teamwork among employees.

Breaking Down Barriers

Expect two problems in implementing the system…

■Unions may balk. Head off opposition by discussing plans early with union leaders. Some unions, for example, see participative management as infringing on their territory. Important: Check, in advance, with the company's labor lawyers to make sure changes in compensation systems or decision levels don't violate any collective bargaining agreements.

■Managers may balk. The simple solution here may be ordering them to try it. In the vast majority of cases, managers almost immediately grow to like the system. Reason: It makes their job much easier because formalities are broken down and a much more easygoing, productive atmosphere takes over.

Caution: Don't fake it. If the CEO isn't temperamentally prepared to operate under a decentralized, participative system, it's better to go ahead and continue managing the company by directive than to make employees believe they have power but actually retain it in the executive suite.

Source: Joseph A. Reres, Joseph A. Reres & Associates, consultants in participative management practice, 3321 S. Stafford St., Arlington, VA 22206.

Workers' Miracle Performances Do Not Have To Be Miracles

Every experienced manager has one great personal tale of "miracle" performance by a team of talented workers who used their ingenuity to brainstorm their way through a major crisis, against tight time pressure and chilling risk.

Rarely, though, do managers understand that this high level of performance can be sustained without employee burnout, without focusing on one task at the expense of others and without keeping the company stirred up in perpetual crises.

Big mistake: Failing to realize that employees thrive on urgency, drama and excitement—even tension—in the workplace. Sure, everyone likes stability. But why, then, does everyone dread coming to work on Monday mornings, complain about drudgery in their jobs, etc.? People want liveliness…they want zest at work.

The "return to normal" after a challenging episode of high-level performance usually depresses most managers and workers. Challenge for management: Create an environment of opportunities to "catch fire." Stop waiting for a crisis to show you what the company is really capable of achieving.

Key: Generating Ideas

Something can always be done right now to improve performance. Organized efforts to solicit ideas from employees on ways to improve productivity and efficiency are always useful. But don't just build up an inventory of ideas. That alone can be depressing—another thing for supervisors to worry about.

Essential step: Identify a breakthrough project based on one especially bright idea. Use it to excite workers into a sense of mission.

The project should be specific and compelling. Everyone involved must acknowledge urgency to arouse the necessary zest to accomplish the task.

Basic Criteria

■The goal must be measurable—on the bottom line. Substitute *Results first!* for the usual habit of *Preparation first!* "Improving inventory turnover on low-end products by 20% in the first quarter" is a good goal. "Improving inventory procedures" is not. "Cutting by half the billing errors on major accounts by July 15" is a good goal. "Improving clerical training" is not.

■People must be able to anticipate that the first successes could be accomplished in weeks—not months or years.

■The project must engage everyone's commitment at the very start, through its easily recognizable payoff. The reaction to be expected from workers is, "It's about time we did this," not, "Oh no. Here they go again!" The project will stall if the supervisor must work at convincing people that they ought to care about the goal.

■The goal must be achievable with available resources and authority. Don't let anyone make excuses by arguing that the only way to make the change is with more people, more advanced computers, or a shift in the way another department works. To cut off such escape routes, keep pressing for a definable goal by insisting that there's definitely something—even something small—that this department can do to improve its productivity or operations without any outside assistance.

No breakthrough success, no matter how notable, is of lasting value unless it is the beginning of a process that continues.

Maintaining Momentum

At first, the most important aim is to establish a pattern of success and a sense of momentum. Pick projects which clearly generate the greatest amount of enthusiasm and energy. Make sure there is recognizable success. Celebrate every time a goal is met. Have fun and create excitement!

Only when momentum is established and managers and workers develop confidence in themselves must attention be given to institutionalizing the new changes—incorporating them into the company's permanent operations. By then, though, the norm for work by both managers and workers should not be institutionalized boredom, but institutionalized zest.

Source: Robert H. Schaffer, Robert H. Schaffer & Associates, management consultants specializing in productivity and performance improvement, 401 Rockrimmon Rd., Stamford, CT 06903 and 67 Yonge St., Toronto, Ontario M5E 1J8. Mr. Schaffer is author of *The Breakthrough Strategy*, Harper & Row, 10 E. 53 St., New York 10022.

How To Turn A Marginal Performer Into A High Achiever

Familiar scenario: After only a short time on the job, a capable and highly motivated individual becomes a marginal performer—a worker who does just enough to get by. Many frustrated managers assume they've made an unfortunate hiring mistake that must simply be tolerated. But it doesn't have to be that way.

Managers can turn around marginal performers and thereby produce large productivity gains for the company.

Problem: Most managers fail to address marginal performance in a constructive way. They automatically attribute performance problems to the employee's lack of ability and/or effort. They respond with punitive measures such as cutting back bonuses or denying desirable assignments.

Result: This only makes matters worse. Something else is usually at the root of the problem—an absence of management support. Even the most hard-working and capable individuals can't maximize their performance if they do not have the necessary support.

Two Types Of Support

Managers must ask if they have done their part to create a physical work setting that supplies employees with opportunities to fully use their abilities. Elements of a supportive work environment:

■Appropriate technologies, tools, facilities and equipment.

■Adequate budgets.

■Clear task goals.

■Responsibility without excessive red tape and other performance obstacles.

■Market-competitive base wage or salary.

■Managers must give attention to other social aspects of the work environment. Recent research into job stress, for example, suggests that social support is critical for sustained high performance. Emotional support from an employee's supervisor and co-workers is considered very helpful in long-term growth in job performance.

Strategy for turning around a marginal performer...

■Bring the performance gap to the employee's attention. Do this politely, but specifically and face-to-face. Give employees with performance problems a chance to express their feelings without putting them on the defensive. Provide them with immediate emotional support by reassuring them that they are viewed as highly capable and dependable workers.

■Ask the employee, in a nonthreatening manner, for an explanation of under-performance. In dialogue with employees, try to identify the causes of the substandard performance. Listen carefully for causes that are beyond the employee's control.

■Describe the implications of the employee's substandard work. Point out that others in the company depend on the employee's work being done well and on time so they can meet their performance objectives.

■Restate the original and still-desirable performance objectives. Do this face-to-face, to reinforce the personal dimensions of the manager-employee relationship, heighten the employee's commitment to improve, and increase the sense of accountability to the manager.

■Offer the work environment support necessary for employees to improve their performance. Managers should invite employees to see them with problems.

■Express confidence that the employees will respond as expected.

■Agree on an appropriate time frame for jointly evaluating future performance. Also agree upon the standards.

■Continue the process until it succeeds—or the individual admits to an employment mismatch that can be reconciled only by a job change.

Immediate positive reinforcement should follow any instances of performance improvements and all above-standard achievements.

Source: Dr. John R. Schermerhorn, Jr., College of Business Administration of Ohio University, Athens, OH 45701. Professor Schermerhorn is author of *Management for Productivity*, John Wiley & Sons, 605 Third Ave., New York 10158.

The Future Value Employee

Identifying promotable employees isn't difficult if managers look at each worker's future value to the company, not just current job performance. Best: Evaluate the individual's initiative, innovativeness, and past experience in the company. In particular, identify areas that have been improved significantly by the employee. Past successes are almost always a strong indicator of future potential.

Source: Daniel Lupton, vice president, human resources management practice, Towers, Perrin, 245 Park Ave., New York 10167.

Older Workers Are Increasingly Important To Business...But...

Special problems arise when young managers must supervise older employees...

...**Communications gap.** There's always great potential for communication problems between younger and older employees, due to differences in attitudes, values, beliefs and career stages.

Solution: Clear the air through frank discussions between younger supervisors and older employees. Have the discussions informally or in goal-setting sessions or performance reviews.

Younger supervisors should state their individual and organizational goals. Older employees must be encouraged to communicate their needs, aspirations and their uncertainties.

...**Role reversal.** In the conventional roles of younger employee and older boss, the employee knows to listen attentively, follow directions, and defer to the boss. The situation is awkward when the roles are reversed and the younger manager must plan, supervise and evaluate the work of older employees.

The discomfort is greatest when the younger manager is required to give negative feedback to the older worker. Two approaches:

■**Tap the older employee's experience.** The manager can say, "We're falling behind schedule on delivery dates. Some of our customers are worried. You've seen these kinds of problems happen before. Based on your experience, what do you think will help get us back on track?"

■**Admit the awkwardness of the situation and then confront the problem directly.** "As a relatively new, younger department manager, I am uncomfortable talking with you, our most experienced senior employee, about performance problems. However, I am very concerned that our deliveries are behind schedule. Late deliveries hurt our reputation for customer service."

...**Skills obsolescence.** Obsolescence happens when employee skills no longer match job requirements either because job requirements change, skills atrophy when they aren't used, or other reasons.

The company may have to retrain older workers to sharpen existing skills or teach new skills.

Problem: Older employees sometimes worry about their ability to master new skills, or they're uncertain about the connection between training and present job demands. Solutions:

■Alert trainers to special concerns of older employees.

■Provide training that views mistakes as opportunities to learn.

■Clearly explain the purpose, objectives and relevance of training for present and future job demands.

■Link successful completion of training to rewards such as new job assignments, bonuses and opportunities for advancement.

...**Overcoming resistance to change.** Senior employees often resist organizational change. They've invested much of themselves in the present system. They feel safe and comfortable with it. Most are confident that they can succeed within the current system. When change comes, they stubbornly cling to old ways. To overcome resistance to change:

■Understand the reasons for resistance to change and then explain logically why the reasons aren't valid.

■Motivate employees to accept the new procedures, with rewards, praise, etc.

■Build acceptance and support for the new procedures among the workforce as a whole, to create momentum.

Source: Joan Larson Kelly, manager, business partnerships and community involvement, Worker Equity department, American Association of Retired Persons, 1909 K St. NW, Washington, DC 20049. The AARP offers free booklets on dealing with older employees. Write to the address above for any of the following booklets: *How to Recruit Older Workers, How to Manage Older Workers,* or *How to Train Older Workers.*

Using Stress To Improve Performance

Many companies are so persuaded that they should try to reduce stress among employees that they forget that some jobs actually require stress. The ones that do are jobs that depend on mental or physical alertness, especially monitoring jobs.

Industrial psychologists who publicly emphasize the need to reduce stress advise company clients privately on how to introduce optimum levels of stress. They use an inverted U-curve to describe the relationship between stress and performance. The horizontal axis is stress; the vertical is performance. As stress increases, performance also rises. But at a certain point, performance declines.

Ironically, some of the signs of too little stress are virtually identical to those of too much stress: Irritability, poor work quality and low quantity, absenteeism, tardiness and the tendency to make decisions either too quickly or too slowly.

Stress researcher Ernest J. McCormick, Ph.D., professor emeritus at Purdue University, explains: *If there are too few stimuli to respond to, a worker doing monitoring, vigilance or inspection tasks may miss even those few signals because of lack of attention. With an increase of stimuli, both attention and performance pick up. Then, if the load gets too high, the person begins to falter.*

Unfortunately, it is often easier to squeeze stress out of a job than to put it in. Jobs with visible responsibility and those that require working on deadlines almost always create their own stress, and little can be done to relieve it. Menial jobs in pleasant surroundings can be stress-free, and there may be no way to change that.

But it is possible for management to create stress in many other types of low-stress situations. The best techniques:

■Design work space so that it is natural and pleasant but not too comfortable. The environment should remind employees that they are in a work situation.

■Keep a healthy amount of distance from subordinates.

■Even though computers handle an increasing amount of analysis, leave some for employees.

■Hire only those applicants who show a reasonable amount of ambition. Too often, personnel departments concentrate so heavily on skills that they all but ignore other traits necessary for top performance.

Exert more than usual pressure when employees:

■Do work with which they are long familiar. Boredom is likely to set in.

■Can reasonably take on more diverse work.

■Need to become more productive at routine tasks.

■Are going stale and must be reminded that the boss is aware of the situation.

General rule: Assign people expected to produce creative work to easygoing supervisors. Put those responsible for more routine tasks under more demanding superiors.

Source: *International Management Consultants, Inc.* New York 10036.

The Magic Of Performance Appraisals

Effective performance appraisals motivate employees to improve performance in specific areas—and boost their self-esteem at the same time. Keys: Take advantage of any training the company offers in performance appraisals. Don't save appraisals for the annual review. Keep a running dialogue with each employee throughout the year. Document all conversations with employees in writing. Keep the appraisals objective—and limited to job performance, not personality.

Source: Loretta D. Foxman, president, and Walter L. Polsky, chairman and CEO, Cambridge Human Resources Group, Inc., Chicago, writing in *Personnel Journal*, 245 Fischer Ave., Costa Mesa, CA 92626.

Why Workers Fail

Besides deliberately slacking off, workers often fail to perform properly because:

■Good performance does not really matter. For example, latecomers are not reprimanded. There is no reward for being productive.

■The safest policy is to do nothing. Workers may shirk their tasks because supervisors, out of a desire to retain power and status, may not tell them how to do a job properly.

■Obstacles erected by supervisors make good performance impossible. Example: A secretary who works for more than one boss and must meet their conflicting demands.

■Negative consequences follow the desired performance. Supervisors might urge their assistants to come up with productivity ideas, but the supervisors' common behavior at staff meetings is to dismiss or criticize suggestions.

Source: Bernard L. Rosenbaum, *How to Motivate Today's Worker*, McGraw-Hill, New York.

Myths About Dealing With Workers

■Managers think they must be nice to their staff. In reality, their job is to meet corporate goals, sometimes at the expense of personal ones.

■Managers and staff must be part of a team seeking the same goals. Not so. Good management often requires making undemocratic decisions. They are easier to make when managers keep some distance from the staff.

■Staff should understand managers' reasons for their actions. But this is often futile. Attempting to win worker acceptance makes managers seem indecisive or unsure of themselves.

■An open-door policy where workers can discuss personal problems is effective. The fact is that knowledge of an employee's personal life will influence managers' feelings about the person's work.

■Managers should be experts on everything in their department or they will lose credibility with the staff. In reality managers who try to keep their hands in every activity are perceived as interfering and robbing subordinates of their initiative.
Source: *Canadian Business*, Toronto.

Complete The Job

For the best staff work, insist that subordinates do the job completely before turning in recommendations or proposals. Often staffers will turn in incomplete work in an attempt to save their time, not the boss's. Break this habit by: Holding the report for 48 hours…then asking the staff person responsible if "this is the very best you can do?" Usually the reply is "no." Tell the staffer to re-do the proposal. Repeat the process until staff members can confidently say the work is their best.
Source: Former Secretary of State Henry Kissinger quoted in *Small Business Report*, 203 Calle Del Oaks, Monterey, CA 93940.

Chapter 2
Better Negotiating

Picking A Negotiator

Chief executive officers should not become directly involved in the early negotiations. Subordinates make fewer concessions and larger demands and have more time available for preparation.

Choose representatives carefully. Choose them for their negotiating skills, not their availability or seniority.

Traits of a good negotiator:
■Sensitive to the feelings of others.
■Knows how to satisfy the psychological needs of opponents.
■Strongly desires to be liked.
■Listens carefully and looks for the hidden meanings in what is said.
■Will be respected by everyone involved in the negotiations.
■Goal-oriented.
■Displays a logical sense and has shown good business judgment in the past under pressure.

Source: Philip Sperber, *The Science of Business Negotiation*, Pilot Books, New York.

The Magic Of Mediators

Hiring a mediator can quickly and effectively solve disputes at low cost, since no lawyers are required. Mediators are helpful when: There are no legal claims (often the disagreements are between neighbors or family members)…you want a solution without sacrificing the relationship (filing a lawsuit can be very hostile)…you want to keep the dispute private (everything submitted or said to a court is public information). To find a mediator: Check the *Yellow Pages* under mediation, dispute resolution or arbitration…or contact your local bar association or social service office.

Source: *Mediate, Don't Litigate: How to Resolve Disputes Quickly, Privately, and Inexpensively Without Going to Court* by Peter Lovenheim, McGraw-Hill, 1221 Ave. of the Americas, New York 10020.

How To Negotiate More Effectively

■Don't allow the negotiations to be hurried by the other side. Clarify everything that seems fuzzy.

■Have the facts to back up every objective. If no facts are available, use opinions from experts as support.

■Maintain flexibility in every position. It avoids making the other side overly aggressive and always leaves a way out of dead ends.

■Look for the real meaning behind the other person's words. Body language tells a lot. Looking away when discussing a key point can indicate a lack of commitment.

■Don't focus only on money. Loyalty, ego, pride, and independence can be more important than dollars to many people.

■Be alert to the other side's priorities. Don't assume that the two sides are going to have the same priorities. Bending on a point that's important only to an adversary is one of the fastest ways to speed the process.

Everything Is A Negotiation

Whether negotiating a multimillion-dollar deal or a used car price, even savvy businesspeople often forget the basics of winning people over. Many mistakes they make are a result of misconceptions about what works at the bargaining table...and what doesn't...

■The tough-guy approach usually fails. Nine times out of 10, friendly persuasion is more productive than intimidation. People usually follow that rule instinctively in negotiating small matters at home. But, too often, they forget it under the pressure of business.

But, put yourself in your adversary's position. Aren't you more likely to agree with him if he's pleasant? I can assure you that he feels the same way.

Example: Fidel Castro is usually paranoid about his own safety. But Ted Turner developed such a trusting relationship with Castro that when the two went duck hunting together, Turner held a loaded gun only a few feet away from the Cuban leader.

■Do your homework. Businesspeople frequently overlook preparation—because it's so obvious. But, in fact, good preparation is really what separates the pros from the amateurs.

Sign of a successful negotiator: Determination to keep digging for information even after assistants say they have all the facts at hand. Top negotiators read periodicals that cover the issue. They familiarize themselves with the background of other negotiators. They also take notes during negotiations. On one level, knowing more than your adversary protects you from getting into deals with hidden traps. On another, it helps you explore compromises that you otherwise wouldn't have thought of.

On still another level, familiarity with your opponent and his business helps build trust. And it's easier to convince someone who trusts you.

■Don't get rattled. The easiest way is sometimes the most difficult—just let your opponent keep ranting. Eventually he'll run out of steam, and you can begin a serious conversation.

But if you interrupt him, or try to trade insult for insult, you might boost your ego, but you'll also reduce the chance of ever finding common ground.

■Choose the right negotiator. When choosing someone to represent the company at the bargaining table, opt for negotiating experience over factual knowledge. A negotiator can usually acquire the needed knowledge, but it takes time to build up bargaining skills.

The negotiator should also have the right temperament for bargaining.

What to look for: The ability to hold ego in check. Reason: During almost every negotiation, there's a potential for egos to clash. The best negotiators are those who won't lose ground by letting that happen.

■Always invite the other party to make the first offer. If he refuses to, you haven't lost anything. If he accepts, there's a chance his initial offer will be better than you expected.

If you make the first offer, you take the risk that it will be too high. You'll know that, of course, if it's quickly accepted.

If the other party refuses to make the first offer, there are some useful ploys for getting him to do it anyway.

Examples: Ask what he's budgeted for…what his last widget cost…what he thinks about a comparable widget.

■Never accept the first compromise offered. Hold out—there's a good chance another offer will follow.

Example: You want to sell property for $10 million. A prospective buyer offers $7 million. Then, he says he'll "split the difference" and offers $8.5 million. It almost always pays to reject the compromise.

Reason: The compromise really means you have a firm offer of $8.5 million. So now offer to split that difference at $9.25 million. If the prospect rejects the offer, you still have a chance to look elsewhere for a buyer. The worst that can happen is that you'll come back and accept the $8.5 million.

■Home court is best. Whenever possible, invite the other party to negotiate at your office. There's a big psychological edge because the other party won't want to spend time traveling to your office only to come away empty-handed.

If it isn't possible to conduct the negotiations at your office, choose neutral ground. Airports are usually good.

If you must go to the other company, make sure you're thoroughly rested from the trip before you start talking. (When the Japanese negotiate at home, they schedule talks for immediately after the other party gets off the plane.)

■Patience pays. I can't explain it, but I've seen it happen time and time again. Negotiations bog down and look hopeless. Then suddenly, the other side gives you nearly everything you asked for hours—or days—ago. It's not a sure bet, but by being impatient, you definitely do lose this opportunity.

Source: Robert Woolf, a professional contract negotiator whose clients include Joe Montana, Larry King and New Kids on the Block. He's president of Robert Woolf Associates, 4575 Prudential Tower, Boston, MA 02199. Woolf is also author of *Friendly Persuasion*, The Putnam Berkley Group Inc., 200 Madison Ave., New York 10016.

Influence Through Negotiation

Most managers don't recognize that they spend a significant share of their working day negotiating with other managers. They are more likely to see what they are doing as persuading or influencing. But, in fact, they are negotiating.

Negotiations are necessary when there is no obvious answer, no obvious decision. Managers often have to ask other departments to change their priorities or to do things differently.

Because managers frequently deal with peers whom they can't order around, and because internal routines and objectives may differ, most managers are forced to negotiate for the resources they need. .

Many managers just assume that most of their business day will involve dealing with bosses or subordinates. Needing to influence peers comes as a shock.

More upsetting still is the reality that their boss will demand things from them that will require getting some critical resources from another department who may refuse or delay. It seems so unfair that they should be held responsible for finishing a project by a deadline when another department can't or won't deliver needed information on time.

Typical reactions are indignation, or even outrage. Seeing the other department's head as an obstacle, a manager may seek to bully him into submission. Of course, such high pressure usually produces an equal and opposite force that doesn't get the need satisfied.

An equally ineffective reply to apparent noncooperation is to accuse the other department of not having the company's interest at heart, or of being inefficient or incompetent. This, too, usually produces friction, not results.

Other typical reactions to not getting the needed resources or aid is to make one of two assumptions...

■It's just a misunderstanding, a communication problem. When the situation is "clarified," cooperation will be forthcoming.

■There must be a clever way of "fooling" the other party and overcoming their resistance.

The first assumption is wrong because it supposes that the organization is really one big happy family and everyone has the same interests and goals. Not so. Other departments you depend upon probably have different interests and get rewarded for doing things that may not be consistent with your needs. Most conflicts over what should be done are not simply misunderstandings—they're real conflicts over goals and tactics.

The second assumption, the "one-upmanship" approach, is doomed to fail, if not immediately, surely in the long run, because it assumes you'll never have to deal with that department head again. And, of course, in organizations, effective managers build long-term relationships and count on friendship or, at least, mutual respect to win them aid and assistance.

Real Negotiations

Since managers can't order cooperation or get it by trickery or threat, at least not without costly reprisals, they must negotiate to gain acquiescence from reluctant sources of aid or supply.

Negotiation simply means give-and-take. It doesn't require going to courses or reading books on negotiating skills. As you explain your needs, you learn about the constraints the other person is facing. Some of the constraints you may be able to alleviate by modifying your request. Example:

If you can't get the project to us on time, what if we get partial specs to you tomorrow and then you'll have three weeks to work on those. When we finish our part of the job, we could contract out the more time-consuming parts and the people in your department would only have to look over the total package when it is complete.

If you've built up some credibility and demonstrated your flexibility, the other side is likely to show some flexibility, too. Example:

There is no way I can get Harry to work on that, even though he is the one you want and could do it best. But, I could get Harry to look over Bill and Jane's work and be sure it is consistent with the way you like things to be done.

Negotiations Take Time

Negotiations are time-consuming and can be destroyed by emotional blame-fixing or threats. If one party in the negotiations becomes indignant, he won't be able to engage in a give-and-take in which the other party thinks he is credible and worth helping. Negotiations assume that both parties want to build a relationship. They shouldn't be approached as a one-shot deal.

Source: Martin Edelston, president, Boardroom Reports, Inc., 330 W. 42 St., New York 10036.

A List Of Negotiating Tactics

■Forbearance. Hold back the threat of negative action until the effect will be greatest. Drop the point immediately once the other party has been convinced.

■Surprise. Shift tactics suddenly to throw your opponent off balance.

■Bland withdrawal. Deny everything. Claim a misquote, an out-of-context quote, or say that an employee was unauthorized to act.

■Apparent withdrawal. Deny the legitimacy or authority of the negotiation.

■Fait accompli. Postpone negotiations until the matter has already been completed, at which time it really doesn't matter who wins.

■Reversal. Shift the subject.

■Feinting. Pay lip service, as long as no concrete acts are required.

■Limiting. Put a deadline on the negotiation.

Signs That Negotiators Are Ready To Make A Deal

It's valuable to know as early as possible that the other side is preparing to settle negotiations. It allows strong points to be pressed home and helps avoid overkill. Clues to look for:

■The discussion shifts focus from points of contention to areas of agreement.

■The two sides are significantly closer together.

■The opposition starts to talk about final arrangements.

■A personal social invitation is made. At this point, agreement is almost always just a formality.

■Other side starts to make notes. Follow through at once, even if nothing but a napkin or envelope is at hand to write on.

But don't handle the signing of the formal agreement through the mail. Both parties should sign it together. This adds importance to the event and helps cement the ties that were formed during the final stage of negotiation.

Source: D. D. Seltz and A. J. Modica, *Negotiate Your Way to Success*, Farnsworth Publishing Co., Rockville Centre, NY.

Negotiation Isn't A Game

Negotiation isn't a game with winners and losers. Both sides can win. Win-lose negotiators look on the other party as an adversary. Win-win negotiators see the other party as a partner in success. Look at agreements from the viewpoint of the people who are going to perform them. Unless they're motivated to perform, you won't get full value from the agreement.

Source: Brian Long, Ph.D., C.P.M., president, Marketing and Management Institute, Kalamazoo, MI, quoted in *Purchasing World*, 6521 Davis Industrial Parkway, Solon, OH 44139.

Beware Of Negotiating Over The Phone

Don't negotiate over the phone if you can possibly do it in person. Reasons: The caller has the advantage of surprise. You can't see the other person's reactions. There's not enough time to think. It's easier to misunderstand. It's less difficult for the other party to say "no" when you can't be seen. It's easy to be distracted. It's hard to avoid being interrupted.

Source: Dr. Chester L. Karrass in *Purchasing*, 275 Washington St., Newton, MA 02158.

Where To Sit To Negotiate Effectively

Seating can have a surprisingly significant effect on the progress of negotiations. Some people still consider the head of the table the seat of power, and opt for it whenever possible. But many people react negatively to the presumed voice of authority in that seat, so sitting there can prove to be counterproductive. Creative approach: Sit on the same side of the table as your opponent. This significantly undermines the us-against-you approach to negotiating and instills a feeling of cooperation from the start.

Source: *Fundamentals of Negotiating* by Gerard Nierenberg, president, The Negotiation Institute, Harper & Row, 10 E. 53 St., New York 10022.

Negotiation Tactics

Use deadlines: Find out the other person's deadline. Conceal your own...put a deadline for acceptance on any serious proposal you make. Give yourself time to think: Arrange to be interrupted by a telephone call, beeper summons or caucus call. A few moments to think can be invaluable during intense bargaining. Keep any person who has final authority for your side out of the bargaining room. That way you have an excuse to renegotiate settlement details later.

Source: Eugene Mendonsa, director of the International and Domestic Negotiation Institute in Red Bluff, CA, in *Sales & Marketing Executive Report*, 4660 Ravenswood Ave., Chicago 60640.

Silence Is Best

When threatened during a negotiation, respond first with silence. This gives you a moment to consider whether the threat is real and credible and, if it is, what your options are. During the silence your opponent may step in to moderate the threat. Perhaps what you heard was merely someone misspeaking, or perhaps you'll get a restatement that introduces some qualification. If the other side doesn't speak up and the silence persists, first repeat or rephrase what you think you heard. You may have misunderstood, or your opponent may now have second thoughts. Only if your opponent sticks to the threat, and you know you've heard it accurately, should you respond directly to it in line with the options that are open to you.

Source: *Negotiate the Deal You Want* by Henry H. Calero, consultant on negotiations, Dodd, Mead, 71 Fifth Ave., New York 10003.

Trading Concessions

Make concessions count by considering each one carefully and agreeing only after a thoughtful pause. This applies especially to concessions that are easy for you to make. If you tell the other side we can easily do that or that's no problem, you lower the possibility of obtaining something in return for your concession. Best: Obtain a concession from the other side in trade for every concession you make.

Source: *Winning Negotiation Strategies for Bankers* by Philadelphia management consultant Linda Richardson, Dow Jones-Irwin, 1818 Ridge Rd., Homewood, IL 60430.

Chapter 3
Managing The Managers

Big Traps In Appraising Managers

Profound mistakes in appraising managers are often made because the company applies the wrong performance standards to its talented people. Two examples of the damage that can be done...

The super-effective non-manager: Some months ago, top management of a securities firm replaced the manager of one of its key commodities trading offices. Reason: He didn't pay attention to the formal managerial aspects of his position. His budgets were late and his reports unfathomable.

The decision to replace the manager was clinched when a top executive made an appointment to visit his office only to find that he was out on the trading floor, working alongside his traders. This convinced top management that he couldn't manage his staff.

Shortly after the firing, a large part of the office staff quit. To this day, the organization has not been able to assemble a comparable group of technically sophisticated traders. The office had been a source of major profits for the corporation. It is now a source of losses.

The mistake, of course, was rigid insistence on the dutiful execution of management formalities.

In this small office, the manager gained credibility as a leader by demonstrating his own technical prowess and by his ability to be immediately available in a very time-pressured environment. "Mixing it up" on the work floor was just where the trading "team captain" ought to have been. But, his bosses missed the point.

The technically talented non-manager: In another company, a new position was created to deal with executive development and succession planning. The first manager to head the group devoted himself to designing and maintaining a computer program that showed every job and every manager, their current positions and what was said about them in their annual appraisals.

But, the manager did nothing to make the system "work." He never learned what the real issues were in getting suitable candidates for current openings or developing people for future openings. He never found a way to manage the selection process or to gain acceptance from senior management. It was easier and "cleaner" to interpret the job as a solely technical one. This allowed the manager to work with his people, undisturbed by the messiness of organizational life. They had developed and operated a beautiful system that just didn't have much use.

Both cases cried out for management to ask itself what it really wanted behind the words, Manager of...

Result: It was impossible to render fair performance appraisals of these talented individuals. Both the managers and the companies suffered.

Source: Dr. Leonard R. Sayles, professor of management, Columbia University Graduate School of Business Administration, New York, and director, executive leadership research, Center for Creative Leadership, Greensboro, NC 27407.

How To Help New Managers Be Effective More Quickly

One of the big impediments to being effective for a newly hired manager is not "knowing the ropes."

Unfortunately, in most companies, little is done to help new managers learn their way around. They're typically left to their own devices, slowly meeting co-workers, and even more slowly meeting people in different departments or divisions of the company. This slows down work and impedes work improvement—contributing substantially to the high cost of hiring new people.

Exception: Corning Glass

Top management at Corning Glass realized the absurdity of leaving new recruits alone to grope their way around their new surroundings. They took a simple, but highly effective step to eliminate the problem. Now, most new managers are given the names of 10–15 veteran managers throughout the company. These veterans are required to schedule a luncheon with the new recruit within his/her first few months at the company.

The purposes are obvious, but almost always overlooked in other companies—to build personal relationships throughout the company, to speed the newcomer's familiarity with the company and to make sure that when problems or opportunities arise, there is always someone to call for information or assistance.

Network Shortcut

New Corning managers rave about the process. They say that they feel comfortable about calling others for help, which in turn makes them feel that they are part of the company and not part of an impersonal bureaucracy. The cross-functional relationships also cut through the red tape of "channels" that often slows down work.

It normally takes years to build up a network of contacts throughout the company. With its simple lunch circuit, Corning short-cuts the process. Now it takes only a few weeks for new managers to build a valuable network of acquaintances in the company.

Bottom line: Meaningful business doesn't get done efficiently when people who must work together don't really know each other. This is a simple way of building the bridges that connect the parts of a company and circumvent the impersonal and inefficient bureaucracy.

Source: Dr. Leonard R. Sayles, professor of management, Columbia University Graduate School of Business Administration, New York and director, executive leadership research, Center for Creative Leadership, Greensboro, NC 27407.

Better Ways To Train Managers

Placing people in jobs that make the best use of their strengths is the key to getting peak performance. Top management must make clear to managers that their priority is to match strengths to job requirements rather than identify and correct weaknesses with training. Correcting weaknesses, if they are major ones, can waste company resources.

Of course, sometimes it is necessary to invest in management training. The trick is to know when training will pay off and when it won't. When that is achieved, constructive training can be provided, and where training won't work, alternative action can be taken.

Management Skills That Can Be Taught

■Leadership skills: Some of these are trainable...
■How to handle interactions with subordinates.
■How to run a meeting.
■How to take disciplinary action against an employee.
■How to plan.
■How to delegate.

Each skill in the leadership spectrum, however, is a separate area. Each must be pinpointed and worked on individually. Beware of courses that promise to make you a leader in all areas in two or three days.

■Communication skills: These management skills become more important as executives rise in the company ranks. Fortunately for a manager who lacks these skills, they're teachable. Skilled coaching may never make lackluster or apprehensive speakers dynamic performers, but they can be brought up to a level adequate for the job.

■Effective decision-making: It usually involves three separate skills...
■Ability to collect and analyze information—which can be taught.
■Good judgment—which usually cannot be taught.
■Decisiveness—which also usually cannot be taught.

Managers can be taught how to identify the data they need to do the job and how to analyze that data. But even with those skills, some people continue to use poor judgment. Others are unwilling to take action, to stand for something. Endless analysis continuously postpones the decision to do something.

Management Skills That Can't Be Taught

■Mental horsepower: The ability to learn. This capacity is usually clearly present (or not).

■Initiative: The high-energy, get-things-done type of person can't be created by training a basically reactive personality.

■Likes and dislikes: The essence of job motivation. Whether a manager likes or hates the types of activities required by a job has a lot to do with his overall motivation.

Experience shows that the biggest cause of job turnover is that people dislike what they are doing—not that they lack the skills for the job.

Example: An engineer may take a job as a manager because of the appeal of status and perks—but hate having to evaluate, train or take action on personnel issues.

Preventing this kind of mismatch is absolutely essential for the company to operate efficiently. And depending upon mechanical techniques to prop people up— "you may hate this, but you can still learn how to do it"—is futile. Managers are much better off learning how to spot poor matches between personalities and jobs than they are trying to force a poor match to do a better job.

■Resilience: Good managers must spring back from a setback without a prolonged period of depression. Salespeople who feel that every lost sale is a personal rejection eventually must get out of sales.

■Tolerance of ambiguity: At the middle levels of management, people can be "experts" at everything they need to know to do the job right. At senior levels, people who can't act unless they "know everything" are doomed to frustration. They injure the company by their efforts to over-control. People either cope with ambiguity—or they don't.

■Personal impact: Managers can be coached into improving the way they dress—and that can help. But self-confidence, enthusiasm, a willingness to pitch in—competencies essential for most management jobs—can't be trained.

Filling The Gaps

Once the areas of weakness are determined, the next step is taking action—either offering training where training can pay off—or making other arrangements.

Caution: Getting high-performing managers to acknowledge that they're deficient in one or more key skills and that they need help is a delicate task. Best way to do it: Collect the data that make the point and present them to the manager, in the hope that he/she reaches the same conclusion.

Example: If the manager needs help in organizing time, cite the number of missed deadlines and meetings in the past month.

Top management's task is to make sure the company has a working performance appraisal system—not an annual formality. Senior managers must be taught how to coach middle managers without destroying esteem and dignity.

Challenge: If a manager acknowledges that he'll probably never master the skill, but knows that other strengths are well-matched to the job. Solution: Make sure his activities are consistently backed up by either:

■A boss who understands the weakness—which has also been acknowledged by the manager. A national sales manager, for instance, may understand that the West Coast manager is no good at getting details under control. When that regional manager makes a recommendation, the national manager takes time to talk through the situation and review the data together. That might not be necessary with the Midwest manager who always prepares the case for a decision in great detail—but who may need the boss's coaching in other areas, such as how to deal with subordinates because of a pattern of being too critical.

■An administrative assistant who is strong in the skills that the manager lacks. A manager who is weak in writing and planning his work should look for an AA strong in those areas.

■Peers can be a great source of help, but can only be effective when they trust each other. If they are in competition for a promotion, for example, it generally won't work.

Source: Robert W. Rogers, chief operating officer, Development Dimensions International, a human resources consulting firm, 1225 Washington Pike, Pittsburgh, PA 15242.

Fit The Manager To The Job

Many companies solve problems short term by opportunistically fitting a manager into an open slot. But the penalties can be long run. Consider a get-things-done executive brought into a troubled department. After setting things right, the executive leaves the company. Meanwhile, the person has alienated so many people that they leave too, and the company is left without an experienced staff. Instead, match the manager to the job.

Lean toward people-oriented managers to keep an already well-run operation in tune. They work very hard and very quickly. And they solve problems pragmatically, though they are not well organized and usually do not like details. Be prepared, though, to work with managers who make decisions at a moderate pace. They need support from superiors. These managers tend to be good at nurturing, but not criticizing, subordinates.

Favor impulsive types for first-line plant managers. They work fast but not hard. They shoot from the hip since they are highly intuitive. Managers above them can expect high performance. But impulsives let everyone know how they feel, whether they want to hear it or not.

Look for sociable and persuasive managers for personnel and public or customer relations. They have a great need to be noticed and stroked by superiors. They also tend to lack clear long-range perspectives and are not especially well organized. But these managers can advance beyond their abilities due to great social skills or the old boy network.

Source: Dr. Gerald Olivero, vice president, Perception and Preference Inventory Division, PA International Management Consultants, Inc., New York.

Matching Managers To Products

The manager who boosts a product's market share in a fast-growing market may not be the best person to manage the product once it matures since managers have widely differing strengths, ranging from entrepreneurial talents to expertise in financial and operational controls.

General Electric classifies its products in three phases: grow, defend, and harvest. The managers who are put in charge of each phase known as growers, caretakers, and, facetiously, undertakers.

Growers are usually entrepreneurial types. They are good at innovation and risk-taking, but weaker on financial controls and organization.

Caretakers tend to be growth-oriented, yet strong on cost-cutting and productivity improvement. They are also good at financial controls and understand the nuances of cash flow.

Undertakers are tough and pragmatic, but not adventurous. They are able to milk every cent of profit from a product after its growth potential has peaked.

But installing a system that matches managers to products has potential hazards. Some of them:

■Bringing in a manager from another division can demoralize subordinates who are expecting promotions.

■Competent managers who are ousted from their positions only because the company's product strategy has changed can become dissatisfied if another challenging position isn't found for them.

■Evaluating a manager's talents can be imprecise and lead to improper assignments. Smaller companies are usually more adept at assessing their managers than bigger ones.

Upgrading Production Managers

Manufacturing management has long been one of the least popular courses in top business schools. But no longer. Companies will soon be able to draw from a bigger pool of talent as more students sign up for production operations courses. The bottleneck consists of a shortage of qualified teachers. Many schools now borrow engineering professors to teach manufacturing operations courses. Another problem is that some courses lack substance in solving practical problems and dealing with production workers and first-line supervisors.

One barrier to recruitment is that many MBAs do not want to start work on the factory floor. And many of them do not want to live in the smaller towns and cities in which so many plants are located. Students from the Midwest generally take to small town living better than most.

To upgrade production managers within the company reward top-notch manufacturing managers equally with top people in finance and marketing; make it clear within the company and outside the company that manufacturing management can be a road to the top; and work with older manufacturing executives to overcome their frequent prejudice against hiring MBAs.

Finding Good Managers

What are the traits to look for in employees who are candidates for promotion? They must:

1. Want to be managers because they're comfortable in the position, not just for money or power.

2. Be able to ease stress for themselves and subordinates.

3. Trust their own judgment enough to work with a minimum of feedback from higher management.

4. Be able to handle different situations well most of the time.

5. Channel other people's hostility to solve the problems at hand.

6. Have had successful experience in management positions.

Source: *The Levinson Letter*, The Levinson Institute, Cambridge, MA.

How To Keep Executive Talent

Important reasons why strong chief executives sometimes fail to hold on to star executive talent:

■They fail to let an aggressive executive know how important he or she is to the organization out of concern that the executive will use that information to bargain. A top-notch executive already knows he is valuable. But he may not know how important he is to that particular company, unless the chief makes that clear.

■They don't always realize the importance of rewarding high performers with both cash and authority.

■They fail to communicate their own awareness of how the organization is changing and what it will mean to aggressive executives' careers.

■They depend too much on feel for talent rather than an executive manpower planning system.

To increase the company's chances of holding on to the best:

■The chief executive must give star performers personal attention and a clearer idea of their potential career within the organization. Speak to them specifically about potential power, responsibilities, rewards, challenges. An exact timetable is not necessary.

■Be sure to employ a balanced approach of outside hiring and inside management development.

■Be prepared. A company needs a systematic CEO-directed procedure for pre-screening and advancing talented people on a five-year time frame. Also necessary is a corporate-wide program for assessing overall need for executives. It is particularly important to identify executives most vulnerable to recruitment by other companies by reason of their skills or their inside information on your company.

Source: Kenneth A. Myers, president, Golightly & Co., International, Inc., New York.

Lessons In Developing Super Supervisors And Super Employees

Unusual dual problem...workers aren't being managed for peak performance ...and managers aren't trained to get the best results from the employees they supervise.

The Core Of The Problem

In 15 years of studying the problem in many different companies, I've seen managers commit a wide variety of simple, but costly, mistakes. Worst examples...and some solutions:

■Workers aren't told why they should perform a task. Take time to discuss the big picture. Tell workers how their contribution is important in moving the company closer to its goals. Explain the benefits of success, and tell them you'll be available to help if they need you.

■No one tells workers what they're really supposed to do. Sounds incredible, but supervisors do get into the habit of leaving out details of their instructions, especially where jobs are routine. In fact, no two tasks are ever absolutely identical.

Better: Don't worry about giving workers too much detail. You can't hurt their performance by being specific. Also tell workers when they're expected to perform a task and what percentage of error, if any, you'll tolerate. Employees often believe they're doing the right thing when they're really not. Solution: Give feedback frequently—even several times a day isn't too often. Whenever possible, ask workers to record their own achievements.

■Workers are regularly told that something else is more important. Assign priorities to each task. When priorities change, let employees be the first to know. Trap: Don't label everything a hot project. Even in hospitals, some emergencies have priority over others.

■The punishment/reward system isn't effective. Some managers actually reward workers for poor performance.

Examples: Giving difficult-to-control workers assignments that give them lots of freedom…or simply correcting a worker's errors whenever he makes mistakes.

Other supervisors punish workers for doing a good job.

Example: Some employees diligently call the boss from the field, only to get bawled out for something.

Before delivering a punishment or reward, consider the consequences on future performance. Helpful: Keep a record of your interactions with workers. Make sure at least half of these are either positive or neutral. If you must assign an unpleasant job, balance it with a reward of, say, some free time.

Management Responsibility

The underlying reason for these forms of mismanagement is most often the belief that management means simply telling subordinates what do. Management, though, really is helping subordinates to do what they're supposed to do…better.

If a manager doesn't believe this, ask him how much work his subordinates get done when he's out. The answer is typically around 90% of what must get done. Then ask how much would get done if his subordinates were out. Answer: Maybe 5%, if he's lucky.

The message: Subordinates are more valuable to their supervisor than he is to them. His job is to help them do their job better. If he doesn't, he's not a manager.

Solutions From Top Management

To help managers get better results from their subordinates…

■Let managers know the responsibility is theirs. When a supervisor tells you one of his people is failing, don't tell him to fire him. Instead, ask the manager what he's specifically doing to correct the situation.

Remind managers regularly that the only reason they're on the payroll is to help the people below them be as successful as the company needs them to be. You'll be surprised at how much better managers perform once they develop this belief.

■Urge managers to praise workers not only when they succeed, but when they fail less. If an employee was habitually four days late in turning in reports, but now is only one day late, acknowledge the improvement. That goes against the grain of most supervisors, but praise of this type is an effective step toward eventually getting the report on time.

■Let managers know that it's cheaper for the company to help a failing worker improve than to replace him. If there's any doubt, ask supervisors to go through the exercise of calculating the cost—including their own time—of firing a worker and training a replacement.

■Instruct managers to stay in close touch with each worker they supervise. That sounds basic, but most managers don't do it. To show them how serious you are, ask them periodically, "Which one of your subordinates has achieved something today?" If they can't respond, tell them you expect an answer the next time you ask. When they do answer, next ask them how they rewarded the achievement.

Let managers know that on performance appraisals, they'll be rated on whether their subordinates generate ideas.

Evidence that a manager isn't doing his job correctly: Constant complaints about his subordinates.

■Use management-training seminars, but choose carefully. First rule: Stay away from seminars built around a catchword that's currently in vogue. Example: "Participative management." (Is there really any other kind?) Instead, look for courses built around training in specific skills—just as an auto-repair course would be.

When you compare seminars, find out what other companies have used the ones you're investigating. Ask executives of those companies what their supervisors are doing differently as a result of the training. If they can't tell you, keep looking.

Source: Ferdinand F. Fournies, president, F. Fournies & Associates, management consultants to companies, including AT&T, Exxon, General Motors and Hewlett-Packard, 129 Edgewood Dr., Bridgewater, NJ 08807. His book is *Why Employees Don't Do What They're Supposed To Do...And What To Do About It,* Liberty House, 1517 14 St. W, Billings, MT 59102.

For Much, Much More Effective Supervisors

Even the most enlightened chief executives will fail in their efforts to create world-class companies if they overlook a vital group of employees whose help is essential for any long-term strategy: Supervisors.

Supervisors are the company's direct link to the work force. They can't and shouldn't be ignored.

Biggest problem with supervisors today: Many are still stuck in the old-fashioned way of doing business, emphasizing the corporate hierarchy. They manage subordinates using commands, deadlines, quotes and reprimands.

Managing "by the book," with no regard for individuality, much less teamwork, is still a major drag on many companies.

Trap: In the short run, such domineering tactics may get the job done by the deadline. But they typically result in subordinates caring little for the company, and resorting to undercutting each other to make themselves look better. In the end, everyone suffers...and so does the company's profitability.

Better Ways

Today, there's no reason supervisors can't stop treating workers like cogs—and boost quality and productivity at the same time.

Key: Workers expect supervisors to acknowledge their basic human needs, dignity and problems. That means, first, learning to listen without being judgmental.

Next: Encouraging people to air their opinions and feelings. This vital communication channel allows teams to form by fostering trust among members of the team. When teams form, and supervisors who lead them are true players on the team, rather than just bosses, effective leadership is the result.

Training Secrets

Top management can start retraining its supervisors by looking at the way they are treated. Does the company typically manage them by command—setting deadlines, quotas, etc.—or does it consult them about proposed goals and incorporate their ideas?

Since they're closest to line workers, if supervisors aren't in agreement with the company's strategic objectives, chances are slim that they will be effective leaders of their own subordinates.

Next, top management must push supervisors to stop thinking of themselves as bosses, and instead to see themselves as team leaders.

Supervisors must understand that producing quality quickly will determine tomorrow's winners. That requires the enthusiastic support of every employee on the company's payroll. Such enthusiasm will never emerge unless supervisors learn to value their subordinates as vital contributors to a common cause—superior performance for the benefit of everyone.

Unblocking Roadblocks

Top management can teach supervisors the tricks of team-building by building teams of supervisors first. Supervisors must be convinced that, contrary to past custom, their own advancement now depends on how well they can lead team members and workers without threats and controlling behavior. This creates incentive for wanting to improve their people skills.

This also allows everyone to hear the same things, so they will begin to develop a sense of common purpose. Talk to them about the company's culture, its philosophy and its intended thrust in the market. If there are changes from the company's traditional way of doing things, explain them thoroughly.

Challenge: Change is threatening to most people. The better supervisors understand the underlying forces, the better they will be able to communicate these to the workers they oversee.

Assume that bad habits can be unlearned. For some companies, it's helpful to bring in outside consultants to teach people-management skills.

By putting supervisors in groups, with a trainer to break the ice, it's easy to demonstrate which ideas work best and which alienate people. Various techniques include classroom instruction, role playing, videotaping and case study interaction.

After the classes, the consultant can fine-tune any areas that may still look weak.

Helpful Tool

We've developed our own Omega Personality Inventory (there are others on the market) which is a simple test that can be administered by anyone in the company. Basically, it explores how a person deals with people and work.

The answers reflect ranges of assertiveness (from leadership to rigid control) ...and responsiveness (from free expression of feelings to cold authority). We use the answers to judge which people might work effectively together on a team—and which ones probably would not.

Additional Prerequisites

Changing the way supervisors function requires two other important steps from top management...

■Strict prohibition of individual power centers or "kingdoms" within the company. These run directly counter to the cooperative arrangement required in today's business climate.

■Encouragement of cooperation among departments. A company beset by interdepartmental rivalry will never establish team cooperation within departments. Nor can such a company ever hope to be competitive against its tough external rivals. Top management can help break down interdepartmental barriers by putting people from different disciplines together on project teams so they'll get to know each other. Rewards should be geared to promoting cooperation among all departments.

Source: William J. Dorgan, III, president, Omega: Consultants to Management, 125 Smith Ave., Greenville, RI 02828. Besides working with individual corporate clients, he designs seminars and in-house training programs for Dun & Bradstreet Business Education Services.

How To Delegate Better

The five biggest delegating problems that managers face and the best and most efficient ways to handle them...

Decision Trap

There's no magic formula that will tell a manager when to ask a subordinate to do a job, but there are useful guidelines...

■Will the delegated task help the subordinate grow in a way that benefits his career path in the company?

■Will delegation move the company closer to its goals?

■Will the extra time you'll have as a result of delegation help you move the company closer to its goals?

Instruction Trap

Many managers aren't afraid to delegate—but they neglect to give adequate instructions to the subordinate. Those managers feel it's patronizing to lay out the job in great detail, so they wind up not explaining it clearly. If the subordinate is brave enough to come back with a question, the manager often says something that the subordinate takes to mean, *You must be an idiot not to know that*.

Solution: Explain the job and its background clearly, but leave the door open so the subordinate feels he can come back to you for clarification later if he needs it.

Dirty-Job Trap

Subordinates resent getting what they perceive as your dirty jobs—only. To head off this problem...

■Make it clear that you're not afraid of tedious, unpleasant tasks. Occasionally do your own photocopying or filing. When you've demonstrated your willingness to do the unpleasant tasks, subordinates will be less reluctant to do them, too.

■When you do delegate one of these tasks, explain its importance, but don't try to hide its unpleasant aspects. Say something like, "We all have to do these jobs, and the quicker we get on with them, the quicker we can move on to something more exciting."

■Give immediate feedback (praise, if possible) to the person you delegate the unpleasant job to.

Priority Trap

New projects come up...priorities change...crises arise. And someone has to respond to them. We all tend to give emergency jobs to our better people, and these are the very subordinates who are already busy. Result: The subordinates resent being shuffled around and productivity plunges.

Encourage subordinates to tell you immediately when they have a conflict in priorities. One way to do this is to avoid showing displeasure when a valued employee points to his work load when you delegate a new task to him.

Instead, work with the employee to rearrange priorities or remove some of the work load to make room for a new assignment. A few employees always try to take on too much work, a trait that's not necessarily good. Before delegating to these employees, remember to ask them about their current work schedule.

Too-Little Delegation Trap

Over-delegation isn't nearly as big a problem as inadequate delegation—nor is it nearly as widespread. The consequences of over-delegation quickly become apparent and need quick attention.

Under-delegation is usually more subtle. Apart from creating bottlenecks in work flow, under-delegation frustrates younger employees. If they do stay with the company, they won't grow, but it's more likely that they'll just move on.

The solution lies with upper-level executives. They must:

■Constantly let managers know what the company's priorities are and how the priorities affect each department.

■Give managers and their subordinates training in giving and accepting delegation. The training doesn't have to be extensive. It should include some of the points we've mentioned here, and it needn't be more than a half hour or so in an orientation program or management training seminar. Delegation becomes much more effective when a training program explains the problems before they're encountered in actual work.

Source: Allan Prager, vice president, Cresap, the general management consulting unit of Towers, Perrin, 333 Bush St., San Francisco 94104.

How To Build Competence Without Missing Work

Unfortunate reality: The task of efficient management requires competencies that many managers haven't yet developed.

Challenge: Training managers at all levels without jeopardizing the output of daily work.

One of the most effective approaches to training is to integrate it with work. It's also one of the most cost-effective ways to develop workers both on the line and in management ranks.

Short-term cost: Some initial slowdown in the work process. Ultimate payoff: Substantial management effectiveness and productivity improvements, as well as cost reductions and profit growth.

Where To Start

Search for opportunities to build competence by identifying in each major task the desired result of the work the individual must perform and the development improvement you want for the individual who must complete the task.

Example: A unit of a major computer company wanted its manufacturing managers to generate new ideas on how the company could better compete in the expanding international and domestic environments it was operating in. Senior management knew it would be difficult to generate those ideas, because these managers were used to operating in a vacuum, working from year to year, getting their jobs done within budget, but with minimal attention to factoring in the realities of outside marketplace trends in carrying out their responsibilities.

Part of each manufacturing manager's job had always been preparing the next-year business plan, with recommendations on how to achieve the goals, budget, capital investment requirements and workforce needs.

To broaden its middle managers' capabilities, senior management added another objective...use the requirement of preparing the annual business plans to develop strategic plans and expertise for the whole business.

That meant getting managers to use information that they weren't accustomed to using in devising their expanded annual business plans, including...

■Long-term corporate priorities.
■What the competition was planning to do next.
■Critical socio-political trends.
■Issues of customer satisfaction.
■Obstacles to getting the product to market in a more timely way.

Senior management suspected that the tunnel vision it had been encouraging in its manufacturing managers (and in managers in other key units) was handicapping efforts to improve performance through change and flexibility.

Many of the manufacturing managers already had a good sense of useful strategic information, but they weren't being asked to use that knowledge in their day-to-day work, including the task of drawing up business plans.

Finding Out The Basics

To quickly discover what the managers already know...

■Divide all the managers of a division (or, in a smaller company, all key managers) into groups of four to six.

■Have each small group spend an hour brainstorming to identify the 10 most significant internal and external trends affecting the company's future operations, financial health and viability.

■For the next hour, have all members from all groups sit together and review each four-member group's output to identify common themes.

Putting The Data To Use

The exercise got the managers to identify how much they already knew about each area. Since they weren't responsible for the knowledge and might even have suspected that they would be criticized by peers for moving off their turf, they generally had not used the knowledge in any systematic way. Now, however, they found that they could put the information to use by thinking of new ideas for, say, marketing the company's products, developing entirely new markets or achieving greater customer satisfaction.

The exercise took the idea of strategic planning from an abstraction to the level of practical usefulness. The managers—whose typical reaction to many classroom exercises is "so what"—could see how taking account of the outside environment could significantly influence what they put into their year-to-year business plans.

If the company decided, for instance, to build a plant in the Far East in no less than four years, managers could begin thinking now about how that move would affect their operations today—and in upcoming years. They could add to their next generation of plans the actions required now for adjusting to the addition of a new Asian plant, instead of just waiting for the plant to be built and then scrambling to adjust. Result: A major new competence—strategic thinking—became integrated into their day-to-day work.

The basic building blocks for competence building...

■Help managers understand what data and trends about the company's competitive situation they already know but are not using systematically in their daily work.

■Provide a system to use that information—with the help of senior managers expert in using such data, or an internal or outside consultant.

■Give managers access to information they need to perform at a higher level (marketing information to engineers and manufacturing managers, for instance; engineering and manufacturing information to sales and marketing people, etc.).

■Find a major task—such as reorganizing the annual budget process—to urge employees to think with a broader base of information.

Source: Charles C.D. Hamilton, president, Charles Hamilton Associates, 236 Huntington Ave., Boston 02115.

Chapter 4
Managing The Work

Principles Of Managing Work

■Myth: Managers get resources and authority to match their responsibilities.

Managers are rarely given the wherewithal to complete assignments and fulfill responsibilities. In most cases, managers have to gain both approval and cooperation from other groups and individuals over whom they have no authority.

■Myth: Jobs and departments operate in non-overlapping compartments.

Inevitably, there is great overlap. One person can't get much done without the cooperation of others. There is no way to establish clear separations. Problems are always arising which "fall between the cracks." Associates who say they won't do something because "it's not their job" are not going to be very successful.

■Myth: Rules, policies and decisions should be mutually consistent.

The manager who expects to get overtime approved because the boss has decreed that "this is a rush order" may well be naive. There can be and often are rules against doing those things which appear to be highly consistent with the objectives one has been given.

■Myth: Employees who "win" get rewarded—consistently.

Even the concept of "winning" may be incorrect for most jobs. Many times upper management views things quite differently and what seems to the employee to be a fine job, well done, is not even going to be noticed. People can't expect to be "rewarded" as they were in school, for every good exam or paper. In any job, much good work can go unnoticed for long periods of time, but of course, in good companies, superior performance does get recognized over time.

■Myth: The "boss" is the focal point for subordinates; work goes through the boss, not around the boss.

Bosses who expect that subordinates will restrict their communications to them are in for a rude awakening. Employees need to access a variety of people in the organization if they're going to work effectively. A manager gets overwhelmed when everything goes through his office and he can never provide the information and the permissions that subordinates need to get by dealing laterally.

■Myth: Organizations are neat "pyramids."

An organization chart tells who works for whom...period. It doesn't pretend to tell how work gets done or how people interact. Those little boxes seem to suggest that everything is neatly compartmentalized when it isn't. Work flows laterally. A great deal of negotiation has to take place that crosses over department lines and job "turf." Tasks are often ambiguous...most can be done in a variety of ways and it takes a great deal of cross-talk to get them done in such a way that they are mutually compatible.

■Myth: Managers who aren't part of top management should be administrators; taking the structure, systems and technology as given and fixed.

Every effective manager needs to be a leader and take responsibility for introducing change. Lower level managers are in the best position to see when procedures aren't working. They then need to negotiate for authorization to introduce changed jobs and different methods of work, even new technology.

Point Of View

Most employees are startled when they discover how differently their bosses see the world. What are "obvious" problems and high priorities to them are often of lesser importance to the boss, and it is not unusual for bosses to give assignments that are contradictory or overwhelming.

Their instructions will often be vague about what problems need attention, and no one rings a bell to announce when to go into action.

■Successful employees eventually become "maze bright," as it is called. They are able to deal with contradictions, vague or implicit requirements and to make sense of a work world that appears irrational.

In a sense, entering the working world mirrors the entrance into adulthood. Children are given clear, understandable rules. And, although they don't always act upon it, children think they know right from wrong—and how to get a reward. Adulthood—and organizations—are much more ambiguous.

Source: Leonard R. Sayles, professor of management, Columbia University's Graduate School of Business, New York 10027.

Getting Results

Telling employees why they do what they do is more important than simply a laundry list of what to do. Such results-oriented job descriptions help focus employees' attention on results, eliminates boredom, and builds motivation. Important: When creating a job description, link duties to results, and then give reasons why work is important.

Source: *Building a Fair Pay Program* by Roger J. Plachy, American Management Association, 135 W. 50 St., New York 10019.

Improving Performance

As managers trim down companies by eliminating layers of managers, staff and assistants, a few significant changes in compensation policy can keep the organization alert, on track, motivated and productive. Key to increasing flexibility and competitiveness: Move decision-making downward and then support that shift by putting more risk in those decision-makers with salaries and bonuses.

A New Way Of Thinking

For compensation to be useful as an engine for company health and growth, it must be contingent on performance at all three levels:

■Overall company performance. This should be the big factor in determining contingent compensation of top executives, but it should carry much less weight in setting incentives for middle managers, and very little weight in setting compensation for employees at the lowest level.

■Performance of a specific unit or department. Heavy weighting here is appropriate in setting the compensation for middle managers.

■Individual performance. More weight due here in setting compensation for the lower middle management of the company—to increase accountability.

For this system to work, of course, employees at all three levels must be clear about what good performance means in their day-to-day work. For top management, the goal could be strictly financial. For middle managers, it could be increasing market share, or more productive operation of the unit they control, or a new product introduction. For hourly workers, performance is likely to mean productivity and efficiency.

Leverage is what makes contingent compensation systems work. The reward for top performance should be generous. In fact, the prospect of a 15% incentive, or more, is generally necessary to produce a major change in the way a person acts on the job or thinks about opportunities.

Rewarding Key Contributors

Companies that depend on innovative research and engineering to keep their competitive edge have to think more sharply now about using compensation to retain—and energize—individuals working on projects that represent the future of the company. The typical reward for good senior managers—base salary and annual bonus—is generally less effective for these technical- or project-oriented individuals. What often does work:

■A major reward—in cash or stock—upon successful completion of a project. For a relatively small project, the reward could be a percent of salary. For a major long-term project, the reward could be three to five times annual salary.

■If the individual works in a fairly independent unit of the company, use an accounting firm or investment banker to set a fair value on the unit, and reward the individual in phantom stock that increases as the value of the unit increases (either in earnings or assets).

Corporate Defense

Protect the company by vesting the reward over time—say 25% a year, which would encourage the highly talented individual to stay on board for at least another four years.

Source: Ira S. Walter, director of executive compensation, Hay Group, New York 10036.

Best Way To Manage Change

Organize a change team made up of: 1. An "inventor"—a top executive who focuses on the broad picture, thereby identifying opportunities for change. 2. An "integrator" who makes sure plans for change don't disrupt important functions in the company and consolidates support for change among employee ranks. 3. An "expert" who acts as a project director in implementing the plan for change. He handles all of the technical aspects of the change, making sure they're understood by managers and subordinates. 4. A team of "managers" who delegate new assignments to employees and ensure that transitions to new ways are completed.

Source: Mary B. Esteves, McBer and Company, Boston management consultants, quoted in *Creative Management*, 817 Broadway, New York 10003.

Creative Criticism

Creative criticism aids subordinates' performance without undermining self-esteem. Important: Be specific about what's wrong—for example, not enough research in a report, careless arithmetic in a market summary, not enough customers called. Outline the changes you expect to be made. Limit fault-finding to one subject at a time. Give criticism in private and allow time for the subordinate to ask questions and get clarification.

Source: *The Levinson Letter*, 375 Concord Ave., Belmont, MA 02178.

The Secrets Of Successful Continuous Change

Problem: Americans are raised on the notion that change is bad. The thinking is if you take care of yourself, do things the same old way and protect your turf, everything will be all right.

Reality: Companies that don't discard this belief are doomed.

Challenge: Getting employees at all levels to feel comfortable taking risks for the good of the organization. In every task the company undertakes—new automation, job restructuring or a drive for better quality—the key to long-term success is having people expose themselves to greater job responsibility and accountability, and possibly to be hurt. The issue always remains the human ego—What will it mean to do something I'm not comfortable with?

Motivator: People basically want to do a good job. They want their jobs and their lives to have meaning. They want their companies to be successful. So, it's almost always the system that demotivates or holds them down.

Before new ways of doing things can be implemented, companies must first confront the real issues that are driving their organization—including the hidden attitudes and assumptions that cause people to talk one way but act quite differently.

Example: While extolling teamwork, some managers may withhold vital information that's necessary to make good decisions. Or one department subtly sabotages the achievements of another. In both cases, change is blocked.

It's important to accept the job of changing the company as a long-term project. You can't get people to accept the virtues of change by simply sending around inter-office memos, or by asking them to read the latest book by a management guru. Changing the company is a slow process.

Starting An Improvement Program

Before initiating a company-wide effort at change and improvement, it's important to create an atmosphere where problems can be vocalized. Management must emphasize and reemphasize the importance of bringing problems out into the open. Only then can constructive change begin.

Some problems come out in meetings where employees are actually asked to state problems. Other issues are sensitive and will be divulged by worried employees only in private one-on-one meetings with a trusted associate or an experienced consultant.

Implementing A Five-Track Program

Once the atmosphere for voicing and solving day-to-day problems is established, it's time to forge the broader foundation for fostering long-term change.

We advise a five-track program, carried out in sequence, with some overlapping. The first three tracks are aimed at behavior...

■Confronting the company's culture—challenging negative attitudes, mistrust, apathy, rigidity, etc.

■Improving management skills. This is best done with separate peer groups of workers and managers to avoid the tendency to play it safe and stick to the status quo—especially in front of one's immediate boss.

■Team building—bringing managers and workers back together, after they have developed more positive attitudes and better skills, to instill teamwork, cooperation and effective problem-solving skills throughout the company.

Example: Hold regularly scheduled work group meetings at which each person must list how he has "lived" the new culture and applied the updated skills on the job since the program began. Then each person shares his list with the rest of the group and asks if they have observed what he describes. If not, the person must come to grips with the fact that knowing what to do intellectually—even agreeing that it's necessary—isn't the same as actually doing it.

The group might say, "You may have thought about being more receptive to new ideas, but just the other day you told us to stop asking so many questions and just do as we were told." After several months of these "gentle confrontations," it will become more difficult for any member to face the group without having made the necessary changes in behavior.

Follow-up is essential. Have the peer group develop a "monitoring system"—a set of actions to be taken if a victory occurs or if further violations persist.

The last two tracks deal with...

■Company strategy and structure—reformulating strategic goals and then realigning divisions, departments, work groups, jobs and resources to best achieve the new strategic direction.

■Revising the company's reward system so that it truly rewards the desired behavior.

Example: Some companies now demand that as much as 50% of a manager's performance assessment depend on how well that manager has fostered team spirit, the new culture and problem-solving skill. The decision can be made by an anonymous poll of subordinates with the results going directly to the manager's superior.

It is critical that senior executives take full responsibility for the improvement program's success—or failure. Leaving it to human resources managers or other staff groups is deadly. Very large companies have found it useful to select a steering committee of top executives and employees—who represent all levels and areas of the company—to oversee the program and make sure it is implemented effectively.

Source: Dr. Ralph H. Kilmann, professor of business administration and director of the Program in Corporate Culture, Katz Graduate School of Business, University of Pittsburgh, Pittsburgh, PA 15260. As president of Organizational Design Consultants, Dr. Kilmann advises major corporations. His book is *Managing Beyond the Quick Fix*, Jossey-Bass, 350 Sansome St., San Francisco 94104.

How *Not* To Undermine Teamwork

The word *teamwork* sounds good to executives, but while voicing their fondness for teamwork, most CEOs do things to undermine it.

Many senior executives still believe management jurisdictions are autonomous. They hire a marketing manager and say, "You do the marketing, but stay away from other functions, like development and manufacturing—and we'll tell them to keep out of your territory, as well."

That's the first step in undermining teamwork. Reason: There's almost nothing one functional head can do that doesn't require either the collaboration of the others or, at least, a good deal of information from them.

Teamwork shouldn't have to be "added" by a company. It should be inherent in the interdependence that exists among all jobs in upper management. Good companies acknowledge this and avoid the common traps that undermine teamwork...

■Moving people too fast. In the naive belief that a good manager can do anything, companies move their executives around too fast. Some executives come to think of each job as only a stepping stone to the next one, not something that needs serious study and mastery. Result: Team members can't really work together, because they don't know enough about their own area to contribute real expertise to decisions.

Example: The marketing manager may want to introduce a new advertising campaign that, if not modified or perfectly timed, will harm the efficiency of the operations department. Only if the head of operations really knows how things work in his area can he make a useful contribution to the decision on how the new campaign should be handled. If he's new at the job, he'll either be blindly opposed or blindly agreeable. Either can be fatal.

■Many CEOs like "horse racing" too much. They frequently let senior subordinates know that they're in a race with one another to be the next CEO or the new EVP. Then, the game senior managers play is, "How can I destroy my competitors?" That's a classic teamwork destroyer.

■Widely dispersed players. When marketing, operations and maintenance are each in different states, it's very tough to promote cooperation and teamwork.

■Underevaluating team skills. Most CEOs don't spend enough time evaluating the team-building skills of their subordinates. Watching people at an executive committee meeting isn't the way to do it. CEOs must penetrate the day-to-day patterns of interaction to see whether the key functional heads can work together.

More Oversights

■Failing to inform. Being a good team player doesn't mean always saying "yes" to peers. It does mean giving full information, as far in advance as possible.

■Failing to stand up for things that are critical, and refusing to compromise when the issue is just as critical to a colleague...as long as the basic integrity of your system isn't compromised.

Effective CEOs learn to observe teamwork in their companies. They give credit (and demerits) for it and stop using fast tracks to encourage people to play "hop, skip and jump" with jobs. They are able to identify subordinates who know their operations and are willing to coordinate their jobs with those of other managers toward common advantage, instead of looking out for their personal bottom line.

Source: Dr. Leonard R. Sayles, professor of management, Columbia University Graduate School of Business, New York, and director, executive leadership research, Center for Creative Leadership, Greensboro, NC 27407.

Teamwork: Why Jobs Don't Fit Together

There's a major impediment to effective teamwork in most workplaces...the managers' presumption that most jobs are neatly bounded or compartmentalized. Managers and their subordinates spend much too much time figuring out who has what responsibility. Result: Employees undermine teamwork, because they're trained not to respond to the needs of co-workers or the good of the organization as a whole. Examples:

■A manager detects a defect in computer software that's creating extra work for his employees. He goes to his counterpart in the computer department and requests that the problem be remedied. He's told that the difficulty represents an "enhancement"—not an actual repair—and therefore must take its place on a long list of priority repair jobs.

■A manager discovers that problems faced by his staff may be due to aging computer disks, which are error-prone. He approaches the disk librarian and requests that the most critical data for his department be placed on new disks, which his budget will pay for. The librarian's response is negative because his job does not specify the management of two sets of disks.

The Solution

Managers need to recognize the broad range of alternatives for how, when and with whom the company's goals will be met. Teamwork is not simply doing the job correctly, but rather doing the job in a way that fits the needs of others whose work is an essential part of the whole. Keys to successful teamwork:

■Demonstrating a willingness to aid others at least as often as you make requests for their assistance.

■Locating people who must make continuous mutual adaptations close to each other and within a work group. People who become friendly and share common goals find it easier to work with each other.

■Learning to patiently explain why a task needs to be done, instead of simply pressuring people to do things your way. Team spirit depends on the absence of high-pressure tactics such as, "You know that senior management will really be on your back when they find out you refused me this request!"

Source: Dr. Leonard R. Sayles, professor of management, Columbia University Graduate School of Business, New York 10027 and director, executive leadership research, Center for Creative Leadership, Greensboro, NC.

Quality Improvement Programs

Many companies know what it takes to improve quality, but they stumble when it comes to putting specific measures into effect. That's true not only of heavy manufacturing companies but of many others as well. The big mistakes...

■Failing to bring together the people responsible for major elements that go into quality—design, engineering and processing, monitoring and inspection. Too often, people responsible for one of these areas don't communicate with people responsible for the others.

Example: Products are rarely designed with the manufacturing process and the inspection stage in mind. When that happens, the design may call for a manufacturing process that's prone to defects. Or the design can result in a finished product that's difficult to inspect or test.

Ironically, it's usually just as easy to design a product that can be manufactured with few defects as it is to design one where quality is a problem.

Key: The design team must work with (not apart from) the engineers and tool designers, the people who actually make the product and those responsible for verifying the quality of the product. And this coordination between workers must begin long before the product goes on line. It's far more expensive to change a design after an assembly line starts rolling.

Useful: Set up cross-functional teams. When the company decides to make a new product, create a team composed of people from each stage of production. The team's goal: To coordinate the design, engineering, manufacturing process and quality assurance of the product.

This approach to quality is a concept that can also be applied in companies that turn out almost any product or service. An ad agency, for example, may design a layout that looks great on the drawing board, but which fails in practice because it poses a difficult printing problem.

■Monitoring the manufacturing process imprecisely. Most companies are fairly efficient at monitoring machinery to verify that such things as numerical settings, motor current and pressure are correct. (New machine-monitoring devices now make the job even easier.)

But companies must go even further now. Very helpful: Periodically take a product out of the manufacturing flow and check it for things that aren't ordinarily checked—things that aren't important to the final product, but that do measure the precision of the manufacturing process.

Examples: In the auto industry, the operator might look at the edges of the panel for burrs, or the presence of die marks on the panel. If there are imperfections in the panel, the operator can immediately pinpoint the source of the problem and correct it. In the paper industry, a mill operator can measure such characteristics as moisture content and color.

These types of overlooked irregularities are almost always symptomatic of bigger problems elsewhere in the manufacturing process. Analogy: When people buy a new house, they often look at the quality of moldings. They're not important in themselves, but poor-quality moldings can be a tip-off of shoddy workmanship elsewhere.

Added advantage: In manufacturing, finding defects in this way can help pinpoint other abnormalities.

Examples: Maintenance problems, machine defects and inadequately trained workers.

■Checking the product imprecisely. In the past, companies typically checked a product or part after it was made. Now, more and more companies realize that in addition to monitoring and controlling the manufacturing process, the product must be checked periodically between all manufacturing steps.

Example: In automobile manufacturing, a door panel must go through several dies as it's stamped out from sheet metal. After each stamping operation, the panel can be monitored to see that all the holes and contours are in the right places.

But even companies that go through this process often make a crucial error. When they measure the part, it isn't always held or clamped in the same position as it was when it was made.

Result: A faulty panel may appear to be correct...or a perfect panel can appear flawed. Moreover, it may be difficult to determine if a flaw is in the tool or in the measurement.

Solution: When the product is checked on the assembly line, have it positioned and clamped as it was in the manufacturing process for accurate measurement. While obvious, this mistake, in fact, occurs often, usually because of the lack of coordination between tool and gauge designers during the product development.

Source: Anthony Lynch, senior consultant, Manufacturing Management Unit, Arthur D. Little, Inc., Acorn Park, Cambridge, MA 02140.

Cooperation Isn't Built In A Day

Biggest mistake managers make in creating teams: Setting up groups of employees based only on the professional skills required to meet a goal, and expecting those individuals to work together toward that goal. That strategy overlooks the most important parts of teams...the individual personalities.

Reality: There's a complex matrix of psychological dynamics that gets set into motion when individuals are grouped together. Though it's difficult to get the dynamics working in complete harmony, ignoring them altogether guarantees that teams will ultimately fall apart or, at the very least, operate well below their potential level of effectiveness. Understanding the dynamics of team psychology is very important and very valuable.

The Vital Components

To function at maximum strength and effectiveness, teams must possess these six essential ingredients...

■Trust. This encompasses the trustworthiness—and the willingness to trust—of each team member. To measure the existence of trust in a group, observe how members of the group interpret what they say about each other.

Example: When comments like, "The guy's out to get me" are made in reference to members of the same team, you know you've got a problem.

Unfortunately, most people are taught at an early age not to trust people. So building a foundation of trustworthiness and willingness to trust among workplace associates requires substantial practice and time.

■Provocability. This element is a form of discipline. It's what follows when one member's trust is breached.

Example: Team Member A says something to management that makes Team Member B look bad in order to cover up his own shortcomings. Team Member B, now provoked, reacts with appropriate anger, and clarifies the unacceptability of this behavior. Result: Member A recognizes the negative results of his poor behavior and is thereby disciplined. Chances are, he'll be less willing to betray a member of his team in the future.

Provocability is a deterrent to unacceptable behavior; properly used, it reinforces positive values in the team's interactions. Danger: Teams that demonstrate ready provocability and no trust. Ultimately, these groups tear themselves apart.

■Forgiveness. It follows incidents of provocation in properly functioning groups. In our example, Team Member B would forgive Member A for his betrayal after venting his anger and eliciting positive problem-solving in the future. It's a signal that cooperation has prevailed...in fact, that the commitment to work together has been strengthened.

■Clarity. This measures the openness of communication among teammates—a critical component of strong team dynamics. Each team member must know exactly what his teammates expect from him. In turn, he must make clear what he expects from others. If anyone on the team characteristically displays reticence or withdrawal, you immediately know you have a problem. If he's not expressing his needs, he's obviously misunderstanding what's expected of him and is therefore unable to be open with his teammates. If only one or two members of a 10-person team display this behavior, it can usually be addressed with confidential one-on-one conversations with the individuals.

If the entire team is reluctant to communicate, the problem is not with the team, but with top management.

■Lack of envy. This is a barometer of how much respect and affection teammates have for each other.

Example: If one team member gets a promotion, his teammates should cheer him, not resent him because of envy.

Lack of envy signifies that the team is mature and its spirit is positive and constructive; it also implies that the system provides adequate recognition for all members of the team.

■Joy. This describes the way teammates feel not only about the work itself, but about the whole idea of coming to work. If they have affection and respect for their teammates and for the company in general...if they look forward to coming to work, it's a sign that they have the joy that properly functioning teams generate.

The presence (or absence) of joy is a measure of whether the other five components of team psychology are properly balanced. If you find there's an absence or low level of joy among individual members of the team, take a closer look at the other elements. Chances are you'll find weaknesses you weren't previously aware of.

Source: Giséle Richardson, president, Richardson Management Associates, Ltd., 2060 Sherbrooke St. West, Montreal H3H 1G5.

Chapter 5
Managing A Troubled Company

Bankruptcy Strategies

When your firm faces insolvency, the first step is to face up to your financial problems early enough so you have time to act positively. Be careful not to fool yourself, which isn't hard to do if you're working hard to fool your creditors. You may be able to forestall the whole complex procedure that, once started, is both expensive and may lead inevitably toward bankruptcy.

What to do: Communicate with your creditors. Let them have the full story. Don't bluff. Credibility at this point may be the only thing that can save you. It buys you time—and even possibly more credit so you might effect a turnabout.

Danger in laying your problem on the line with creditors: One or more nervous creditors can reject your request for cooperation and rush to court to force you into bankruptcy. But if you can get the major creditors behind you, they'll be able to use their leverage to get cooperation. In my experience, they can be very persuasive, so play it straight with these big creditors—you need them.

Even if you can't forestall court action, the same general rule applies: seek creditor cooperation. Try to work with the committee of creditors in establishing a practical plan to keep the business operating. Don't wait until you're in court to do it. Emotions may be calmed and the credibility factor is much higher before you get into court.

It may sound self-serving, but it's vitally important: If you think you're going to face insolvency—get yourself into the hands of competent bankruptcy counsel—fast. Your corporate counsel will be the first to admit that this is a very specialized field that shouldn't be handled by general counsel.

There are three major forms of bankruptcy:

■Straight bankruptcy, which is limited to liquidation proceedings.

■Chapter 11, a voluntary proceeding in which the debtor seeks court protection while it continues in business as a debtor-in-possession and tries to work out an arrangement with unsecured creditors.

■Chapter 10, generally for large firms with public shareholders and public debt, and affects the rights of all classes of creditors, secured and unsecured, and of stockholders. It may be voluntary or involuntary.

What the bankruptcy lawyer does: His first job is to explore the reasons for your problems, possible cures, and to determine how you should act. Whether you should seek court protection, the timing and how and when to confront the creditors with your situation. These are critical decisions that can affect the final outcome of the proceedings and may determine whether the firm can stay in business.

Once those decisions are made, he'll be your key liaison between the court and the creditors' committee in either establishing a financial plan to keep the business operating or in dealing with the intricate steps of insolvency.

Straight bankruptcy liquidations vary in length, depending on such things as size and nature of the assets involved, potential causes of action to be asserted by the trustee. Chapter 11 proceedings also depend on the complexity and can last anywhere from several months (rare) to a few years. Chapter 10 proceedings are generally involved and go on for years.

If your customer faces insolvency, speed and good information are vital. If you wait too long, you may end up at the end of the line, holding out your hand with scores of other creditors for a share of a fast-shrinking pie.

If you have even the slightest hint your customer is in trouble, investigate that very day. Many lawyers advise checking with credit-reporting agencies and trade associations. I'm not so sure you should stop there. Better: Go to the firm's customers, suppliers and lenders—and do it personally, or have one of your trusted people do it. It requires a person with knowledge of industry insiders, a person who can deal in confidence and a person who is sensitive to people's reactions. Reason: Many executives hesitate, except in the strictest confidence, to report someone's financial plight. That's because such a person could face a defamation of credit suit if he's challenged by the firm he's reporting on.

If you determine your customer, to whom you may have just shipped $100,000 worth of goods, is in trouble, then you may be in trouble, too. What to do: Call your lawyer. Check whether you have liens on the goods. Have the liens properly filed (many aren't, for a multitude of reasons, mostly carelessness). Types of errors: Name of firm (using the trade instead of the corporate name) isn't exact, dealings were actually with a subsidiary or some other affiliate, chief place of business is in another state, etc.

Retaking shipped goods. Determine what the customer's chances of rehabilitation are. If bleak, move fast to get your goods back.

The Uniform Commercial Code gives you certain rights to demand return of goods delivered on credit while customer was insolvent (customer may refuse, but you should pursue anyway). You must make the demand within 10 days of receipt of goods. Another possibility: Every purchase agreement should contain the customer's written representation that he's solvent. If you can show he misrepresented his solvency within three months before delivery, you can demand the return of the goods, and you aren't bound by the 10-day limitation. Warning: These rights of reclamation may be cut off if not acted upon before a bankruptcy petition is filed. However, if you are able to retake the goods before the filing, you may have an excellent tactical advantage, because there's a serious legal question on how a bankruptcy court can overrule the de facto return of your unpaid-for-goods.

If, on the other hand, you determine your customer is in financial difficulty, that by itself is no reason to stop doing business with him. But be prudent. Maintain all shipments on a cash basis—or, if you're willing, grant him credit, but demand collateral or some security. Keep checking the customer's condition on a frequent basis and keep the level of credit within control.

Filing proof of claims: If you determine to file a claim, after consulting counsel, do so in time so that your claim isn't barred. The time within which a claim must be filed depends on the type of proceeding. If you aren't independently advised by counsel, you should monitor the proceedings and check with the court or creditors' committee attorney to be sure you are fully aware of all critical deadlines—and do not lose tactical advantage or forfeit your claim.

Warning: Don't be too quick to file a claim. Check first to see what, if any, claim the insolvent firm has against you. If it does have such a claim, and you make a filing, you now fall under the full summary jurisdiction of the court. It may end up costing you more than you could possibly get back.

If your supplier becomes insolvent. You may, for sound business reasons, want to protect your supplier from bankruptcy. You may just want him to stay in production to satisfy your supply needs, or you may want to buy him out. Don't be hasty. If you decide to assist him in remaining in business first check with the creditors' committee. Get their approval; they could give you trouble. But chances are they will support you.

Warning: If one form of your assistance is helping the insolvent supplier cover his payroll so he can keep operating, be sure provision is made for payroll taxes. If tax isn't paid, IRS may hold you liable.

If you wanted to acquire the insolvent firm, your main problem is establishing, to the satisfaction of court, creditors and shareholders, that you're paying fair value. Once again, check with the creditors' committee and preferably try to work out the arrangements under the court's umbrella.

Source: Joel B. Zweibel, partner, Kaye, Scholer, Fierman, Hays & Handler.

Alternative To Bankruptcy

A small paint manufacturer came close to bankruptcy during the last recession. The owner paid off the small creditors, then calculated that if the business was liquidated the major creditors would get only six cents on the dollar. Instead, he began negotiations with major suppliers for:

■Two years to make good on the debts. During that time, they would be paid in installments.

■Continued flow of supplies, to be paid for COD.

The creditors had nothing to lose. Profit on current COD transactions would be equal to or greater than the interest they would earn on the money they received from a forced bankruptcy. The owner also promised to close shop and liquidate immediately if ever behind in these payments on the debt.

The plan succeeded. Using time effectively, the company was in shape to prosper when the economy recovered.

"Creative" Accounting Devices Can Conceal Corporate Problems

"Creative" accounting devices are not causes, but symptoms, of corporate failure. If you're an employee (or an investor, vendor, or customer) and suspect your company has problems, look for these creative accounting devices as possible warnings of trouble ahead:

■Delaying the publication of financial results as long as legally possible.

■Capitalization of research costs, basing the write-off against existing or expected orders.

■Continuation of dividend payments from new equity or loans.

■Cuts in routine maintenance until repairs are so overdue that it becomes necessary to renovate.

■Consider leasing agreements as capital rather than as what they are—loans.

■Dividend increases from subsidiaries to the parent company and consolidation of more and more subsidiary results, from wholly and partially owned subsidiaries, into the parent company account.

■Retention of the main asset of the business in the owner's name (or that of the owner's spouse) rather than the company name (thereby removing it as a source of payment to creditors).

■The valuation of assets at whatever figure is wanted, since nobody may notice.

■Capitalizing interest charges, training expenses, computer installation costs.

■Using inflation as a cloud to hide asset revaluation.

■Paying company debts out of the proprietor's pocket to improve profits before he sells his share.

■Inventory valuation at latest market selling price rather than at actual cost.

■Deferment of current expense to the following year improves this year's sales and profits.

■Inadequate provision for depreciation by failing to revalue assets.

Source: *Corporate Collapse* by John Argenti, John Wiley & Sons, New York 10016.

How To Hide Debt

Until accounting rules are changed so that corporate balance sheets reflect the true value of assets, the only way many companies can expand their borrowing capacity is to use off-balance-sheet financing.

Keeping new debt and debt-like obligations off the liability side of the balance sheet enables a company to maintain a debt/equity ratio that's in line with the expectation of rating agencies and lenders. As long as lenders believe that a company's assets are undervalued to begin with, they're usually willing to go along with off-balance-sheet financing. This is especially true of money-center banks that are more aware that current accounting standards don't paint a true picture of a company's worth.

Off-balance-sheet financing techniques:

■Leasing. Rather than borrowing funds to purchase new equipment, a company can lease the same equipment without weakening its balance sheet. Even though the lease is a contractual obligation, accounting standards don't require it to be listed as a liability.

■Take-or-pay contracts. These can be good alternatives for companies that plan to take out a bank loan in order to finance quantity discounts. Instead, a company and its supplier enter into a pact that lets the company pay a lower price for its supplies if it guarantees to buy a specified quantity. Advantage: Avoids a loan which would show up on the balance sheet. Risk: If a company doesn't need all the items it contracts for, it must remain overstocked or sell the supplies, probably at a loss.

■Joint ventures. If two companies invest a small amount in a 50–50 joint venture and then borrow a far larger amount to complete the project, only the investment need be included in the asset/liability equation. Under accounting rules, the debt obligation is included only as a footnote. It's listed fully on the balance sheet of the joint venture itself, but that ledger isn't part of the sponsors' financial statements.

■Establishing a financing subsidiary. The subsidiary uses the accounts receivable of the company as collateral for a bank loan that's used to purchase the accounts receivable. This provides the company with cash, but the bank debt doesn't have to be shown on the balance sheet. The newly created financing subsidiary will then pay off its debt as accounts receivable are paid by the company's customers.

■Defeasance. This procedure, which is gaining in popularity, strengthens the balance sheet and provides a one-time boost to earnings. How it works: A company with long-term bonds uses cash to purchase government securities that will be put in an irrevocable trust. Interest on the government securities is then used to repay the principal and interest on the bond obligations as they come due. Because the trust guarantees the payments, the bond debt can then be wiped off the balance sheet. And since the old debt is at a lower interest rate then the new government securities, a lesser amount of face value of government securities than old debt is needed to cover the obligations. This difference is considered a gain and can be taken as a one-time increase in earnings.

Source: Arthur Wyatt, director of the Accounting Principles Group, Arthur Andersen & Co., 69 W. Washington St., Chicago 60602.

Practical Alternative To Chapter 11

Though filing under Chapter 11 of the Federal Bankruptcy Code is meant to protect the company from creditors while working out a plan of reorganization, for many companies filing for bankruptcy simply speeds up their collapse.

Pitfalls Of Chapter 11

■High costs: Fees must be paid to bankruptcy lawyers, accountants and consultants. Total cost ranges from $50,000 to $250,000 for a company with annual sales of about $5 million. It flies way up for the tangled bankruptcies of larger companies.

Many small companies find that so much of their revenue is spent on the filing that they don't have enough resources left to successfully reorganize.

■Delay and distraction: A company can be under the court's protection for as long as 18 months. During that period, its owners and managers are likely to spend more time handling the bankruptcy proceedings than running the business in a way that would get it out of trouble.

■Disruption of business. The bad publicity of a Chapter 11 filing may encourage customers, suppliers and employees to cut their losses by abandoning the company and taking their business elsewhere.

Healthy Alternative

Fortunately, there is an alternative to Chapter 11...negotiating an out-of-court settlement for the payment of debts with the company's creditors.

This is the solution that all professionals who work with troubled companies actively seek. The goal is to achieve the same result as Chapter 11 filing in face-to-face, out-of-court negotiations with creditors.

Key to negotiating a nonjudicial agreement with creditors: Early recognition of the problems that could lead the company to file for bankruptcy. Early warning signs: A continuing trend showing inability to make financial projections. Difficulty in meeting a bank's debt repayment plan.

Advantages Of A Nonjudicial Settlement

■Saves money. The fees paid to professionals are kept to a minimum, leaving more assets available to reorganize and revive the company. The same professionals are involved—bankruptcy lawyers, accountants and consultants—but in a much more efficient, hands-on and productive way.

■Less threatening to creditors, who are well aware that Chapter 11 proceedings will dissipate the company's assets.

■Resolved more quickly than Chapter 11 agreements—usually. That leaves company principals more time to work on solving the company's problems.

Reasons why nonjudicial settlements work well for small companies:

■Small companies have fewer creditors than large companies. The fewer parties involved, the easier it is to negotiate an agreement. Big companies must answer to large groups of shareholders…they often have no choice but to go to court to sort out conflicting claims.

■Small companies typically have a closer relationship with lenders and suppliers than do big companies. This closeness makes it easier to reach an agreement.

Last resort: Negotiation of a nonjudicial settlement to a company's problems should be part of the process that may ultimately lead to a bankruptcy filing. Only when the parties agree that there can be no agreement, should they file under Chapter 11.

Source: Joseph J. Giordano, partner and national director of the business reorganization services group, Coopers & Lybrand, CPAs, 1251 Ave. of the Americas, New York 10020.

Dealing With A Company In Chapter 11

With soft spots scattered throughout the economy, many companies are coming up against customers or suppliers in severe enough financial difficulty to file for Chapter 11 rehabilitation, which is far more common than actual bankruptcy that results in liquidation.

Suppliers should use extreme caution in reopening lines of credit with a Chapter 11 company. It is easy to identify such a firm, as it must have DIP (Debtor in Possession) after its name. Although new debts have priority over old debts coming under a Chapter 11 proceeding, there is no guarantee that the company will have enough money even to pay current creditors. Operating problems are not corrected just because the company has filed under Chapter 11.

A good general rule is to extend no credit at all unless there is reason to believe that the company will survive and confirm a plan. Then, whatever credit line the supplier extended before the Chapter 11 filing should be greatly reduced until the company proves that its cash flow is adequate. For example, a pre-Chapter 11 credit line of $100,000 might be reduced to $10,000.

Stay out of the picture during the first 30–60 days after a filing under Chapter 11. It takes that long to learn whether cash flow is sufficient and whether the creditors will stick by the company.

One risk to a supplier is that secured creditors may have a lien on all liquid assets of the company. If this is so, their claims have priority. Such a creditor may choose to cease financing the company, causing liquidation of the company's assets.

Another problem is that payroll, attorneys' and accountants' fees, taxes, and certain claims take priority over repayment of trade debt. Sometimes one current creditor gets a superpriority. For example, a key supplier refuses to grant credit unless it gets special consideration, and without the supplier the company cannot do business. The court and the creditor committee may agree to give that supplier priority over other new creditors.

Even if a company confirms a plan and is discharged from Chapter 11 (at which point it can erase the DIP from its corporate name), the danger period is not over. The credit risk is still high immediately after the company comes out of Chapter 11. In a common situation, a company scrapes together every last penny by refinancing its assets with the creditors' blessing, then it faces going out of business within 90 days after confirmation because of insufficient cash flow. Many of those companies that do survive remain weak for years.

Use the prudent approach. Do not take the company's own cash-flow projections at face value. Instead, assess its debt-payment schedule and its cash requirements, and then determine if cash flow warrants the granting of new credit. In addition to the company itself, sources of financial information about the company are members of the Chapter 11 creditor committee; the creditor committee's accountant (who supplies reports to the committee); and to a lesser extent, the company's bankers. If the bankers will not talk, assume the company's problems are serious.

Customers of a Chapter 11 company face less danger in dealing with it than do suppliers who are waiting to be paid. If the relationship has been a long and fruitful one, stick by the ailing company. But play it smart. Hedge with alternate suppliers in case the company does fold after all.

Source: Malcolm P. Moses, Malcolm P. Moses Assoc., Merrick, New York.

How To Deal With—And Avoid—Crises

The precipitating cause of most company crises is lack of cash, not lack of sales or profitability. Crisis points now arise with astonishing speed as companies do business with 20% or more interest rates and high volatility. The key is faster and more frequent review of basic company controls on credit, purchasing, inventories, taxes, and spending.

■Beef up credit departments. Call the customer at the same time that a 30-day statement is mailed. The traditional practice of three collection letters and a phone call is obsolete for effective cash management under today's conditions.

Reduce the time lag between the day a shipment is made and the day it is invoiced. The current average is seven days; most companies can do better.

Eliminate cash discounts. They are ineffective for stimulating cash flow, when customers are stretching payments because of high interest rates and their own liquidity concerns. Charge interest on the past-due accounts. It's becoming increasingly commonplace.

■Run the company's payables to produce the maximum amount of cash flow, not for the convenience of the company's billing department. Relate payments to due dates of the bills.

■Scrap excess inventory. The tax benefits and cash flow may make it worthwhile. The company will also save on rent, utilities, and insurance.

Should the company cut down on its customer-service guarantees? The era of shipping within 24 hours after receipt of an order may be at an end. The cost in inventory is just too much for most firms. And if the company can't afford it any longer, its competitors probably can't either.

■Minimize inventory buildup. Spend the money necessary to install data-processing systems that project the best inventory level. They should be able to update that projection rapidly and often.

■Update production costs. Revise the standard costs that the company uses to measure profitability. The usual practice is to update data once a year. Labor and materials are rising too fast for that now. With computers, it should be possible to revise every three months.

■Going public is an option for many companies right now. Venture-capital groups are eager for sound, growing businesses. And the company does not have to be in high technology. (One nonglamour company found that a stock offering at seven times earnings made more sense than more bank loans.)

Convertible debt has virtues: 15% locked in for 15 years may be a sounder deal for the company than bank loans at three points over the prime interest rate.

■Defer taxes. Use the new installment sales rules as much as possible to defer taxes (and to hold on to current cash). Look for opportunities to use the same technique in overseas subsidiaries, especially in countries where rapid inflation means the taxes will eventually be paid in depreciated currency.

■Get top management involved in monthly and quarterly cash planning. It need not be detailed. But top management should know how much cash is coming in short-term from cash sales, collection of receivables, and other sources, and how much cash is going out short-term to suppliers, for loan repayments, and for other purposes. And it should immediately incorporate potential cash surpluses or deficits into the company's overall strategy.

■Push suppliers to stockpile low-turnover items. Or pool inventory needs with nearby firms.

■Purge customers lists. Eliminate the slowest-payment accounts. Offer to sell them for cash only.

■Stratify suppliers into three categories, those that must be paid currently, those that accept late payment occasionally, and those that take late payment as a matter of informal policy.

■Improve cash management by reducing balances in low-interest-bearing savings and checking accounts. Have banks apply funds in company checking accounts against the company's revolving line of credit to reduce interest payments.

■Pay insurance on a monthly basis. The added service charge this incurs is less than the financial advantages of avoiding prepayment of insurance premiums.

Borrow against life insurance policies the company holds on its executives in order to capitalize on low interest rates.

■Toughen tax planning: Accelerate depreciation where possible. Reevaluate the remaining life of company property annually.

■Keep earnings projections current to estimate tax payments more accurately. (Companies in cyclical businesses are thus able to delay tax payments until the high point of their cycles.)

■Buy new equipment late in the year to make maximum use of the 10% investment tax credit.

Source: Nicholas Gallopo, partner, Arthur Andersen & Co., New York, James Wicker, partner, Peat, Marwick, Mitchell & Co., St. Paul.

Putting The Business Up For Sale

There are four kinds of potential buyers for money-losing businesses:
1. Large public companies with a specific need for products or assets.
2. Risk-playing entrepreneurs with expertise in the industry.
3. Foreign companies looking for a toehold in a market in the United States.
4. The business' own management, backed by venture capital.

To find a buyer, figure out which one of these groups will most logically profit from acquiring the business. Then quietly send out feelers to candidates within that group to see if they express interest in acquiring.

If word gets out that the business is for sale, capitalize on the publicity. Use it to flush out as many potential buyers as possible, then pit them against each other.

But publicly putting a business on the block hurts employee morale. If a business is labor intensive, it's generally best not to publicize the intended sale. Labor-intensive companies on the block get raided. The loss of their top talent depresses the business' value.

Make sure you know the strengths and weaknesses of the business. Address both openly when negotiating. Don't spread false turnaround tales. When an owner tells a prospective buyer that the business is about to turnaround, the buyer will wonder why the owner wants to sell it. This casts doubt on the owner's credibility.

Price the business at least 30% higher than the final acceptable figure. Don't overbluff, however. And keep marginal prospects in the picture to foster competition with the serious potential buyers.

If the sale is not made, liquidate or remove the business from the market for the time it takes to revive it and increase its salability.

Recovering From A Bank Turndown

Common mistake: Giving up after the first try. Instead, immediately prepare a new thrust.

What works:

■Asking for specifics on why the loan was refused. Common causes: The bank is overextended or doesn't know the company's type of business.

■Inviting the loan officer and one of the officer's supervisors to visit the plant. Purpose: To build confidence by showing off equipment, facilities and personnel.

■Soliciting ideas on how the application can be made more acceptable through financial or accounting changes, tax regulations, government programs or production changes.

■Applying for another type of loan or a different credit basis. Possibilities: Pledging machinery as collateral, using a third-party guarantee or borrowing against seasonal receivables.

■Reapplying when the timing is better. Use an upswing in sales or profits to obtain a line of credit or get close enough to the banker to be informed when the bank has excess funds to loan.

■Changing banks, particularly to one that is newly chartered and looking for customers. Possibility: Splitting a loan between the old and new banks.

■Reminder: The way the loan proposal is presented can be critical. A friendly banker will advise the company on which documents to present and the best ways to compile financial data.

Source: *Finding Money: The Businessman's Guide to Sources of Financing* by J. G. Hellmuth, Boardroom Classics, Springfield, NJ 07081.

How To Save Money On Consultants

Some companies gird for recession by cutting off all outside help. A better strategy is to negotiate to cut the consultant's costs. Now is the time the company may need the consultant.

To start, "hire" the company's own employees to work with the consultant.

Before signing a contract, ask the consultant for a detailed proposal of the services to be performed, including a breakdown of how the consultant expects to spend his time. This way you will pay for the consultant's expertise but avoid having an expensive staff collect routine data and figures that the company's own people could readily provide.

Then, take the consultant's detailed proposal to the company's managers and ask which tasks could be performed by their subordinates. Go back to the consultant and negotiate to remove as much work as possible and reduce the fee accordingly.

For example, many times, consulting firms are engaged to gather data for decision-making. Frequently, much of that data is internal. In fact, employees often complain that consultants are being paid for presenting information that they themselves supplied or could have supplied.

If a consultant is someone the company needs badly for either his independence or his special expertise, leverage will be somewhat weaker.

Next, take a hard look at peripheral areas (copying, typing, telephone charges). See how much of this could be done on company equipment and regular staff time as opposed to having it billed (with a markup) by the consultant. Try to renegotiate the proposed fee without these ancillary costs.

With staff participation, employees develop a stake in the work, viewing it as a joint effort instead of something imposed from the outside. Assigning the company's own employees to work under a consultant's direction gives valuable training to the company's people (rather than the consultant's), and it provides a constructive way to take up slack time.

Source: Norman Kobert, *Inventory Strategies,* Boardroom Classics, Springfield, NJ 07081.

Repossessing Property Without Court Permission

Repossessing property without going to court is legal if the peace is not breached. In one case, the buyer of a truck missed payments, so the seller had an agent follow him. When the buyer left the truck unlocked with the keys in it, the agent got in and drove away. Court's decision: The repossession was legal. There was no fraud, trickery or threat of violence involved.

Source: *Piercey Ford Motor Co.*, 373 So. 2d 1113.

Protecting Records From Federal Eyes

The Right to Financial Privacy Act protects bank records of individuals and partnerships (of five or fewer individuals). The protection is limited, however.

Where the problems are: The law doesn't apply to Internal Revenue Service subpoenas. Nor does the law apply to state investigators. And any federal agency can examine financial records for 90 days or more without telling the individual, if the agency can get a search warrant first.

The new law also does not apply if the target of inquiry is the financial institution itself, if the records are sought in judicial or administrative proceedings involving a bank and its customer, or if the federal government is considering or administrating a loan or loan guarantee to the individual or partnership.

There is also an exemption for national security matters.

How the law works: In matters where the law does apply, the government must notify the customer before asking a financial institution (bank, credit union, savings and loan, consumer finance company, or credit card issuer) to disclose personal records. The notice must name the records, the agency involved, and the purpose of the disclosure. Key point: The federal official wanting the records can have the customer served with a subpoena giving notice that the material will be examined after ten days. Or the official can simply ask the customer to consent to an examination within ten days. The simple request can be refused without going to court. But a journey to federal district court would be needed to try to quash a subpoena. If the court refuses to deny access, the ruling cannot be appealed. It may, however, be contested in later proceedings. Persons believing that the statute has been violated may also sue the government and the institutions involved.

Source: C. Westbrook Murphy of Wald, Harkrader & Ross, 1300 Nineteenth St. NW, Washington, DC 20036.

Business Diagnosis Formulas

Here are a series of ways to analyze a firm's capital position if it has been declining and you want to identify the causes and find correctives.

■Be sure there are no changes in the statements you are studying that are attributable to changes in accounting practices.

■When comparing two different time periods, be sure to allow for any seasonal factors, and always use the same basis for measurement. If an average inventory figure is used, calculate turnover in one period; don't use opening inventory as a basis in the following period.

■Compare trends rather than just one period. A decline in working capital between two periods could be an extraordinary occurrence. But a trend of a year or more indicates the probability of a basic problem.

Current ratio (working capital ratio): In the analysis of working capital, this is the basic analytic ratio used:

$$\frac{\text{Current Assets}}{\text{Current Liabilities}}$$

This ratio describes a firm's ability to meet its short-term liabilities. As a rule of thumb, a 2:1 ratio is considered desirable.

Quick ratio (acid test ratio): Measures a company's immediate liquidity:

$$\frac{\text{Cash + Marketable Securities + Accounts Receivable}}{\text{Current Liabilities}}$$

A ratio of at least 1:1 indicates that the firm is in a highly liquid position.

The following ratios measure the factors that make up working capital, and are useful in determining the reasons for changes in a firm's working capital position.

Cash to sales ratio: This ratio can be expressed either as a percentage derived from cash divided by net sales, or a percentage derived from dividing net sales by cash. The latter gives dollars-of-sales per dollar-of-cash. Either figure permits measurement of the amount of cash balances a company requires to maintain its sales level.

Days' receivables outstanding:

$$\frac{\text{Accounts Receivable}}{\text{Net Sales}} \times 30^*$$

As the days' receivables outstanding increases, so does the working capital needed by the firm. An increase can also indicate that a greater number of the firm's customers are becoming delinquent in paying, or that sales efforts have resulted in longer terms than usual being given on sales.

This ratio can also be applied to accounts payable, where an increase in days' outstanding would indicate a reduction in working capital requirements. A decrease could indicate a change in suppliers' terms, or an overzealous accounts payable department, which is paying invoices long before they are due.

Inventory turnover:

$$\frac{\text{Net Sales}}{\text{Inventory}}$$

In most firms, inventory represents the single largest working capital item. Its efficient control is usually a major factor in the profitability of these firms.

The higher the number of inventory turns per year, the greater the efficiency of inventory management. The efficient firm is reducing the amount of inventory required in order to maintain sales volume. A decrease in inventory turnover is a warning that it's time to examine existing inventory for slow-moving or obsolete items. Or it could be time to check for overstocked conditions.

The use of the above ratios gives management insight into the key relationships that exist between the operating and the financial aspects of the firm. Aim: Using these relationships to increase efficiency and profitability.

*If using monthly sales. When using annual sales, the multiplier would be 365.

Chapter 6
Increasing Productivity

How To Stay In Control
Of Business Operations

Trap: Thinking that to stay in control, every piece of information generated by the business must cross your desk. Executives who insist on knowing everything that goes on in their company at all times ultimately become swamped by reports, memos and computer printouts to the point where they simply can't effectively manage anymore.

A Better Way

Set up a monitoring system that allows you to track only the information you need to stay in control on a regular, but not constant, basis. Set up a schedule of when you need what. Resist the temptation to delve too deeply beyond the reports you get. Rule of thumb: The more detail you devour, the less return on invested time you get.

Example: Accounts receivable can pile up quickly. But insisting on weekly or even daily reports only adds clutter to your desk. Monthly accounts receivable summaries are the only tools useful in making decisions about which customers are good credit risks and should receive credit, and which tardy accounts should be pursued.

The chart below is an example of an efficient monitoring system...

	Frequency		
Type of report	Daily	Weekly	Monthly
Total sales	•		
Sales by product group		•	
Sales by territory			•
Average sales prices of major products		•	
Gross profit margin (total)		•	
Gross profit (per product)		•	
Production costs			•
Direct expenses			•
Other income and expense			•
Net profit			•
Cash flow		•	
Accounts receivable			•
Inventory		•	
R&D status and expenses			•

Source: *The Best of Inc. Guide to Business Strategy,* Prentice Hall Press, One Gulf & Western Plaza, New York 10023.

Cutting Product Delivery Times

To cut product delivery times: Increase stocks. This is simple, but can be costly. The company must forecast needs correctly and invest in more inventory. It may be stuck with unwanted stocks if forecasts are wrong. And it may not be able to modify products to meet changes in demand until stocks are used up. Alternative: Adopt just-in-time production. This cuts inventory and improves the company's response time to market changes. But it may have to redesign the entire production process to make production both quicker and more flexible.

Source: Walter E. Goddard, president, Oliver Wight Companies, writing in *Modern Materials Handling*, 275 Washington St., Newton, MA 02158.

How To Make Your Company Into A Great Place To Work

All about making your company a great place to work, from Jerry Winters, whose company was named one of the "Ten Best to Work For" by the *Business Journal of New Jersey...*

■Job advancement. The company offers on-the-job training for workers who excel in their jobs and wish to grow with the company. A manual worker on a packing line can advance to a job in sales, accounting, telemarketing, even management. Workers know that they're not in dead-end jobs. They know that they can have careers here and a chance to make a better life for themselves and their families. Benefit to the company: Increased productivity. The opportunity to advance to a better job provides an incentive to work hard and prove yourself quickly.

Bottom line: A good job is much more than the money it pays. A good job is a reason to get up in the morning. I make sure that the people who work for me have a chance to grow to their fullest potential.

■Substantially above-average pay. Most companies start their packing workers at the minimum wage. We start them at $4.50 an hour, move them to $5 within two weeks, and to $6/hour within six months. Benefit to the company: We get top productivity because we pay top wages. Workers know that there's something unique about a company that pays well. They also realize that the company will only be able to pay this extra money if the employees work extra hard.

■Travel incentives and trade shows. On the whole, our benefits are only slightly above average. But we do offer a unique fringe benefit for production workers— free trips to trade shows. Benefit to the company: Better-made products. Employees who go to the trade shows come back proud of the product they make, and that leads to better work on the line.

Example: We had a problem with sloppy packing of products for counter displays. To correct the problem, we set up a program to send packing workers to trade shows where they quickly learned how important it was to have the product properly packed. Back on the production line, they told other workers why it was important. The problem was quickly solved.

■Family atmosphere. People here talk about being part of a family. The boss works on the production line with them during the peak season and he eats in the lunchroom with them. Workers know that they're playing important roles in a growing company that cares about them. The attitude is "we're all in it together." Benefit to the company: Workers are willing to pitch in to help in an emergency. For instance, they're willing to work overtime to fill large orders for important customers. As in a family business, they know that if they benefit the company, they benefit themselves.

■Weekly and daily cash incentives. We used to have a high absentee rate on Mondays. It didn't seem to matter what the hourly wage was, Monday was a bad day. We corrected that by giving a bonus—an extra $10 pay—to everyone who put in a full five days' work. We also give cash incentives and free lunches and dinners to groups of workers who exceed standards of production.

■Open to suggestions. We're always asking employees to suggest ways to do things better. And we listen to those suggestions. Many of them have been implemented. Some have greatly increased productivity.

Example: At the suggestion of a group of employees, we added an old-fashioned conveyor belt to our state-of-the-art production line. Products that formerly had to be carried by hand back to the beginning of the line now move by conveyor belt. This increased productivity. Bonus: Employees work harder when they know that their suggestions for a better workplace will be listened to.

Source: Jerry Winters, president, Winters Original Chocolate Liquor Bottles, Inc., Box 709, Garfield, NJ 07026.

Training Trap

Many companies that provide training for new workers neglect to provide adequate training for experienced workers. But improving productivity requires keeping current employees up-to-date on new production techniques and project objectives. However, almost 25% of workers in a survey described their training as inadequate for their jobs.

Source: Gwen Stern, Wyatt Company, quoted in *Management World*, 2360 Maryland Rd., Willow Grove, PA 19090.

Productivity Basics Checklist

Before starting a drive to improve productivity, review the company's basic foundation. Any weakness in it could hurt the productivity campaign. Fundamental questions:

■Are there clear, basic company goals? Are they translated into specific long-range objectives?

■Does the chief executive have time for planning and meetings with employees and public contacts? The CEO shouldn't be swamped with details.

■How do rivals compare in technical development? Management strength? Market share? Overall profitability?

■Are there detailed formulas to measure performance? Mere forecasts and budgets aren't enough.

■Do decision-makers have access to full information quickly?
■Is management structured to handle emergencies smoothly? To implement new programs?
■Do customers get quality service on time?
■Are policies for minimum orders and customer credit up-to-date?
Source: Brooks International Corp., Montvale, NJ.

Worker Productivity Is Only The Beginning

Workers alone do not boost productivity. Encouraging increased productivity by labor is still vital, but it should be regarded as routine. The most successful companies: 1. Increase the payback from raw materials, equipment, technology, and capital; 2. Emphasize effectiveness (meeting market needs) over efficiency; and 3. Measure performance against goals, not merely unit output.

How Quality And Low Cost Can Work Together

"Keep the line moving," the primary operating rule for production managers in most American companies, no longer works well enough to keep all those companies competitive. The key problem is the assumption that quality and low cost are mutually exclusive and one must be traded off to get the other. Japanese firms have demonstrated that both are attainable, and they are gaining market shares as a result.

The push for more productivity in a company today must be directly related to a push to upgrade quality. If a company achieves greater output per hour or per dollar of cost, but that production is of poor quality, it gains nothing. If the defect rate is cut by improving quality, however, a company can accept lower productivity and still be ahead of the game. The main reasons for this:

■Reduced rework and repair. Rework can be a huge drain on manufacturing productivity. One manufacturer estimates that 21% of its labor cost goes to correct production mistakes.

■More cooperative workers. They take more pride in their work and feel management is sharing its prerogatives with them.

Behind the new recognition of quality as the key to productivity is W. Edwards Deming, an American statistician whose ideas were adopted in Japan 30 years ago. Deming's work centers on the use of statistical techniques to identify and reduce defects. Much of what he says now has been known for years, but has not generally been applied by U.S. firms the way Deming recommends.

In many American companies, quality control is a separate function from production and is the domain of experts who are usually industrial engineers. When a quality problem arises, the line managers call in the engineers rather than become intimately involved in solving it themselves. Deming's approach is to integrate quality control into the production process itself. Teach workers basic sampling techniques and how to use control charts. Make both workers and managers responsible for quality. If necessary, a worker should be able to stop the line to correct a quality problem. It is essential to get away from the idea that quality is an issue solely for experts.

In the U.S., the tendency among managers is to put the blame for quality problems elsewhere—on suppliers or the workers. Managers often say that if the workers would just work harder or pay more attention to what they are doing, the company would not have this problem. Deming's approach is to assume that the problem is caused by the system, not the suppliers nor the workers. This is true 85% of the time. It may be that workers are not trained properly, or they are poorly supervised, or something else. But usually they have no direct control over the fundamental cause of the quality shortfall.

Some of Deming's other ideas are intriguing, but they are also controversial:

■Eliminating numerical goals. Deming believes these are disincentives if they are not accompanied by detailed plans on how to achieve them. Also counterproductive, in his view, are slogans (such as "zero defects") and posters. They are a lazy way out for managers who do not manage.

■Doing away with mass inspections. Many U.S. companies inspect 100% of output, often at several points in the production process. Most have to do this because their defect rate is so high. Deming says that a company using high-quality parts in a high-quality production process with well-trained personnel should not have to inspect everything.

■Eliminating excess suppliers. The conventional wisdom is that several sources are necessary to avoid overdependence on any one supplier for critical parts. In Japan suppliers are tied into virtually permanent relationships with their customers. They are secure in knowing they will not be cut off in bad times, unlike even key suppliers to a U.S. company. One U.S. automaker that now has 4,000 suppliers has embarked on a five-year program to cut the number to 800. Toyota has only 380 suppliers, according to Deming.

The new rule for American production managers: quality, productivity, and costs are completely linked.

Source: Dr. David Dannenbring, associate professor, Columbia University Graduate School of Business.

A Better Way To Measure Productivity

Measure productivity for each product line separately, even though it entails more detailed record-keeping.

The practice enables managers to focus maximum attention on lines that account for the bulk of sales, and allows them to calculate product strategies more easily because more information is available to them.

Use the specific data to plan the use of company resources more effectively.

Source: David J. Sumanth, University of Miami, *Manufacturing Productivity Frontiers*, Illinois Institute of Technology, Research Institute, Chicago.

Measuring Company Productivity

■Choose a convenient measure of productivity.

■Tailor the measure to the activity being evaluated. For the production area, consider physical output per worker-year. Alternatively, one large manufacturer tracked real value added per worker-hour and per unit of capital input. For sales consider net sales per payroll dollar.

■If the company is using more than one productivity measure, it should be able to convert units of one measure into other measures. For example, know how many worker-hours are worth one hour of machine time.

■When dollars are used in a productivity measure, keep them constant by making an adjustment for inflation.

Source: Irving H. Siegel, *Company Productivity*, W.E. Upjohn Institute for Employment Research, Kalamazoo, MI.

How Japanese Productivity Methods Work With U.S. Employees

It is often said that the management strategies that have boosted Japan's productivity aren't transferable to the United States because of cultural differences. In reality, Japanese companies with U.S. operations have applied their ideas to the United States extremely successfully. As proof, Sony's best production line for color TV is in San Diego, not in Japan.

Sony's San Diego workers are trained to understand how a TV functions, and to point out production problems. Managers are required to know employees' career backgrounds and goals, meet with them regularly, and listen to their complaints. And workers are guaranteed lifetime employment.

Another Japanese company with operations in California, Fujitsu America, an electronics maker, cites these differences between Japanese management practices and those used by most American companies:

■Job mobility is encouraged in the United States, wasting training efforts.

■Most U.S. workers are unprotected against sudden dismissals.

■Japanese firms have predetermined wage structures with graduated increases. They do not reward on whim, as U.S. firms often do.

■U.S. firms rely on profit-sharing and incentives. Japanese companies disdain these benefits.

■Japanese firms provide greater benefits, including health checkups, company vacation resorts, etc.

Another difference is that Japanese unions organize by company rather than by industry, encouraging identification with corporate goals.

Source: *World Business Weekly*, New York.

Business Forms Can Block Productivity

For every dollar a company spends on business forms, an additional $40 goes for expenses such as clerical costs, storage, and disposal. A company can save substantially by reducing the number of forms, designing them more effectively, or retaining a forms management company that will eliminate common mistakes:

■Too many forms. When different departments use several forms that relate to the same subject, consider using a single form, perhaps with separate sections that can be routed to the various departments.

■Using copy machines for reproduction. When business forms are produced on copying machines, the price is 10¢–12¢ each, compared with about two cents for printed forms.

■Too much paper per form. Companies often order $8^1/2$- by 11-inch forms when a smaller size would do.

■No inventory control. Business forms are usually ordered in volume to get quantity discounts. There is no analysis to see which ones have become obsolete and no system to warn of impending stock outs.

■Rush printing. It's very expensive. And frequently there are design errors.

Professional forms management companies handle printing, storage, and computerized inventory control. Printing is done at competitive prices, but there is usually a 15% fee for the forms management service. The service includes analysis of company forms to determine their effectiveness and the public image they convey. The process makes executives focus on the problem for the first time. Also, use it to raise morale by including employees in the redesign of the form. For example, secretaries know when forms aren't aligned for typewriter settings and appreciate being consulted.

Conventional forms suppliers traditionally rely on a network of salespeople who are paid straight commissions. They often sell companies more rather than better forms. Business forms management companies are paid to improve and reduce the number of forms that a client uses.

Source: Alfred Jay Moran, Jr., president, TJM Corp., New Orleans.

Ergonomics And Productivity

Today, when even slight productivity gains are crucial, more and more businesses are taking ergonomics seriously.

Ergonomics—the science of matching people, machines and environment—has demonstrated that better design of offices and office equipment can boost productivity dramatically by...

■Increasing work performance.

■Decreasing turnover because people who work in ergonomically designed offices are usually happier in their jobs. In one study, turnover dropped from 35% to 5% a year. And if workers do leave, it's much easier to attract new applicants.

■Decreasing employee health complaints relating to repetitive motion syndrome—and other consequences of poorly designed offices.

Ergonomics is far from a cure-all for productivity woes. Poor performance obviously may have causes that have nothing to do with design, such as faulty supervision, training or hiring. And, ergonomically designed work areas are expensive. They can cost up to three times as much as standard ones.

How It Works

In the vast majority of businesses, chairs, desks, filing cabinets and other types of office equipment—not to mention offices themselves—are almost always the choices of interior designers and decorators. They might look great, but they're not designed with function in mind. In fact, they're often designed in ways that make efficient use almost impossible.

Example: Non-adjustable chairs that require workers to lean forward from the waist. Result: Workers are likely to strain in the lumbar, or lower, region of the back—the point where it's the weakest. As the body slumps to compensate for the extra load, the weight shifts from muscles to tendons, which are not developed to support weight in the first place. The worker develops muscle aches, becomes fatigued, and performance inevitably deteriorates.

What To Expect

A study at the National Institutes for Occupational Safety & Health (NIOSH) demonstrates potential productivity gains from properly designed work areas. In the study, a group of data-entry workers alternated between working at ergonomically designed work stations and traditional ones.

Result: The average individual's performance increased 24% on the better-designed work station. Other research has revealed gains at least this high.

The NIOSH study included basic elements of office ergonomics most companies should be considering today. Key examples:

■Chairs that can be adjusted by height and seat surface angle for lumbar support.

■Work surfaces that can also be adjusted for height.

■Computer keyboard support heights that are adjustable so the operator's arms and hands tire less quickly during a day of heavy use.

■Computer monitors whose angles can be adjusted for better vision and that have anti-glare screens.

■Devices to hold the copy upright, so the worker can easily see the copy as well as the computer keyboard and monitor.

■Overhead lights that give off soft, non-glaring light.

■"Task lighting," that illuminates the employee's specific work area.

Comparison

In the study, the traditional office had pre-1980 non-adjustable chairs and desks. For many in the study, the desk surface was at an uncomfortable height, and they had to twist back and forth to see first the copy and then the monitor. The screen reflected glare from an overhead fluorescent light.

Cost Factor

The majority of companies are still getting by with these kinds of office arrangements. Main reason: They're expensive to change.

Good starting points: A good ergonomically designed chair costs $600–$700, compared with about $200 for less-efficient ones. A desk with adjustable height costs $1,200–$1,500, compared with $450 for a traditional model that may or may not be appropriate for the height of the user. And it may cost more than $2,000 to overhaul the lighting system in a single office.

Making The Changes

But, a better-designed work area can pay quick dividends. After the Army Corps of Engineers introduced ergonomic work stations, it estimated that its payback period was nine months.

Ergonomics is a new field, and only a few major consulting firms can offer help.

Resource: The Human Factors Society, a professional association of ergonomists. The group will help businesses find a top consultant in their area.

Recommended: Since the price of properly designed equipment is high (and since many business people are still skeptical), experiment with ergonomics in only one or two work areas and then measure the gains.

Begin by modifying work areas for employees whose work is intense.

Examples: Any worker who must perform the same tasks for more than three hours at a stretch, especially data-entry workers who must work with a monitor and keyboard for this length of time.

Source: Dr. Marvin Dainoff, Dept. of Psychology, Miami University, Oxford, OH 45056. He is also author of *People and Productivity: A Manager's Guide to Ergonomics in the Electronic Office*, Gage Educational Publishing. U.S. Distributor: MDA Books, 8606 Empire Court, Cincinnati 45231.

Improving Productivity

Improve productivity by encouraging workers to look for problems. To do this successfully, workers must receive more than just rote instruction on how to do their jobs. They must be shown how their jobs relate to the entire business. Payoff: Line workers who understand how their tasks relate to others will come up with suggestions that management would never think of. Workers who see themselves as an important part of the whole business take greater pride in the company and in the jobs they do, and are better motivated to search for problems to solve.

Source: *The Idea Book* by the Japan Human Association, Productivity Press, Box 30007, Cambridge, MA 02140.

Productivity Improvement Programs

Productivity improvement programs are often defeated by the resistance of line workers and middle management. Trap: Fear that authority and prerequisites will be lost while responsibilities are increased. To overcome that resistance: Educate the workforce about the goals of the plan, why it's necessary, and how they'll benefit. Install the program in "do-able" steps to show employees that the job can be done and that they'll benefit as a result.

Source: *American Business and the Quick Fix* by Michael E. McGill, Ph.D., professor of business, Southern Methodist University, Henry Holt, 115 W. 18 St., New York 10011.

How To Increase Output Without Sacrificing Quality

Major management mistake: Not looking for ways to speed up production until the company is faced with tougher customer demands and/or competitors who offer more reliable deliveries and shorter lead times.

All businesses should look for opportunities to speed up the processes and flow, while increasing quality, before the crunch comes…

■One electric equipment maker was able to cut a 16-week lead-time on one product to three weeks, and an average eight-week lead-time for the entire plant down to three days.

■Set-up times for machines were reduced by 30%, which meant that lot sizes for efficient production could be cut in half.

Best candidates for significant improvement: Discrete or "repetitive" manufacturing plants that make similar products in volume, with many distinct operations such as milling, drilling, welding and other machining or assembly processes.

Major improvements are also possible, however, for "process flow" plants common to primary metals, food and beverage, and pharmaceutical and medical supply industries, to name a few. They often have "hybrid" operations, particularly in finishing or packaging, that can resemble batching processes as far as non-productive time is concerned.

Achievable goal: No finished-goods inventory at all. All production is made to specific customer order. The end of the production line is the shipping dock with a truck waiting to be loaded.

Happy Outlook

The more the company works to cut manufacturing lead times, the more opportunities will be uncovered.

Example: One company had a standard 10-week lead-time to produce aluminum coils for the beverage industry. By methodically breaking down the production process, company engineers and outside consultants cut excess, non-productive time throughout the process down to four weeks. But that opened up a whole new opportunity. If the lead-time could be reduced to three weeks, the plant could be driven by firm customer orders.

Gain: Little or no finished inventory and a reduced need to rely on sales forecasts to plan and schedule production. This had a favorable impact on work-in-process inventories as well. (The longer the lead-time, the more inaccurate the forecasts seemed to be.) The team searched for spots in the production process where there were build-ups of inventory or bottlenecks. At one point, about 400 giant coils of aluminum were arrayed on the plant floor, cooling down for two days from the previous hot rolling process before they could be moved to the next step. The consultants suggested using giant fans to speed the cooling. That simple, inexpensive idea cut five shifts ($1^1/_4$ days) more out of the lead-times and reduced inventory 45%.

Then the team began working with customers, asking if they could provide "semi-firm" order releases four to six weeks ahead of delivery, followed by firm orders (with specifications and delivery locations) within a week or two of shipment. Most customers agreed to that if the supplier guaranteed that the specs would be followed—and delivery schedules met. That cut more time out of the cycle and, together with other small improvements, brought the lead-time down to the crucial three-week period.

Once plant lead-times are cut, managers can look at the ordering process for even more productivity. A three-to-five day period to translate a customer order into a manufacturing order may be justifiable with a 10-week lead-time—but it can be a real show-stopper once lead-time is down to three weeks.

Big Change Needed

Management must learn to give up the traditional way of measuring plant effectiveness—by looking at the efficiency of each separate operation, workstation by workstation. They must begin measuring the entire operation.

Look for ways to cut down machine set-up times, and produce only what's needed immediately. Ultimately, short production runs may lead to greater overall productivity.

The search for opportunities begins with a team that looks for areas of lowest productivity or highest inventory. Find opportunities (such as the big fans that cooled the aluminum coils). Start small with one area of operation. Show that the new technique—a faster way to set up a machine, for instance—will work. Then, one by one, continuously go system-wide.

Source: Gerald J. Bose, senior consultant, Operations Management, Arthur D. Little, Inc., Acorn Park, Cambridge, MA 02140.

Wall Colors And Productivity

Repetitious office work is quickened by a backdrop of reds, yellows and beiges. The walls of a chemical manufacturing company were changed from gray and blue to cream and red. Result: Typing speeds increased by 12% and transcription speeds went up 20%.

Source: *Making Your Office Work for You* by Jan Yager, Ph.D., Doubleday, 666 Fifth Ave., New York 10103.

Chapter 7
Improving Managers' Productivity

Improving Managerial Productivity

The nationwide push to boost productivity has led to a rash of new shop floor programs. But in many cases, companies can best improve profits by concentrating on their executives' output.

The most elusive but crucial causes of executive ineffectiveness are failure to set objectives and to establish procedures to make sure those objectives are met.

Management-by-objective is a buzzword. To make the process real, the company chief executive must commit the company to year-to-year objectives; get departmental objectives in numbers; master the details of senior managers' activities. Then, challenge their plans, steps and timing for meeting the objectives. And be able to measure where the company and each department stand month-to-month in relation to its full range of objectives.

Source: Joseph Eisenberg, president, Profit-Improvement, Inc., New York.

Strengthening Middle Management

Business managers commonly agree that one of the vital keys to improving productivity is upgrading the performance of middle management. How to do this:

■Develop a new frame of reference for the company's middle managers. Bring in a new middle manager from the outside whose work is clearly superior to the standards presently in force.

■Instruct senior management to stand back as the newcomer learns his way around. Let the new middle manager publicize his superior performance standards himself. Give him an opportunity to describe what he's doing in reports that are generally circulated and in oral briefings at staff meetings.

■Separate the company's middle-management ranks into two groups: Those who have responded by raising their own work standards, and those who haven't.

■Recognize the improved work being done by the first group of veteran managers. Give those in the second group capable of improving their performance, but who have not, an ultimatum—pick up speed, or else. Transfer veteran managers not capable of improving their performance to different functions. Maybe transfer this last group to customer service because veteran managers' familiarity with operations will make them effective in helping customers.

■Once the company's middle management has begun to improve performance on its own, formalize the higher standards with a more demanding budget and sales targets than before.

This approach should be continual. Top management should periodically inject new blood into the middle-management ranks. Simply transferring old managers to new jobs is not enough.

To make this approach work, top management should not transform each new outsider into a prima donna. To do so will isolate the newcomer from the people whose work he should influence.

Fitting Priorities Into Categories

Even some of the most efficient managers sometimes lose ground because they haven't accurately weighed the relative importance of their activities. To prevent this, categorize activities carefully according to priority, and revise the categories on a daily basis.

How to classify work activities:
- Category A. Important and urgent.
- Category B. Important but not urgent.
- Category C. Urgent but not important work. This category is usually the big trap because the crisis nature of the activity makes it seem more important than it is. (Crisis management vs. management by objectives.)
- Category D. Neither urgent nor important. For example, cleaning drawers, straightening files.

Since activities will vary in urgency as time passes, it is important to revise the priorities list each day. Most managers don't have enough time to complete all tasks. They should tackle the A and B priorities, and then the C tasks if they have the time. If they never get to the D jobs, what has been lost?

Source: Milton R. Stohl, president, Milton R. Stohl Associates, Farmington Woods, CT.

Productivity Gaps At The Top

Computers, word processors, desktop terminals, and other kinds of information-automation have not yet made a big impact on the way managers gather and analyze essential business information. The frustration level is still high, according to a recent survey.

Some 25% of top managers' time is usually spent in nonproductive chores such as traveling, filing papers, or trying to get information by conventional means.

Almost half of their time is spent getting information via the telephone or in face-to-face meetings.

Time wasted on the least efficient ways of gathering information means top managers don't devote enough time to analyzing and planning company operations.

Source: Harvey L. Poppel, senior vice president, Booz Allen & Hamilton, Inc.

The Secrets Of Big Gains In White Collar Productivity

Banks are ideal places to go to study management techniques' effects on white-collar productivity. Waino Pihl and Michael Wamby completed an in-depth survey of productivity in 73 banks across the nation. Many of the techniques that they found for boosting white-collar productivity at the banks they surveyed are equally applicable to the white-collar operations of businesses in any industry...

The payoff for taking just a few basic steps to improve white-collar worker productivity in service businesses is tremendous. We found that high-productivity banks, on average, were twice as productive as low-productivity banks.

Comparing similar operations, bank to bank, we found departments in high-performing banks using only one-half the staff to generate the same volume of work as the low performers.

These 100% differences in productivity were not chiefly the result of automation. Often they were the result of steps managers took before automating to streamline operations and systems.

What Works Best

Concentrate on just a few techniques to increase productivity.

The key to boosting productivity is to focus on one or two short-term modifications of department procedures and activities likely to produce the biggest bang. Once you have a crisp, clean-running department, you can automate or then go after other ways to produce further, usually smaller, gains.

Example: Bank auditing departments have discovered that by using risk-based auditing techniques to identify the most likely areas for major trouble, together with computer-assisted audit programs, they can reduce their accounting and clerical staffs by as much as 75%. Risk-based auditing allows staffs to focus time on chronic or high-volume transaction areas, such as the securities trading desk, custody and loan documentation, while computer techniques will confirm, on a broad basis, accurate accruals and fees through the system. Internal audit staffs, therefore, are able to focus their time on critical areas.

Best: Pick one or two techniques that have high-productivity payoff potential and concentrate on making them work in the department. There's time enough for these enhancements after the big gains are achieved.

Standardize operations by focusing on the key variables to provide cost-effective, high-quality service.

Use McDonald's, the pre-eminent fast-food company, as a standard for providing efficient and consistent service across the country.

Key: Standardize business functions. If the same function is performed in a number of branches where workers meet face-to-face with customers, look for ways to standardize those functions by using techniques often found in a manufacturing environment...

- Simplify
- Integrate or centralize
- Automate

The easiest and least-expensive technique is to simplify functions by removing unnecessary and redundant tasks. For example, reducing the number of required signatures on a document can improve both employee productivity and customer satisfaction. Simplifying the workplace often provides the greatest increase in productivity and worker enthusiasm.

After simplifying, the next step is to look for opportunities to centralize functions that don't require face-to-face customer contact (e.g., telephone customer service or budgeting and bill-paying for branch offices). This allows the customer-contact people to focus on their job of serving customers and moves administrative functions away from customer-contact areas.

Once these administrative functions have been centralized, additional productivity gains can be made by automating routine functions, such as bill-paying or handling routine customer service questions through a touch-tone-activated voice-response system. Banks have also developed automated credit scoring and document preparation to enable lenders to focus on selling and more quickly closing the deal.

Trap: The drive to improve productivity can sometimes lead to lower-quality customer service. Safeguard: Survey customers frequently as changes are made.

Measure productivity. It's not too complicated.

More than 25% of the banks surveyed did not attempt to track productivity. They relied simply on financial information to assess operating effectiveness. That's no longer enough. Managers must now measure operating statistics, results and levels of accuracy—as well as calculate the bottom line.

Financial measures alone often confuse workers. Clerical workers who are told their raise or year-end bonus depends on how much the company increases its market share or profits rarely can see a way of relating that to doing their own job more efficiently. Managers, on the other hand, often make the task of measuring productivity too complicated. There's no "perfect measure," but the following works best...

■Use the simplest measure that correlates most directly to the prime output of a particular work area. If keypunch operators are supposed to produce accurate data, use a ratio of total output to accurate output.

■Make sure people understand the measure, why it's being used and what you expect from them.

■Make clear that you're willing to pay for increased productivity. (Keypunch operators put under a clear incentive compensation program consistently improve their accurate output by about 40% for about a 20% increase in compensation.)

Source: Waino Pihl, partner, Andersen Consulting, and Michael Wamby, partner, Arthur Andersen & Co., 33 W. Monroe St., Chicago 60603.

Chapter 8
Improving Employee Productivity

Improving Productivity
From The Bottom Up

In the rush to upgrade U.S. productivity, many companies are mistakenly pushing only for harder work from their employees. In the right corporate environment, employees can be sources of creativity and intelligence about organizing production for more efficiency.

Managers, particularly those in production, should ask for and expect more than increased effort. Since most U.S. production workers have at least a high school education, after six months on the job, they understand the details of their work at least as well as their supervisors do, and often better. As a rule, within a 25-foot work space, no one knows how to do the job better than the worker on the spot.

To encourage worker involvement, move away from a top-down, overenergized, aggressive style to a more democratic and bottom-up approach. Some common-sense ways to do this:

■Pay more than lip service to the notion that top management listens to employees. Follow through on good suggestions. Explain why those not used will not work. Take production managers into close confidence. Then let them know they are to do the same with lower-level workers.

■Set practical goals. Make sure production supervisors and workers know what par is for each activity or operation. Then provide some leeway for differing work skills and styles.

■Strip down management layers. The world's oldest and largest organization, the Catholic church, gets along with just four layers. Two are ideal for a company. The goal is to help people do their jobs, not to multiply the number of their bosses, company reports and meetings.

■Communicate directly and clearly. Explain the bad news with, and even ahead of, the good. Communicate face-to-face if possible. Take time to send well-written messages to employees, using nonbureaucratic language.

■Do not let managers throw their weight around. Titles rarely have much to do with getting work done. Managers must lead, not push.

■Resist relying on inspectors to ensure quality. Quality should be the natural aim of every employee. If resentment, misunderstanding, bad judgment, or miscalculation is causing a falloff in quality, quickly open up a new line of communication from bottom to top to remove the block.

■Do not insist on a single way to accomplish something. Many more ways may be acceptable. Let the employee figure out how best to reach a goal.

Training programs can be a powerful incentive. But rely on a manager's instinct that a training program offers a benefit, rather than demand a formal cost justification. When business is slow, retrain in order to ready production for an upturn.

Then promote or reward the workers who gain most from the training as an added incentive to increased productivity.

The value of job security is also often underestimated. In fact, workers concentrate best on the task at hand when they are reasonably sure they will have a job tomorrow. Set up a reward pool. Make it uniform for the entire company and distribute the reward as a percentage of income without regard to rank.

Reward employees quickly, preferably monthly, for rising above the average. Let them vote on the payment method. Key to effectiveness—if 70% of the employees do not approve of the incentive plan, change it.

Source: Rene C. McPherson, Stanford University Graduate School of Business, Stanford, CA.

Motivating Employees To Better Productivity

It's important to get workers involved in any campaign for greater productivity. The strategy:

■Good planning. Start the productivity campaign with a flair. Finish the effort before employees tire of it. Kick off the campaign with a letter from the boss. Create some excitement, and avoid talking in management terms.

■Settle for immediate gains. Don't press workers for input on a continuing basis. Thirty days is about the limit for a successful campaign.

■Implement good ideas quickly. The same day if possible. Action, not words, convinces employees that management is serious.

■Ask employees for ideas on even the most modest items. Many have ideas from previous employers. One company discovered from an employee that its competitors were recycling corrugated containers. Adopting the idea resulted in an annual savings of $120,000.

■Informality. Complicated employee-suggestion rules should be relaxed for a month. Encourage everyone to take a fresh look at the job. Open direct links to management.

■Recognition. Substitute recognition for money rewards during the campaign. Money prizes can promote jealousy and undercut motivation when they're stopped. Encourage immediate supervisors to recognize contributions. This puts line managers on notice that improvements are expected.

As a result, apart from productivity gains, a successful campaign is likely to renew spirit and improve morale. Most workers want the security that comes from being part of a profitable organization.

Source: George J. Schmidt, president, Industrial Motivation, Inc., New York.

Productivity Boosters

Seven insights to help improve an employee's overall productivity:

1. Most employees want to see others succeed—but never at their own expense.

2. Employee change and development are usually slow and subtle. Change is most often visible over a period of months, not days.

3. Each worker has one or two specialties. The manager should learn something about each of those.

4. Some employees will always be jealous of others' success.

5. Every employee, to some degree, resents changes in work patterns or changes in situations.

6. Ease the stress of change by offering the employee more reassurance and encouragement than usual.

7. Most employees have some emotional problems that stymie their progress at different times and in various ways.

Source: Charles C. Vance, *Boss Psychology*, McGraw-Hill, New York.

Mistakes That Undermine Productivity

■Not giving employees enough to do. Common causes are failing to delegate or to capitalize on an individual's initiative.

■Overworking the best people. Reward employees who carry more than their share of new responsibilities or a bigger staff, not only for a bigger work load. A tip-off that someone's pushed too far is a change in mood or a rash of sick days.

■Failing to live up to promises. A typical case is promising ambitious new workers they will receive training and a promotion for filling a dull or low-level job, but never delivering on the promise.

■Being inflexible. Make exceptions to rules when it's necessary and sensible.

■Moving too quickly with new policies. Changing departmental operations without investigating or explaining them properly can anger and frustrate workers. The biggest problem often lies in calling in outside consultants who promise easy answers to deep-seated problems.

Source: *Supervisory Management*, AMACOM, New York.

Informal Ways To Measure Employee Productivity

Alternatives to elaborate, costly time-and-motion studies:

■Short-interval scheduling. Work is assigned and measured for clearly defined intervals throughout the day. It works best in companies with an almost continuous backlog of routine work. Supervisors must ensure a steady flow of work. Both supervisors and workers may object to meeting such rigid schedules.

■Work sampling. Managers make random observations of the work and pay special attention to how long each step takes. It is the most accurate of the informal productivity-measurement techniques. Best used to measure nonrepetitive tasks, determine how much time is unproductive, examine work distribution within a department and find causes of delays. Workers must be told that management is trying to establish standards and that it is not spying. Of course, it's only useful for jobs that are visible.

■Time-ladder studies. Workers keep logs of the time they spend on specific aspects of their jobs. But employees must be persuaded to report their activities honestly and completely. The logs are easy to conduct and understand—applicable to many kinds of jobs. But data may be inaccurate. Results can sometimes be difficult to analyze.

Source: R.E. Nolan, *Improving Productivity Through Advanced Office Controls*, AMACOM, New York.

Why Flextime Is Paying Off

Allowing employees to individually decide when they'll start their work day was first thought of as a morale booster. But flextime is paying another big dividend. Companies using it report sizable productivity increases. Other benefits:

■Lateness and absenteeism (because of personal business chores) are reduced.

■Employees fit their work hours to their own best work times. Output increases because workers are functioning at their peak.

■Employees become more time conscious because deadlines, absences, and meetings have to be individually coordinated.

And flextime forces supervisors to be more careful about work assignments and scheduling.

Source: *Chronolog*, Orinda, CA.

Secrets Of Motivating Hourly Workers

The same basic motivators work for nearly every type of employee—ego boosters, compensation and recognition of lifestyle. The trick is to modify them for hourly workers and to tie them to productivity.

Because the lowest level of workers may be earning only $3.50–$6.00 an hour, the thought of waiting a year—or even six months—before they can expect a raise can be deadening.

Solution: A performance review after the first month that can result in a small increase…followed by the chance of receiving small quarterly raises for the first few years.

The cost to the company: Four raises in the first year may total 14% for a worker who starts at $3.50 an hour. But to make these increases effective motivators, they must be tied to productivity increases.

If a worker fails to satisfactorily reach each new plateau, he receives a very small raise in hopes of inspiring him to try again…or he receives none at all. Workers who exceed output standards will be eligible for bonuses from the first day they begin their new job.

It's essential to explain the program to workers when they're hired and at any time the policy changes. Nothing kills productivity like a change in standards.

Single out individuals who show a capability for handling more difficult tasks and a desire to do them. Even if there aren't any openings for those better-paying jobs, it often makes sense to train workers for new responsibilities in advance.

Hourly workers can also be motivated by public recognition of their contribution to the company's efforts. Naming an employee "worker of the month" costs the company nothing, or very little if you present a plaque or a small gift or cash award to the employee, and it pays off in a continued strong effort.

Other recognition motivators: Some method of recognition for the number of years worked, appointments to worker councils, preferred parking places near the factory door, invitations to special company events.

Source: Sigmund G. Ginsburg, faculty, Graduate School of Business Administration, Fordham University, New York, and vice president, finance and administration, Barnard College, New York 10027.

What's Wrong With The Four-Day Week

Four-day work weeks haven't been widely adopted. Only 2.2% of full-time employees work fewer than five days a week. The main problem is that most plants and offices can't close on the fifth day because customers and suppliers would be inconvenienced. And worker productivity was found to drop in many fields because of fatigue from working 10-hour days.

In some companies, employees work nine-hour days every two weeks, taking the tenth day off. A bonus is frequent three-day weekends.

Source: *U.S. News & World Report*, New York.

Worker Participation Pays

Letting production workers have a voice in company management is a radical idea. But it's been tested and has produced good results in certain cases:
■ Long-term labor peace.
■ Productivity gains.
■ Easier introduction of new technology.
■ Reduction of the adversarial relationship between workers and management.

These advantages are prompting companies—including General Motors, Polaroid and many smaller ones—to let employees have a voice in management's traditional decision-making power.

How It Works

One way is to recruit workers into committees to work with top managers (not their immediate supervisors). The committees—usually made up of three or four managers and 10 or fewer subordinates—meet regularly on company time to discuss work and how it can be improved.

Manager members help refine subordinates' suggestions on ways to improve the functioning of their own areas. Once the committee decides on a course of action, it makes a recommendation to top management.

When it sets up the committees, top management makes clear that it intends to follow all committee recommendations unless there's a compelling reason not to. That obligation gives the committees strength.

Management-worker committees can be more influential than quality circles, which make suggestions only about matters concerning quality…and whose recommendations management isn't necessarily obliged to follow.

Committees usually meet once a week and report directly to a top manager such as the vice president of the division. Because top management makes the final decision, there's no chance that management-worker committees will cause disruption in the plant or office.

Example: At one U.S. auto plant, committee members suggested that the repetitive nature of assembly line work depressed productivity. Their solution: Instead of performing one repetitive function on an assembly line, the committee recommended that employees should do their jobs at work stations where they could perform several tasks. Management tested the idea. Result: Workers became conscious of the reality that they were involved in making a car, a fact they lost sight of when they performed only one task. There was a big increase in production and quality.

Caution: If recommendations are ignored too often, employees will feel their efforts aren't being taken seriously…and their commitment to productivity will be undermined.

Most ideas that come from the worker groups are valid because they have the most detailed knowledge of how things are actually done. If an idea must be rejected, management should give a detailed explanation.

Unless workers feel that management is serious about involving them in improving the factory's functioning, the committees will quickly turn into complaint groups where individual problems will supplant overall factory improvement as topics of discussion.

Meeting Union Objections

To get the most benefit from management-worker committees, most companies don't name union leaders or middle managers to the committees. Reason: These groups of people will inevitably try to manipulate committees to protect their own authority.

If workers are unionized, expect objections from the union regardless of whom you name to the committees. If objections are forceful, it's probably not worth the effort to pursue the idea. Besides, unless these committees are agreed to by management and unions, a union might be able legally, or as a practical matter, to force the company to abandon worker participation in decision making.

To sell unions on the idea, point out that management-worker committees are an effective way to achieve improved productivity, which, in turn, may pave the way for higher compensation. If the union still objects, challenge it to come up with a better way to raise productivity.

Selling middle managers on the idea is sometimes even harder than convincing unions. To head off objections, tell middle management of the plan before it's announced. Present the committee as a device to help middle managers.

The line to middle managers: You're doing a great job, and it could be even more effective with a system that's working elsewhere—letting people on the assembly line take more responsibility.

Explain that the majority of committee recommendations will increase efficiency and therefore make life easier for middle managers. If you suspect that one or two middle managers will almost certainly oppose the idea, tell them about it first. Try to incorporate some of their ideas into the plan...and get them on the team.

Source: Management labor lawyer Alfred T. DeMaria, a specialist in employment law, and partner, Clifton, Budd, Burke & DeMaria, 420 Lexington Ave., New York 10170.

High Productivity Performance Formula

High productivity performance formula—1. Be hard on work. Set demanding standards for worker attendance, product quality and number of units completed per hour. 2. Be easy on workers. Don't bark at employees, and don't wait until the last minute to announce mandatory overtime, etc. Instead, listen to their suggestions and complaints, show respect and ask workers to do jobs according to their needs and interests. Result: Productivity will go up as workers begin to feel more positive about the job.

Source: Jim Hamerstone, TRW, Inc., Human Resources, Cleveland 44124.

To Prevent Paperwork Disease

Nearly 70% of all working hours are spent preparing, reading, recording, interpreting, filing, and maintaining over 30 billion pieces of paper. To spend your day on more productive tasks:

■Read fast during uninterrupted scheduled reading times. Have an assistant pre-read and flag items that need a response.

■Respond informally by using notes. Not every response has to be a letter.

■Confirm by telephone unless there's a legal reason to confirm in writing.

■Avoid writing reports, especially when the information is already available.

■Substitute reports with a visual or oral presentation. Pictures are often more effective than words.

■Speak when you want immediate feedback or a reaction, to negotiate or persuade, to listen to the other person, when what you have to say is boring, to give a reprimand, when "how you say it" is important, or when you don't want your words coming back to you.

■Write when you want to stay out of court, persuade a hostile audience, praise subordinates, send complex information, or think through ideas.

■Ignore documents that don't require a response.

■Remove your name from irrelevant distribution lists.

■Give papers a destroy date. If you must save certain papers, write on them the date when they're no longer needed.

■Use electronic message systems. It's better than playing telephone tag.

Better Management

■Create an atmosphere of trust. Staff shouldn't be required to put everything in writing to protect themselves.

■Give commendations for undocumented achievements. Otherwise, employees will spend their time stuffing their files with written memos about what they've accomplished.

■Listen to talk seriously. This will discourage people from feeling compelled to put everything in writing.

■Reward ideas that cut down on paperwork.

Source: Dianna Booher, president, Booher Writing Consultants, 12337 Jones Rd., Houston 77070. Ms. Booher is author of *Cutting Paperwork in the Corporate Culture*, Facts on File, 460 Park Ave. S., New York 10016.

Chapter 9
Training Programs

Getting The Most From Employee Training

■Be sure training takes place in an environment that is free of distractions. Most common mistakes are bad food, no coffee, incorrect equipment, time limitations, and telephone interruptions.

■Reinforce the initial training. It's estimated that people retain only 10% of what they have learned. Their retention rate can be boosted to 60% with the help of ongoing programs.

■Determine whether it's best to do the training in-house or out-of-house. In-house is good for on-the-job training, one-day job introductions, quick hands-on experience with equipment operation. Out-of-house serves best for intense seminars of more than one day, management training, planning sessions, and for sales, marketing, and product demonstration seminars. Even companies with training centers are going out-of-house for concentrated sessions with no interruptions.

Training Rules

Break down training actions into a number of small steps:
1. Tell what the operation will achieve before showing how to do it.
2. Explain the first step before doing it.
3. Demonstrate slowly.
4. Repeat the demonstration and then have the employee try it.
5. Ask if there are questions before moving on to the next step.
6. After it has all been explained and demonstrated, perform the entire procedure at top production speed to give the worker a goal to shoot for.
7. If the training is interrupted, start over.
8. Follow up by letting trainees know how they are doing. Assist slow learners with the steps that are giving them trouble.

Source: *Executive Action Series*, Bureau of Business Practice, Waterford, CT.

Problems With Management Training Programs

Managers usually find supervisory training courses stimulating and enjoyable. But there is little evidence that the supervisor's overall effectiveness improves as a result of the training. Usual reasons for failure:

■There is no agreement on what supervisors should be taught. It's not yet clear which supervisory style is best and under what circumstances. Focus on identifying those who seem to know intuitively how to lead.

■Managers find it difficult to transfer training from a classroom to real situations. Usually the course becomes nothing but a fondly remembered experience.

■Supervisors often have little personal control over their management techniques. A dictatorial style is often the solution when the competence of subordinates is low.

The best use of training is to identify those with supervisory skills, teach them the basics, and weed out those who lack leadership potential.

Source: *Work Redesign*, Addison–Wesley, Reading, MA.

Quality Circle Trap

The toughest resistance to quality circles and similar quality-improvement programs in a company often comes not from workers, but from supervisors who feel threatened when workers get more say in managing their own jobs. Hostile supervisors who undercut worker suggestions just to show who's boss can cause the whole program to fail. What to do: Follow the lead of IBM, which 25 years ago taught its factory supervisors that their job is to help workers find ways to be productive, rather than order them to be productive. Get this idea across by involving supervisors in their own quality circles before applying the technique at the worker level.

Source: *The Frontiers of Management* by Peter Drucker, Harper & Row, 10 E. 53 St., New York 10022.

Chapter 10
Time-Saving Techniques

A Systematic Approach
To Time Management

Effective time management involves an internal and external component. The internal aspect requires heavy doses of self-discipline. The external, a systematic approach to keeping track of how time is spent and how plans to spend it actually work out. A sample system to follow:

■Weed out anything that can be delegated.

■Rank the remaining tasks in order of their importance. Give priority to those items where immediate action will reduce the total amount of work.

■Schedule sequentially enough time for each task.

■Keep a careful log of the actual amount of time spent.

■Once a week, compare the log with the schedule. Evaluate the discrepancies to learn whether enough time was allowed and, if so, what happened to interfere with the schedule.

Hard-Nosed Approach
To Managing Time

■Concentrate on the best ways to spend time, instead of worrying about how to save time.

■Keep an accurate log of activities to identify and define work patterns.

■Have only one chair (besides yours) in your office. Keeping people standing saves time.

■Each meeting should have an announced time limit.

■Have all calls screened. Make a list of who should be put through immediately.

■Arrange office with back to door.

■If someone asks, "Do you have a minute?," say no.

■List tomorrow's priorities before leaving the office today.

■Don't rush needlessly. It takes longer to correct a mistake than to avoid making a mistake.

Source: Merrill E. Douglass, director, Time Management Center, *Marketing Times*, New York.

How To Develop Good Time-Use Habits

Managers can make more of themselves and their life if they take the trouble to cultivate good time-use habits until they are second nature. Habits automatically steer everyone's lives. When habits become time-thrifty, managers will get better use of their time for the rest of their lives, automatically.

To develop better time-use habits, managers should:

■Pick those habits that are good and drop bad ones. Make a list of times and places to substitute a new habit for an old one. It takes a month or more until a new habit is second nature.

■Concentrate on using the new technique as often as possible. Every time a new habit is used, a mental pat on the back should be given. Otherwise, a mental kick is in order.

■Put weekly reminders of resolves to change habits on a calendar. When the reminders come up, evaluate the progress. Then list additional times and places to apply the new habit.

■Announce intentions to develop new habits to other people. This strengthens the motivation to finish the job.

Source: Robert Moskowitz, time-management consultant, Canoga Park, CA.

Setting The Right Order For Tasks

When managers feel overwhelmed they react by leaving many tasks untouched or unfinished. They fail to communicate that the jobs are undone. And then they do low-priority items first.

The root of the problem is that they have no master plan for sorting out their tasks. Their work lacks direction.

To regain control:

■Inventory available resources. Include people, equipment, money, or prospects for financing.

■Identify the ways to measure results. Examples: Profit, sales, units produced, letters sent out.

■Be realistic about expected accomplishments. Consider both personal and business goals.

Have a close associate ask the questions. Write down everything important. Be specific. Ambiguities often result from hidden assumptions.

Many offices are snagged by bad communication. Openness is a must in making viable plans, and in changing them if mistakes are made.

Distribute copies of goals to associates to coordinate plans. Ask them to use these as a basis to work out their own objectives in the same way. Many employees do not understand their boss's plans and expectations, so they work at cross-purposes.

Update plans and goals on an ongoing basis. Spend half a day every month with associates, identifying goals and planning how to achieve them.

Once goals have been established, define the specific steps that must be taken to achieve them. Set deadlines for those goals and for intermediate ones, too. Ask:

■How long will it take?

■What will it cost?

■What resources are available?

■From whom can I get the information?

Keep a summary of goals close at hand. Read through it every day and use it. Before scheduling an appointment, be sure its purpose fits in with goals. Focus on productive ideas by noting which techniques and activities were successful during the day.

Source: Howard Schor and Mariana Somer, Creative Communication Corp., New York.

How To Find Another Hour In The Day

To add at least 60 minutes to each day:

■Make a list of points to be covered in meetings or telephone calls. Focus on the major concerns of the customer, spouse, boss, or subordinate. The sooner the other is satisfied, the quicker you can move on.

■Set deadlines. Then meet or beat them. Setting specific plans for an evening or a weekend gives incentive to get office tasks finished promptly.

■Identify time buffers, the built-in mechanisms to delay that everyone uses (driving around the block a few times before facing a tough customer, overcommitments, miscommunications, accommodating others unnecessarily). Rather than putting off staff training, for instance, do it. This will free more time later, since you can then delegate more.

■Use your own prime time (most productive period in the day) for your prime projects. Zero in on accomplishing highest-priority goals.

■Be prompt. It minimizes problems with customers, supervisors, peers, and subordinates. And it saves time apologizing and explaining.

■Communicate clearly. It saves time spent in clarifying misunderstandings, correcting errors, rewriting, redoing, explaining delays, and worrying. Use words that are easily understood. Avoid double meanings. Emphasize important points.

Source: David K. Lindo, *Supervision Can Be Easy*, AMACOM, New York.

Dealing With Details

When your mind is cluttered with details, use one of these techniques to redirect energy and improve organization:

■Take a mini-break. A short walk, or a minute of relaxation. Or, simply breathe deeply for 30 seconds with your eyes closed (this can help concentration when you shift from one subject to another).

■Keep your schedule on paper. Resist the temptation to keep it in your head.

■Avoid interruptions. Work away from the office and keep your distance from the telephone.

■Delegate details. Rely more heavily on your secretary. Let subordinates handle routine jobs. Let them attend most of the less important meetings.

■Set time limits. If a task isn't completed within an allotted time limit, come back to it later.

Source: *International Management*, New York.

Use Commuting Time To Plan The Day

Questions to get started:
■What are the priority items in the current work load?
■What problems can be expected today?
■Which jobs from the previous day need to be cleaned up?
■What special opportunities exist that are particularly challenging or call for special skills?
■What personal contributions to company goals are likely or possible today?
It's best to plan tomorrow the night before.

How To Spot Time Wasters

To identify nonproductive executive time, do a careful analysis of a typical week's activities.

Make daily time sheets on which each line stands for a 15-minute period. Keep a running record of how each period is spent. It is time-consuming to do, but saves many hours later.

Then, using hindsight at the end of every day, "grade" each activity 1, 2, or 3, according to this guide:

1. The right thing at the right time.

2. The right thing, but at the wrong time. The task might have been more effectively handled later, after something else occurred.

3. The wrong thing, something not worth doing or that could have been done by someone else.

The key to winning the battle against time wasters is to know exactly which high-priority activities to undertake when a time-waster is eliminated. Otherwise, the free time that is created will quickly be dominated by another low-payoff task.

And bad use of time often has an overlooked secondary impact. The negative feelings that result from being forced to carry out a trivial task often create more wasted time (in griping or slacking off) than the original chore.

Source: *Effective Time Management*, Prentice-Hall, Englewood Cliffs, NJ.

How Managers Waste Time

■Doing others people's work. Most managers could improve their efficiency up to 30% if they delegated work more effectively.

■Spending time on phone calls that could be handled by a secretary.

■Working on a favorite chore that might not mesh with the company's priorities.

■Repeating instructions. Give instructions orally to as large a group as feasible, then follow up with a written version of the same instruction. This way, questions can be answered at one time and misunderstandings are less likely to occur.

A simple time-saving axiom: Do it now. About 75% of a manager's work can be done right away.

Source: Norman Kobert, Norman Kobert & Associates, Ft. Lauderdale.

Chapter 11
Communicating Your Ideas

How To Write Clearly

The "Fog Index" measures how clearly letters, memos, and reports are written.

■Count off a 100-word section.

■Count the number of sentences and divide 100 by that number, which gives average words per sentence.

■Count the words with more than two syllables. Add this figure to the average words per sentence.

■Multiply the total by 0.4 to get the Fog Index (indicating the minimum school grade level a reader needs to comprehend it).

The lower the index the better. A score of 11–12 is passable for most business writing. (The Fog Index for this item: 7.6.)

Source: *Time Talk*, Grandville, MI.

Pitfalls you should avoid:

■Using popular but vague modifiers, such as exceptional or efficient, without defining precisely what is meant. For example, an exceptional record can be either exceptionally good or bad. Describing something as efficiently designed does not say enough. It's better to use facts, numbers, details.

■Exaggerating. Overstating a fact is acceptable (and common) in conversation, but it destroys credibility in writing because readers take it literally. For example, thousands of people attended the noon rally in the park. In reality, only a few hundred attended. The others were there eating lunch or passing by.

■Generalizing. Words to avoid: All, right, wrong, true, false, always, never. Instead, say this is true under such-and-such conditions.

■Surface reasoning. For example, "No routine inspection program has been established because of the personnel change every two years." The real reasons for the lack of inspection actually are any number of other factors.

Source: William C. Paxson, *The Business Writing Handbook*, Bantam Books, New York.

Write As Clearly As You Think

Concentrate on simplifying sentence structure in business writing. It's the easiest way to say what is meant and to make sure the message gets across. Remember three basic rules:

■Keep sentences short. They should be no more than 17–20 words. If an idea has multiple parts, use multiple sentences.

■Vary the length of sentences. The 17–20 word rule is the average. When sentences drone on at unvarying lengths, the reader's attention begins to wander.

■Vary the punctuation. Include plenty of commas, as well as a sprinkling of semicolons, to go with the necessary periods. This improves clarity of communication. Well-placed punctuation is a road map, leading the reader comfortably and accurately through the message.

Source: Paul Richards, "Sentence Control: Solving an Old Problem," *Supervisory Management*, New York.

Communicating Basics For A Long Memo

Before preparing a long memo, ask yourself if this information is:
■Needed at the other end? (If you are not sure, call and ask.)
■Being sent to all the people who can do the most with it?
■Already on hand in another form?
■Generated too frequently?
■Issued not often enough?
■In the simplest and most useful format?

Source: Auren Uris, *Memos for Managers*, Thomas Y. Crowell, New York.

How To Sell Ideas

Creative people often find it easier to do original thinking than to sell their ideas to others.

Before presenting an idea to a group:
■Look for reasons why others might oppose the idea.
■Seek out early supporters.
■Decide on goals. Ask yourself if the acceptance of the idea is more important than getting credit for it.
■Downplay originality. Instead, discuss similar concepts that have been successful. Never assume that others want innovation because they say they do. Most people prefer the status quo.
■Play politics. Get an unpopular staffer to oppose the idea. Or point out that competitors might use it first.
■Be detached and appear uninterested. Depriving opponents of a victory reduces their joy in taking the idea apart. Or be the first to point out the idea's flaws, then listen as others solve them.
■Make sure that others' perceptions of the idea are accurate. Otherwise they may reject what they think the innovation is, not what it really is.
■Throw out decoys for opponents to shoot down. Once their negative impulses have been satisfied, bring up the real idea.

Source: Thomas J. Attwood, managing director, Cargill Attwood International, *Management Review*, New York.

How To Give More Effective Instructions

■Be highly specific, never general.
■Focus on the task at hand, not the circumstances surrounding it.
■Select a time when there are no distractions.
■Don't overload listeners. Present instructions that are complicated or long in a simplified or graphic way.
　■Have the employee repeat critical portions of the instructions in his own words.
　■Be considerate of the feelings of those receiving the instructions.
Source: Randall S. Schyuler, Ohio State University, *The Personnel Administrator*, Berea, OH.

Speaking With Authority

When giving orders:
■Avoid weak expletives. Don't use: Darn, golly, gee whiz, or other trivial expressions. They reduce credibility.
■Don't invite a subordinate to agree with your instructions. The wrong thing to say: "This has to be done today, doesn't it?" The right way is to confirm authority by saying: "You'll get this done today, won't you?"
■Don't confuse politeness with authority. Wrong: "Will you please do this report?" Right: "Please do this report." Repeatedly asking employees if they're willing to do their job costs a manager credibility.
■Don't use disqualifying phrases when giving suggestions. Avoid saying: "I don't know if this will work, but try it anyway." Instead, simply state the suggestion.

Making The Most Of Office Confrontations

One of the most unpleasant parts of being a manager is confronting subordinates who fall short of your expectations. As a result, many executives bottle up their feelings of displeasure until their working relationships with problem employees have deteriorated beyond repair.

Instead, as soon as a subordinate's work falls below standard, have a talk with him about his job performance, with the objective of achieving the necessary improvement in performance from the subordinate and coming out of the talk with both sides feeling better and the relationship intact.

How to do it:
■Prepare for the confrontation. Review beforehand the specific criticism; how it will be presented; what it should accomplish. (It is best to write it out, at least in outline form.)
■Come to the point as quickly as possible.

■Talk about the subordinate's performance in descriptive terms. Don't evaluate. Don't say: "You're not trying." Say: "You're not producing enough."

■If the employee's behavior provokes anger, tell him or her so.

■Make all statements personal. Don't talk about top management's displeasure. Don't say "we." If the boss personally accepts responsibility for the confrontation, there's a better chance that the subordinate will accept the responsibility for improving his or her performance.

■Take the trouble to understand the subordinate's point of view. That perspective provides a clearer picture for you of why the subordinate's performance is unsatisfactory.

■Be as specific as possible about the improvement required. Don't say: "Change your attitude." Do say: "Please stop trying to interpret my instructions. Just follow them."

■Don't conclude the talk until there's agreement on what's been said.

■If something specific should result from the talk, tell the subordinate what it is you're expecting. If this talk is the subordinate's final warning to shape up, let the individual know it.

■Before ending the talk, say something sincere and complimentary about the subordinate.

Learning to express feelings before they become explosive will not end all problems with subordinates, but many executives who learn to speak their minds more freely discover that their fear of confrontation was unfounded and they take more pleasure in their work relationships.

Source: Aubrey Sanford, vice-president, The Atlanta Consulting Group, Atlanta.

Becoming A Better Listener

Becoming a better listener is not easy. Simple techniques that help:

■Relax yourself and the speaker. Give your full attention to what's being said. Stop everything else you're doing. Maintain eye contact.

■Don't let the speaker's tone of voice or manner turn you off. Nervousness or misplaced emotions often cloud the message the speaker is trying to get across.

■Prepare beforehand for the conversation. Take a few minutes to read or consult information pertinent to the discussion. That also helps you to quickly evaluate the speaker and the subject.

■Allow for unusual circumstances (extreme pressure or disturbing interruptions). Judge only what the speaker says given the conditions he's faced with.

■Avoid getting sidetracked. Listen very closely to points you disagree with. (Poor listeners shut out or distort them.)

■Mentally collect the main points of the conversation. Occasionally, ask for clarification of one of the speaker's statements. This shows your interest and helps the speaker better organize his thoughts.

■Restate what you've heard at the end of the talk to avoid misunderstandings. Emphasize important issues brought up in the discussion.

Source: George De Mare, *Communicating at the Top*, John Wiley & Sons, New York.

Bad Listening Habits

■Thinking about something else while waiting for the speaker's next word or sentence. The mind races four times faster than does the rate of conversation.

■Listening primarily for facts rather than ideas.

■Tuning out when the talk seems to be getting too difficult.

■Prejudging, from a person's appearance and speaking manner, that nothing interesting will be said.

■Paying attention to outside sights and sounds when talking with someone.

■Interrupting with a question whenever a speaker says something puzzling or unclear.

Source: John T. Samaras, University of Oklahoma, *Personnel Journal*, Costa Mesa, CA.

Less Time For Listening Means More Time For Work

Listening is usually a very inefficient way to get information. The reason is that most people don't talk efficiently. They don't organize their thoughts. They ramble on, taking about three times as long as necessary. Also, it builds a subordinate's ego when his superior listens to him.

How to save time when listening is unavoidable:

■Insist that appointments and meetings start on time. If people are late, don't wait for them. Do something else.

■For complex problems, insist on written background material beforehand.

■When the speaker rambles, interrupt with questions to bring out the point.

■If a decision can't be made immediately, say, "I'll think about it." Then move on to other matters. Don't waste time rehashing the problem over and over.

Sounding Better On The Phone

■Make a better impression on the phone by opening your mouth wider as you speak and moving your lips. Most people move their lips too little, flattening the voice tone. Do not squeeze the phone between your neck and shoulder. This tenses your throat and makes you talk from one side of your mouth.

■Speak in your lower vocal range. Telephones transmit lower pitches more truly than high ones.

How To Prepare A Speech

Decide exactly and precisely what your subject is. Then logically think through your subject. List the ideas and conclusions to stress. Become thoroughly familiar with the important books, speeches and other literature on the subject.

Prepare an outline of the speech: Introduction, main body (usually divided up into two or four sections) and the conclusion.

Start by writing the speech. Be complete.

Prepare a brief introduction. Various ways in which you can introduce your speech: 1. Attack the topic head-on by simply announcing it. 2. Begin with a human interest story, an illustration or a funny anecdote relevant to the topic. 3. Startle the audience by beginning with an exciting question or an arousing statement. 4. Use a quote or an idea from somebody else. 5. Explain in factual terms why the topic is important to your audience.

The main body of the speech should make it apparent to your audience that you have a thorough knowledge of the topic. Back up your points with facts, numbers, examples. If you want to convince your audience of the wisdom of your view on the topic, begin with material that agrees with those views. Don't argue. Just explain your points. Those points should be clearly defined either at the beginning or the end of the speech, or as they develop within the speech, or any combination of those three.

Conclude: Briefly go over the points you've made. Use a quote. Strive for a big climax. You can compliment the audience. Or end by being encouraging and optimistic, or by telling a particularly dramatic story, an historical anecdote or a joke. You can also recommend that your audience take some action. Another ending would be to suggest that they change their view to yours.

■Type the last line of each page on the top of the next page.

■Don't have speech typed in all capital letters. Word recognition is easier when normal upper- and lower-case letters are used.

■Have speech typed triple-spaced.

■Don't hyphenate words.

■When gesturing, keep a finger (or pencil) on the line being read (so place won't be lost). Gesture with other hand.

■Don't staple speech manuscript. Allow completed pages or large cards to be casually (and noiselessly) slid off to side.

■Memorize important points. Then eyes can lift from text to look directly at audience when these points are being made. Memorize both opening and closing lines.

■Use a slant-top lectern so manuscript can be read by dropping eyes only slightly—but not your head.

■Write words "slow down" in large letters at top of each page. That compensates for general tendency to speak too rapidly.

■Speaker who writes on blackboard or easel pad as a visual aid should keep it on his left (when he's facing the audience) if he's right-handed, and on his right if he's left-handed. Prevents turning back on audience or blocking what's written.

■When your remarks are scheduled for the end of a program, have two versions ready: One regular length and the other much shorter. If the programs runs long, go with the short one.

■Most people speak several tones too high. The reason: They don't hear their voices as others do. The sound reaches them through the head rather than through vibrations in the air, distorting the tone. Speak low. Use lots of jaw and lip movement. This will improve tone, make you look more animated and slow your delivery, giving you more time to think of what you want to say.

■Prespeech stage fright can be turned into a vitalizing force with exercises that actors do in private, just before going on: Flop hands and legs, and roll head and shoulders…stretch facial muscles (shut eyes tightly, with nose and mouth practically touching, then release into a silent scream with eyes and mouth wide open)…finish by stretching while walking (big, indulgent, lionlike movements). Then face the crowd energized and free from tension.

Speeches With Impact

■Remember that your audience is interested first in people, then in things, finally in ideas.

■Only rarely is it possible to change deep-seated attitudes or beliefs. Aim no higher than getting the listeners to question their attitudes. Avoid alienating an audience by pressing points too hard.

■The most successful speeches state conclusions and call for action.

■When you have to speak extemporaneously, develop a theme early and stick to it throughout your speech.

■Use silence to underline a point.

■End a speech with a short, emotional, conviction-filled summary of the main points.

Source: Michael Klezaras, Jr., director of research and planning, Roger Ailes & Associates, Inc., New York.

Using Humor Successfully

1. Avoid humor when speaking out-of-doors. The laugh tends to get lost, leaving people with the feeling it wasn't funny at all.

2. Avoid puns, even though they may go over well in a parlor. They almost always cause the audience to groan more than laugh.

3. Leave enough time for the laugh before proceeding. Audiences sometimes react slowly, especially if the humor was unexpected. To a nervous speaker, a second's delay seems like an hour.

4. Be prepared to carry on smoothly and self-confidently if the audience doesn't laugh. The audience will quickly forget that the speaker laid an egg if he remains calm and composed.

Source: Paul Preston, *Communication for Managers*, Prentice–Hall, Englewood Cliffs, NJ.

Chapter 12
Running Effective Meetings

How To Take Control Of A Meeting

"I'll write a summary" is a masterful way to take control of a meeting, especially when the discussion is going against the position you favor. Reason: Like taking minutes, writing up a document gives immense powers of emphasis and omission. The writer can shade the argument or even the decision and give it almost whatever tone he wishes. Few will insist on corrections.

Source: *Meetings, Meetings* by Winston Fletcher, William Morrow & Co., New York.

Getting Your Ideas Accepted At Meetings

1. Don't be the first presenter.
2. Never present your best idea first. The energy level is too high at the beginning of a meeting, so you are apt to get clobbered.
3. Never be enthusiastic about your idea. Presenting it modestly, even doubtfully, disarms hostile forces.
4. Be courteous to the ideas of others and you may get the same treatment.
5. Don't count on friends or best buddies.
6. Don't present your ideas too slickly. If you do, your opponents will get suspicious and seek even its slightest faults.
7. Listen carefully to comments on preceding ideas for clues to a negative response to something in your idea.
8. Don't be the first (or last) to arrive. Don't sit too close to the table. Don't drink too much water. (It may be mistaken for a hangover—or illness.)

Ways To Save On Business Meetings

■Deal with hotel sales offices, not reservation centers. Hotel sales reps can be more flexible about group discounts.

■Before setting a date for a meeting, find out when the hotels under consideration have the least business. As a general rule, big-city hotels have the most vacancies (as well as the most negotiable rates) from Wednesday to Friday.

■Pay for open bars at meetings by the bottle rather than by the drink. Request that bartenders pour one-ounce shots rather than free-pour the drinks.

■Ask hotels about their complimentary-room policies. Hotels generally offer one free room for every 50 rooms booked. The policy is negotiable.

■Serve a light buffet lunch rather than a heavy meal. Buffets are cheaper and the lighter fare helps keep employees from falling asleep at afternoon sessions.

■Organize meetings on days of the week that enable the company to take advantage of any available discount air fares.

Source: Stephen Moran, president, Meetings Planners, Inc., Boston.

How *Not* To Run A Meeting

■Call a nonemergency meeting during nonbusiness hours or on a weekend.

■Have secretary leave surprise short-notice invitations on desks.

■Invite people without regard to their duties or priorities.

■Fail to distribute an agenda in advance.

■Don't announce the subject of the meeting.

■Never reveal who will be there.

■Neglect to bring records along or bring obsolete data. Then it will be impossible to document anything.

■Use technical terms that no one understands.

■Argue and frown a lot to show seriousness. Challenge every statement.

■Always blame someone else for problems (especially in front of customers).

■Run out on the meeting, leaving everyone else wondering what they're supposed to do next.

Source: David K. Lindo, *Supervision Can Be Easy*, AMACOM, New York.

How To Chair A Committee

■Be aware of every member's interests, hopes, and suggestions for the committee. Meet privately beforehand with invitees to ascertain their points of view. This will insure against unpleasant surprises during the session.

■Handle housekeeping details efficiently. Be sure agendas and supplies are distributed on time. Welcome members at the door to relax them.

■Don't let talkative members dominate and quiet ones fade into the woodwork. Privately urge quiet people to speak up. Or get permission to pass on their views.

■Remain neutral. Avoid granting individual favors or advancing narrow causes. Chairpersons are judged by how their committee performs as a whole, not by personal contributions they might make.

■Stress the blending of divergent opinions into a consensus. Be wary of advancing too many opinions from the chair.

■Check the final report with the full committee before submitting it to make sure it accurately represents the group's findings.

Source: Dr. John E. Tropman, professor of social work, University of Michigan, *Directors and Boards*, McLean, VA.

To Keep The Meeting Lively

■Don't ask questions that can be answered with a simple yes or no, for example, ones that begin with do you, have you, will you.

■Never open a session with "I think." Employees won't offer new ideas when leaders state their positions right away.

■Steer members back to the point whenever they wander. Summarize periodically. A meeting won't go anywhere unless the focus is always on a solution.

■Stress the importance of getting different points of view. This makes it easier for everyone to participate.

■Bring disagreements out into the open so they can be discussed.

Source: Michael Renton, *Getting Better Results from the Meetings You Run*, Research Press, Champaign, IL.

How Breaks Improve Meetings

Well-planned coffee breaks allow informal one-to-one chats so that meeting participants can work out disagreements and clarify misunderstandings in some privacy. To make breaks effective:

■Organize the agenda so that controversial or complex items will be interrupted by a break. It reduces logjams during the discussion.

■Schedule as many breaks as needed (up to one hour). But avoid late afternoon breaks. Some participants may wander off.

■Locate the refreshment table as near to the conference room as possible (outside the door) so that the meeting atmosphere isn't disrupted.

■Duration of the break should be slightly less time than needed for a trip to a coffee shop or back to the desk for a quick task. Remember, breaks are part of the meeting, designed to expedite (not interrupt) the discussion.

■End breaks on time. Get participants back into the formal session by closing conference room doors, ringing a small bell, or both.

Source: William T. Carnes, *Effective Meetings for Busy People*, McGraw-Hill, New York.

Meeting Dimensions

■Committee meetings: 30 minutes to 3 hours; 3 to 15 people in attendance.

■Training meetings: 1 to 30 days; 10 to 30 people.

■Planning meetings: 1 to 5 days; 6 to 15 people.

■Information meetings (in which participants are introduced to a new concept or practice and are motivated to use it): 1 to 5 days; attendance can be unlimited.

Too few persons at meetings limit the number of ideas that can be generated. But too many people make agreement and decision-making cumbersome.

Source: Coleman Finkel, president, National Conference Centers, East Windsor, NJ, *Successful Meetings*, Philadelphia.

Part II

**THE GREAT BOOK
OF BUSINESS SECRETS**

Financial Analysis
And Control

Chapter 13
Smarter Budgeting

Secrets Of Much Better Budgeting

Year-end is when managers gear up—usually with little enthusiasm—for their annual budget ritual.

Traditionally, a standard spreadsheet is used for measuring performance, generally on a monthly basis, against budget—cost to cost and revenue to revenue. This is the manager's chief road map for performance.

This traditional, inward-focused budget, however, lacks any relation to the company's performance for its customers. True, order processing costs may be down 10%, for instance, but are errors up significantly? Are customers defecting to the competition?

The company may be living well within its budget, but top managers who content themselves with this, while quality, service and customer loyalty deteriorate, are in for serious long-term trouble.

That big gap between budgeting and actual performance is now being closed by companies that look beyond their annual and quarterly financial numbers to performance-monitoring.

How To Do It

There's no need to completely dispose of the way the company now prepares its budgets. But companies need a parallel stream of information on their actual performance in delivering products and services in order to get an honest view of the budget numbers.

Key: Interview customers—by survey, focus groups or one-on-one—to find out what performance criteria are key to their continued loyalty. What are the main irritants to the relationship?

Then, the company can begin to develop performance measures for these key activities.

Next step: Design the company's parallel information system to highlight weaknesses in the quality and performance goals set as a result of determining what is important to customers.

Example: How often was delivery to customers later than the promised 24 hours? Are returns higher than specified? What is the error rate on invoices?

Impact on budgeting: With this hard data on performance, the company gets an important new dimension on its budget information.

Example: A department that operates within or substantially below budget would traditionally be rewarded for outstanding work. In reality, the quality of the department's products may be terrible. The parallel performance-monitoring exercise tells management that the department is in desperate need of quality improvement and that the impressive budget performance is therefore meaningless, because customers are ultimately being lost.

By contrast, a department that is over budget may actually have incredible performance improvement to show for it, and this improvement may generate future savings that justify the budget problem today.

Once budgets are looked at in connection with performance this way, the company can collect historical data to see if its overall performance is truly improving—continuously.

Budgeting will no longer be a sterile quarter-by-quarter review. It will become part of the company's continuous process of improvement.

Source: David Y. Schwartz, managing partner, Chicago audit and financial consulting practice, Arthur Andersen & Co., 33 West Monroe, Chicago 60603.

Taking Gamesmanship Out Of Budgeting

Most executives will recognize the two classic top-management budgeting traps: The add-10%-to-last-year's-expenses-and-press-for-a-20%-increase-in-sales trap; and the slash-10%-off-all-requests-and-forecasts-submitted trap.

These almost automatic responses to the budgeting process inevitably destroy the real function of budgets, which is to pinpoint opportunities (and threats) for the company and direct the use of its resources most effectively. Worse, subordinates recognize the automatic response and skew their numbers accordingly.

Begin the next budgeting process now, nonquantitatively. The first challenge for top management is to set guidelines for what the company must do to survive in the year ahead, grow in the short term and flourish in the long term.

In practice: A specialty chemicals firm that traditionally pegs research-and-development expenditures to the industry average decides it needs to add a high-margin item to its product line to bolster gross margins. Options: Scuttle R&D spending for the year, and retain a patent attorney to license a product from the outside. Or dramatically boost R&D to develop the product inside. First decide on the strategy. Then start budgeting.

The next step is to project sales for the year. Subtract the fixed costs (such as rent and taxes) and the desired profit margin. Then separate the balance remaining into two sets of expenses:

■Those required to keep the firm operating. Example: Salespeople's salaries and commissions.

■Those earmarked to help the company grow. Example: Advertising.

Think about the sum earmarked for growth as investment money. The goal in budgeting is to get maximum return on this investment.

The big goal of such budgeting: It allows the company to focus its discretionary expense money, rather than spread it thinly across all departments.

Having determined basic objectives and targets for discretionary spending, set guidelines for departmental budgets. Within those guidelines, negotiate final numbers. Middle managers will work harder to make negotiated budgets work than those imposed from above.

Avoid slashing departmental requests across the board. Selective additions to requests, along with acceptance of some requests untouched encourage departmental chiefs to submit honest numbers.

Monthly financial checkpoints should be salted with nonfinancial checkpoints. Example: If the specialty chemicals firm plans a June introduction for its new product, check to see that advertising is ready by April.

In the weeks following the annual budget go-round, review the company's reporting system to make sure managers get the right information to make the budget work.

Ask key managers two questions:
- What information do they need?
- How often do they need it?

Sample result: The company may find that its plant managers need daily information on plant output and direct labor hours. Central-office operations managers may need this information only monthly. But central-office operations managers may need company profit and loss statements weekly, while plant managers may need them only quarterly, or not at all.

Point: By pinpointing needs at each managerial level, the company can reduce the information overload that causes managers to stop focusing on their budgets.

Source: Albert A. Fried, president, Applied Strategies, Inc., New York.

Trimming The Fat Off Budgets

The greater the detail in budget, the greater the waste. The problem is that managers allow a little extra for each item in the budget. As the number of items mounts, the more fat "cushion" accumulates.

This cushion is seldom left in the budget at the fiscal year's end. It gets spent. If it were left over, managers would have to worry about budget cuts the following year.

To trim the fat, require less detail. Allocate expenditures by broad categories. Leave managers some freedom to shift money from one category to another in accordance with need. This cuts the temptation to overbudget. It also reduces the paperwork and administrative efforts associated with budgeting.

Four Ways To Make A Budget More Useful

1. Each budget sheet comes with accompanying instructions. Everyone who fills one out follows the same rules.

2. Costs are grouped into categories so that all operating results can be analyzed fairly.

3. There is a clear procedure for midstream revision that includes a definition of what changes justify it.

4. Preparers are accountable for compliance. Their results are periodically examined to judge progress and performance.

Source: *Evaluating Accounting Controls: A Systematic Approach*, report of Ernst & Young, New York.

When Formal Budgets Don't Make Sense

Many companies operate—or strive for—a system of strict, annual budgets. This is usually counterproductive. The companies that benefit most from rigid budgetary controls are old or well-established firms with a consistent rate of sales growth and a relatively unaltered product line from year to year. Firms that are inhibited rather than helped by strict budgeting:

■Are growing rapidly or erratically—fast one year, slow the next.

■Do not always know which segment of the business will produce the most growth in the coming year.

■Serve widely varying markets, some of which may be very strong one year, while others turn quite weak.

Example: A chemical company supplies products to the automotive and electronics industries. When the auto market is weak, the firm's auto business will be lower than budgeted. Meanwhile, electronics may be doing better than the budget anticipates. To shift more capability into electronics may mean hiring more personnel because electronics is more people-intensive than automotive, which relies more on capital equipment.

Under rigid budgeting, such sudden shifts can be difficult. Managers are normally held accountable for what they had budgeted several months earlier. They would most likely be in trouble if their sales were 5% above or below their projections. They may actually be penalized if they exceed their targets (the electronics manager) as well as if they fall short (the automotive manager). In the final analysis, the budget is keeping the company from taking advantage of changing opportunities.

The chemical company's alternative is ad hoc budgeting. A formal, detailed budget is prepared each year as in other companies, but it is not continually revised with every shift in business conditions. Instead, changes are made in succeeding years' budgets.

One benefit of this approach is that managers know they are not going to be forced to live by the old budget when circumstances change. This permits them to respond to external events and capitalize on opportunities without having to spend time revising budgets.

Another is that the company avoids getting top-heavy in its management. The company in question, for example, has a small management group and wants to stay that way. By not repeatedly revising the budget, there is no need for a huge financial department.

And the real world, not the budget, becomes the true control mechanism. Both the board of directors and management use the budget as a guide, not as a bible that tells managers what they can and cannot do.

Ad hoc budgeting lets fast-acting managers change operations without going through numerous formal budget revisions. It gets around the common problem of managers who try to live with out-of-date assumptions rather than go back and change projections.

For example, a company's raw-materials costs soar far beyond the budget. Unless the budget is revised (perhaps several times), the purchasing staff goes on buying as scheduled. Meanwhile, the marketing department keeps pricing the product on the basis of the budget because it does not know the actual costs. In extreme cases, marketing may sell more and more and think it is doing a great job, while margins narrow or even disappear entirely.

The company's ad hoc budgeters prevent this by preparing detailed, monthly cost sheets that keep all top managers informed of changes as they occur. Direct manufacturing costs account for 60% of the company's sales dollar. So, the changes reflected in the cost sheets are what the managers use to shift tactics. But this continually updated information is not used to recast the budget, because it would keep managers working on budgets instead of on real tasks.

If a company does not pay attention to the budget, why bother to go through the exercise at all? The answer is it should pay attention to the budget, but as a planning tool rather than an operational control. This company uses its budget to plan in the following way:

■Marketing forecasts where sales will come from in the next year.

■Production determines whether enough capacity is in place to fill those orders.

■Selling prices are determined and costs are estimated to see what is happening to margins.

■Managers project overhead, staffing, and expenses.

■Financial managers project cash flow and figure out whether internally generated funds will be sufficient to finance or whether to borrow.

The key requirement of ad hoc budgeting is an active, attentive management. Managers cannot simply rely on a computer to punch out numbers and put up a red flag if the figures stray a certain percentage from the budget. Managers must look at the monthly cost, production, sales, and other figures intelligently and ask the right questions. The best control is management by people, not by mechanism.

Source: Dr. Herman W. Andre, vice-president for finance, and Norman L. Ritter, treasurer, Great Lakes Chemical Corp., West Lafayette, IN.

Chapter 14
Credit Management

Smart Credit Policies

Tightening credit in response to high borrowing costs should be done without antagonizing good customers or losing sales. Credit should be more liberal for high-margin products than for low-profit items. If the customer cannot be approved for credit, encourage bank letters of credit, personal guarantees, consignment sales, partial shipments, or liens on assets. Allow volume discounts only if payment is prompt. And maintain a bad-debt ratio close to the industry average.
Source: BDO/Seidman, CPAs, New York.

Better Credit Checks

Most businesses rely exclusively on Dun & Bradstreet's services for credit information on customers, suppliers and competitors. But there are other ways to check the creditworthiness of companies you do business with, and these methods may give you even more complete, and up-to-date information on a company...

■Check industry specialists. A number of credit agencies specialize in gathering information on businesses in certain industries—the garment industry, retailing, automotive parts. The information you get from these agencies will be more reliable and complete. The reports are written by industry experts. However, there's always a disclaimer in the report that makes it virtually impossible to sue an agency for giving inaccurate information about a customer.

■Do your own investigation. This is a good way to protect against inaccurate agency information. How to do an investigation:

■Call the customer's bank. Ask to speak to the officer who handles the company's account. Be frank. Tell the officer that you're checking credit on the company and tell him how much credit you're planning to extend. While banks won't give out specific financial information about a customer's business, they will supply information in ranges. It's up to you to interpret this information. Questions to ask:

■What is the average balance in the company's account? If the response is "low five figures," it may not be prudent to give credit on a $60,000 order.

■How long has the company been a customer of the bank? If the company has been with the bank for only a couple of months, it really doesn't have a credit history with that bank. In that case, it doesn't matter what the bank officer says.

■Has the company borrowed from the bank? What kind of loan? How much? From your standpoint, the best kind of loan is an unsecured loan. That means the bank considers the company a good enough credit risk to lend it money without asking for collateral.

■If the borrowing is secured, ask the bank which of the company's assets the liens are filed against. In most cases there are blanket liens against all the assets. There also may be liens against the company's accounts receivable. This information is important because it tells you that the bank considers the company less creditworthy than one to which it would make an unsecured loan. It shows that the company is borrowing on a revolving basis as fast as it needs the money.

■Does the bank officer personally know the customer? Has he been to the company's place of business? If the answer is "no," you can assume that the bank doesn't value the customer highly.

■Call the company's accounting firm. Generally, an accountant will only give out detailed credit information on clients who are in good shape financially. The questions to ask:

■What is the company's net worth?

■How is its cash flow?

■What is the current ratio of assets to liabilities (working capital)?

■Have the officers been drawing large amounts of cash out of the company that have been treated as loans?

■Ask for references from suppliers. Call the suppliers and ask if the customer pays promptly.

■Do a lien search. Search the county clerk's records for Uniform Commercial Code (UCC) liens on the company's assets. Your firm's accountant or lawyer can file the forms necessary to facilitate the search. The search will show if creditors, including the IRS, have placed liens against the company or its assets for unpaid bills.

■Ask the company for a financial statement. Many companies don't give information to credit agencies because they don't want their competitors to get their hands on it. If the company's credit is good and you're checking for a legitimate purpose, they should be quite willing to give you financial statements and any other pertinent credit information.

Source: Edward Mendlowitz, CPA, partner, Mendlowitz Weitsen, Two Pennsylvania Plaza, New York 10121. Mr. Mendlowitz is the author of *New Tax Traps/New Opportunities*, Boardroom Books, Box 1026, Springfield, NJ 07081.

How To Make Better Use Of The Credit Department

An effective credit department assembles much information that other departments can use—at very low incremental cost. Credit data can help other departments to:

■Forecast liquidation of receivables (finance department).

■Keep top management up-to-date about business conditions and trends.

■Profile customers demographically and geographically (marketing department).

■Identify or rate prospects before sales force solicits them.

■Provide specialized data about new markets.

■Evaluate vendors, and find new sources (purchasing department).

■Screen merger candidates.

■Train managers in financial controls.

Source: Dr. Harold W. Fox, professor, Ball State University, Muncie, IN.

Tightening Credit Controls In A Recession

A recession is no time to continue the standard business practice of making the sales now and worrying about collection later. During a recession, stretched-out accounts receivable weaken cash flow, and borrowing to stay liquid cuts into profit margins that are already thinned by weak sales. One result is higher unit costs.

For example, if a company has $5 million in accounts receivable, borrowing $1 million of that at 12% to cover accounts payable costs $120,000 a year. But if the company tightens credit controls at a cost of less than $120,000, and in the process reduces its accounts receivable by $1 million, it will come out way ahead.

The key to tightening credit controls is not altering credit policy, but improving its execution. This involves analyzing the risk in extending credit to each customer, improving the coordination between the company's credit and sales operations, and clearly establishing the credit manager's authority in regard to how much credit he can extend without management's approval. Also important is how much bad debt he can pass on to a collection agency or write off on his own authority.

Recommended steps:

■Have the credit manager report to the chief operating officer, not to the controller, in order to draw him into the management process.

■Periodically send credit personnel into the field with salespeople. This gives credit analysts a feel for sales problems, and fosters better working relationships.

■Take a critical look at the company's methods for gathering credit information. Review the questions credit analysts ask when calling a customer's bank to see if those questions can be sharpened still further.

Source: Myron J. Biggar, management consultant, Nazareth, PA.

How Flexible Credit Terms Boost Sales

Requiring every customer to make full payment of a bill within 30 days may shut out some otherwise good accounts. Instead, consider offering cash-short customers with good credit ratings a payment plan that lets them pay within an average of 30 days. Flexible formulas include:

■One-third down, one-third in 30 days, one-third in 60 days. The average time is 30 days.

■One-half down, one-half in 60 days. This also gives a 30-day collection average.

■One-half down, one-quarter in 30 days, one-quarter in 60 days. The collection average falls to 22.5 days.

Source: Thomas J. Martin and Bruce Trabue, *Sell More and Spend Less*, Holt, Rinehart & Winston, New York.

Nine Ways To Spot Credit Scams

Scam operators drain $110 million a year from U.S. businesses by buying goods on credit, then declaring bankruptcy or simply vanishing.

Typically, a scam operator will study an industry until he understands its credit policies. He's most likely to look for situations when credit checks are most perfunctory, for example, any season rush period. Also, he will place and pay for small orders. Then, when the time is right, he will place a bunch of big orders, take delivery, and disappear without paying.

Alternatively, a scam artist will buy a small but reputable firm, place large orders, take delivery, and declare bankruptcy.

To avoid getting bilked, check:

1. Unsolicited orders, especially those unrelated to a customer's direct line of business.

2. Trade-show orders, especially the ones taken by suppliers who forgot or couldn't bring their credit files with them.

3. Rush orders from strangers or new customers.

4. Companies that haven't been in business for three years or more.

5. Recent change of ownership.

6. Sudden, large orders.

7. Companies whose names are similar to those of reputable companies in the same area, or use impressive titles such as worldwide or federal.

8. Companies that supply too much unsolicited credit information. Their hope is that this creates instant credibility and won't be checked. Also, check phone numbers of credit references to ascertain their genuineness, as well as letters from CPA firms and other references.

9. Unknown companies that enclose partial payments with first-time orders.

Source: Les Kirschbaum, president, Mid-Continent Adjustment Co., Morton Grove, IL.

Credit-Checking Trap

Relying solely on Dun & Bradstreet for information on customer creditworthiness can be dangerous because its credit reports are notoriously incomplete and sometimes very dated. Alternatives: 1. Join the National Association of Credit Management (520 Eighth Ave., New York 10018). The trade group has 75 affiliated organizations across the country and can provide basic credit reports on specific businesses for about $10. Membership costs $100–$300 per year, depending on your location. 2. Ask your banker to do a bank-to-bank check. For a small fee you'll receive a report on the customer's credit line, minimum balance and extent of borrowing. Drawback: Because of banking regulations, the information will be vague but still useful—a report might say the customer's line of credit is in the mid six figures, probably meaning about $500,000.

Source: *Inc.*, 38 Commercial Wharf, Boston 02110.

Spotting A Bad Credit Risk

Now more than ever before a company must be sure of the financial health of its suppliers and credit customers. How: Arrange a meeting between the company's accountant and the other company's accountant and banker.

Ask the banker: Has the company borrowed against its accounts receivable? Be cautious if it has. Reason: Interest rates on these loans are so high at present that the companies borrowing in this manner are short of cash. Be especially wary if:

■Either customer or supplier sales have gone down. Since the company borrows against receivables, its credit line has probably gone down as well. Cash may be very tight.

■The company's credit line has increased, but sales have not. Significance: This may indicate that the company has been unable to pay the interest on its debt. The lender has added the interest to the principal, a very bad sign.

Also ask the banker:

■How long has the company been with the bank? If not long, ask: Why did it switch from its old bank?

■Is the company a secured or nonsecured borrower? Importance: The bank considers the company trustworthy if it has extended an unsecured line of credit.

■How often do customer or supplier overdrafts occur?

■Is the bank's relationship with the company satisfactory?

Take the time to gather firsthand information about a new customer:

■Visit the company's place of business. Does it look like a reputable and aboveboard operation? Does the company produce a quality product?

■Use a Uniform Commercial Code (UCC) search to uncover creditor or tax liens filed against the company. How: File for such a search at the office of the local secretary of state. Cost: Between $2 and $10 in most states.

■Obtain credit reports on the customer's or supplier's top officers. Key question: Have the officers recently transferred personal property to other family members?

■Examine the company's financial statements. If they have not been audited or reviewed by an independent certified public accountant, be cautious.

■Obtain credit information about each company separately, if the customer or supplier does business through more than one corporation.

Danger signal: The company's lawyer is one who is known for bankruptcy work.

Ask the accountants:

■Does the company pay its payroll taxes on time? Significance: Late payments often indicate that the company uses the tax money to meet operating expenses.

■Are payments to a company pension or profit-sharing plan up-to-date? Importance: These are corporate tax shelters that are more likely to be used by a healthy business.

When these queries raise doubts about a potential customer's or supplier's financial status, and that company's business is sound, it will offer a debt guarantee. If not, the company probably doesn't deserve further credit.

Other ways to guard against credit risks:

■Ask for a lien on the customer's inventory.

■Ask for the company owner's personal guarantee.

When a company that owes your company money seems like a candidate for bankruptcy, immediately demand payment on the debt. Threaten a lawsuit. Point: The customer or supplier will not want its other creditors to find out about its shaky financial situation. It may pay just to avoid the suit.

Rule for this situation: The first to sue is the first in line to be paid. The rest may get nothing. Reason: After the first creditor is paid, there may be no money left for any other creditors.

Source: Edward Mendlowitz, partner, Mendlowitz Weitsen, CPAs, New York.

Checks Marked "Payment In Full"

If there's no dispute as to the amount, a check tendered for less than the amount due and marked "payment in full" (or the like) may be cashed without prejudicing the right to recover the balance.

If there's a bona fide dispute as to the amount owing, the creditor must be wary. Alternatives: Reject the check and demand full payment. Or: Accept the check but run the risk that payment will be deemed to have settled the disputed claim for the lesser amount. It's easy enough for a debtor who wants to pay less than the amount for which he's billed to create a dispute on the basis of quantitative or qualitative deficiencies in the goods or services supplied.

Stamp the check with a statement to the effect that "Check is accepted without prejudice and with full reservation of all rights under Section 1-207 of the Uniform Commercial Code." The effectiveness of this technique is untested in the courts, but it may help protect a creditor's rights and provide leverage in a settlement.

Spotting False Credit Cards

1. Compare the signature on the back of the credit card with that on the driver's license and sales slip. 2. Hold the card up to the light to see if the area around the name and numbers is dull or scratched. Some thieves iron over the original name and numbers to repunch them. 3. Check the card's corners. Counterfeit cards are usually cut with a paper cutter and have square corners or rough edges.

Source: *Check & Credit Card Fraud Prevention Manual* by Robert Cekosky, Publishers Services, 6318 Vesper Ave., Van Nuys, CA 91411.

Why You Should Avoid Acknowledging A Debt

Acknowledgement of a debt extends the legal time period in which the creditor can collect it. Case: In the course of his practice, a lawyer incurred a debt to a doctor. Two years later he acknowledged the debt in a letter. Two years after that the doctor sued to collect. But the lawyer said that the three-year statute of limitations had run out. Court: The lawyer's letter restarted the three-year time limit. So the doctor could press his case.

Source: *Heffelfinger v. Gibson,* 290 A2d 390.

Ways To Show A Credit Bureau Your Company Deserves A Higher Rating

It's not necessary to live with a poor credit rating. Steps may be taken to convince the rating services that your firm deserves an upgrading.

The key is to be aggressive. Tell your story to the services if you believe it has merit. Many of the rating categories overlap—especially in the middle ranges. Thus, your company may easily fit into a higher range than the one it has been assigned. The intangibles, the reasons behind the ratios, make the difference. It's important that you put these factors—quality of management and long-range planning—into the best perspective.

What to do: Keep in touch with the rating services. Make regular presentations using top executives (including the boss). Emphasize how the firm is positioning itself for the future. Explain why store assets may not appear on balance sheets. Help the rating services to know and understand the business. Point out special advantages, such as able leadership and tight cost control program.

Additional pointer: Present future plans as realistic projections. Plot alternatives; discuss management depth, market leadership, and how the firm has taken advantage of its position (if not a leader, can it react quickly to changes).

Hold a practice session to throw unanticipated questions at executives. (Ask your investment banker for help here.) Evasiveness or lack of preparation can hurt you. Also a drawback: Gimmicky accounting techniques. Expect queries about how you're preparing to react to current trends and future economic problems.

Note: The services pride themselves on consistency. If you can show that your ratios compare well with those in the next higher category, you might get a boost. Or, if you're about to be downgraded, stress that your ratios have held steady or are moving up.

The communication shouldn't be one-way. Ask the services for feedback. You may discover that by making a few changes, you can move to a higher category.

Source: *Institutional Investor,* 488 Madison Ave., New York.

Chapter 15
Collections

When Should Overdue Bills Go To A Collection Agency?

Focus on collecting past-due accounts within the first 90 days. After that time, in-house collection efforts are almost totally ineffective. It's usually more productive then to turn over unpaid accounts to a collection agency, even though the creditor ends up with an average of only $10 back from each original $100 debt. Pay the agency a fixed fee rather than on a percentage basis to discourage it from pursuing only the largest and easiest accounts.

Source: Richard D. Schultz, National Revenue Corp., *Financial Executive*, New York.

How To Find The Best Collection Agency

As receivables lag, the pressure to turn past-due accounts over to a collection agency grows. Make sure the agency is equipped to handle the job. Key questions to ask:

■Do you specialize in accounts of a certain size? There is a clear difference in the ways that accounts of different sizes are handled.

■What is your collection record? A 75% success ratio is excellent; 50%–75% is average. Ask for an audited report of the collection record. Keep expectations realistic. Do not expect miracles with the company's worst deadbeat accounts.

■May I observe your operation? Spend several hours watching and listening to agents work on the phone. Judge their persuasive abilities. Abrasive or threatening techniques can reflect badly on the firm or open it to harassment charges.

Fees: Expect to pay 20%–40% of the amounts collected. The agency should provide monthly reports on its progress. Additional charges are likely for more frequent or detailed reports, personal visits by agents, skip-tracing (following a debtor who leaves town).

References: Ask for five. Almost any firm can come up with three satisfied customers, the number usually asked for.

To protect your company, put a cancellation clause in the contract. And the agency should have hold-harmless insurance, which protects the company from harassment suits that can arise.

If the company has numerous small debts that are difficult to collect, it may be desirable to buy a collection agency series of dunning letters. Cost: $2–$5 per letter in a four- to six-letter series. Caution: The agency will not follow up.

Shrewd tactic: Create the company's own dunning letters, using a dummy company letterhead that seems like a collection agency's. Use legal-sounding language, with words such as heretofore, notwithstanding, etc. Red flag: It is illegal to display the dummy agency name anywhere on the envelope.

Source: Horace Klafter, lecturer on collection techniques for the Business and Professional Research Institute, Westport, CT.

Getting More Out Of Collection Agents

Some corporate managers instruct their accounts payable departments not to pay bills until they hear from suppliers' collection agents. That buys time because small suppliers can't afford to pay these agents the 28%–50% commission for collecting until it's the last resort. As a result, those suppliers find their cash flow positions seriously undermined. A solution is to find an agent willing to collect accounts on a routine basis for a fixed fee, rather than for a percentage of the bills that they collect. Under this arrangement, the company routinely forwards data on accounts as they become 60 days overdue. The client invests a low fee for a block of the collection agent's services, then keeps 100% of the payments. The company thus pays less for the service, but still impresses its customers with a strict payment policy. And using the service allows the company to use its best inside collectors to concentrate on key accounts.

The collection agent must offer the full range of dunning techniques, give reasonable guarantees, and agree to protect the credit-grantor's goodwill. Without such precautions, some agents might write letters that make the problem worse or alienate future business.

Source: David Allburn, vice-president, National Revenue Corp., Columbus, OH.

Collection Methods That Work

Make calls early in the week. Customers who promise on Friday to pay on Monday often "forget" over the weekend.

Be persistent. If customers are out, leave a name and number and request a return call. Ask when they are expected, then call back again, and again. When writing a letter for payment, tell customers these messages have gone unanswered.

Encourage the debtors to commit for a partial payment. Then use that amount to arrange a payment schedule.

When customers agree to pay, send a letter formalizing that agreement.

If a letter threatening use of a collection agency or legal action is sent, don't follow up immediately. Silence makes customers edgy. They will call.

After setting a deadline for payment, stick to it.

Source: Wayne A. Dugger, senior credit representative, Union Carbide Corp., New York.

The Embarrassing-Pause Trick

Identify your company and say that the purpose of the call is to ask about the overdue account. Pause, and say nothing further, no matter how long it takes. Usually it won't take long for the embarrassed debtor to start apologizing and promising to pay. The caller should then insist on a date (it should be one in the immediate future) by which the check will be mailed.

Collections Game

With the economy slowing and bankruptcies increasing, it's especially important now to take a close look at the company's system for collecting from slow-paying accounts.

Too often, the collection system is an improvised process in which no one is really responsible and there are no written policy guidelines...that's a big mistake.

Delinquency in paying bills almost always signals the beginning of a customer's financial difficulties. Picture the accounts payable clerk sitting at a desk with a six-inch pile of payables and a one-inch pile of cash.

Challenge: Getting your company's invoices to the top of the payables pile.

Solution: Make a lot of constructive noise. The company that gets paid earliest is the company that shows the greatest determination to be paid. Customers respect companies that are serious about collecting what is owed them.

Develop A System

Since nobody likes to make dunning calls, it won't happen unless someone is made responsible and given specific guidelines and procedures on how to do it. Formulate a clearcut policy on payments that the credit department, the CEO and the sales department can all agree on.

Example: 30 days after the original statement goes out, if payment has not been received, send another statement, with a firm but polite letter expressing how much the company would appreciate payment on the past due amount.

After 60 days, start telephoning. Important: When phoning, try to set up an appointment with a person responsible for authorizing cash payments, to work out a schedule to pay the outstanding bill. Key: After 60 days, it's clear that the customer will have difficulty paying the bill in full. Often, customers can pay if the vendor allows them time to pay in installments.

If that doesn't work, wait no longer than 30 more days before bringing in a third party—a collection agency. After that long, a letter or a call from a collection agency gets more attention than another bill on your company's letterhead.

Mistake: Waiting too long before bringing in professional help. A recent study by the Commercial Law League of America demonstrated how receivables become less and less collectible the longer they age.

Three months past due...73.6% are collectible.

Six months past due...57.8% are collectible.

Twelve months past due...26.6% are collectible.

Recognize that a customer who normally pays promptly but is now delinquent faces some financial difficulty. Chances are that the condition will get worse before it gets better. Your technique should be to move in fast and collect before all available cash goes to pay other creditors and before the situation deteriorates into bankruptcy.

Why Companies Hesitate

The reasons most companies hesitate to use a collection agency are cost and fear of alienating customers. Most collection agencies charge fees that can range as high as 25% to 50% of the balances they collect. Often such high fees are reasonable because the collection agencies are given only the toughest, most delinquent accounts. The trail may have grown cold and/or the customer's financial condition deteriorated to the point where collection becomes extremely difficult...and costly.

That's why it often pays to bring in an agency early when it can do a better job for its clients—and do it at much lower cost.

Our average fee, for example, is as low as 2% of the total amount owed...because we generally start our work no later than 90 days after the initial statement was mailed. Our success rate in collecting is therefore quite high.

Fear Factor

Companies—and especially their salespeople—worry much too much about offending customers when they have a collection agency push for payment. But, when they have received five or six progressively more pointed statements and phone calls from the company, delinquent customers can hardly be too surprised to hear from a collection agency.

Professional collections people today understand the need for sensitivity in dealing with valued customers. They're not nearly as heavy-handed as they used to be. For one thing, the Federal Fair Debt Collection Practices Act, passed by Congress in 1978, outlawed abusive practices in collecting from consumers. The law doesn't apply to business collections, but the tenor of the industry is considerably more sophisticated than it was in the past. To find the right agency...

■Ask managers in other companies for names of agencies.

■Call the American Commercial Collectors Association, a trade organization of agencies, for the names of agencies in your area. (The ACCA also publishes a useful booklet about collecting, *Collection Guidelines*.)

■Ask the local Chamber of Commerce for several names, and interview them and companies they've worked for.

Source: Lou Bishop, president, Parson Bishop Services, Inc., 7870 Camargo Rd., Cincinnati 45243. He got into the collections business after running an auto rental service that had a number of slow-paying corporate customers.

Smart Collection Tactic

When a customer who suddenly has trouble paying bills offers to pay part of the outstanding balance, decline the initial offer. Reason: The customer's first offer is usually not his best. Better...say, *I wish I could accept your offer, but the company won't allow it.* When the customer then asks what you will accept, ask for at least three-quarters of the full amount and the balance with a post-dated check. If that is not possible, gradually loosen the demands. But let the customer struggle until you feel you've gotten all you can.

Source: *The Check Is Not in the Mail* by Leonard Sklar, Baroque Publishing, 4 West Fourth Ave., San Mateo, CA 94402.

Make Debtors Pay Collection Fees

Credit applications should contain an agreement by the debtor to pay reasonable attorney's fees for collection, in case of default. (Without an agreement signed by the debtor, collection fees usually can't be recovered.) That should be clearly spelled out in the agreement, in the same print as the rest of the application. Put it right before the signature line, so the debtor can't claim he didn't know what he was signing at the time.

Source: Theodore P. Sobo, Sobo, Wellens & Balocco, lawyers, 7500 NW Fifth St., Fort Lauderdale, FL 33317.

Delaying-Payment Ploys That Hurt Suppliers

Retailers, including some of the most prestigious in the country, are being harsh with suppliers to delay paying them. The most severely affected are vendors so dependent on the retailers that they cannot fight back. A common example is the lost-invoice or lost-proof-of-delivery-document game. One of the biggest and most prestigious retailers kept it up for six months with a particular company.

The cancellation-and-delay play is even tougher. The retailer places an order, then asks for partial shipments, delaying the balance, often more than once. At the end, it may cancel the unshipped portion. The supplier has to finance the undelivered part of the order for months, and then perhaps absorb a loss at closeout.

The suppliers' defense is to tighten operations. Be prepared to reduce sales to major retail customers. Or accept the retailers' terms and be squeezed.

Source: Malcolm Moses, financial consultant, Merrick, NY.

Words That Produce Faster Payment

Calculate the true discount for prompt payment as an annualized rate of interest. This may be all that's needed to remind a customer of the substantial advantage of paying within 10 days.

Instead of marking the invoice with the standardized code (such as 2%/10 days, 30 net), translate the savings into plain English. Sample: This is our offer of 36%

interest. That's the true annual interest rate in the 2%/10 days, 30 net discount this invoice offers you, if you pay 10 days from now.

Other quick payment offers translated into annualized interest rates:

■2%/10 days, net 90 days, equals 12% annual interest.

■3%/10 days, net 60 days, is 22% annual interest.

■1%/10days, net 30 days, is 18% annual interest.

If the bill isn't paid promptly, send a photocopy a week later marked: Your discount period ends tomorrow.

Source: *Sell More and Spend Less* by T. Martin and B. Trabue, Holt Rinehart & Winston.

Writing Good Collection Letters

Effective collection letters are polite, straightforward and concise. Ideas that might apply to your company's particular situation:

■Always include the date, debtor's name and address, a description of the merchandise involved, the amount due and a self-addressed reply envelope.

■Address letters to a named individual. Don't address the Accounts Payable Department or some other anonymous entity.

■If the goods were shipped in response to an oral or telephone order, don't mention this in the letter. It may tempt the debtor to deny that the order was placed.

■Appeal to the customer's reputation, sense of fair play, self-interest or fear of legal problems. Escalate these appeals as the collection series progresses. (Avoid form letters late in series.)

■Send the letters in close sequence. Keep the debtor's attention with changes in letter format.

■Successive letters should be signed by executives of increasing rank (assistant collection manager, manager, president). Intersperse with telegrams or phone calls.

■Use certified mail, return receipt requested.

■Encourage the debtor to respond, even if he can't pay in full.

■Imprint envelopes with "address correction requested" so the post office will supply a forwarding address if the debtor has moved.

■Maintain intensity of the collection effort. If the debtor has several creditors, chances are the most insistent will be paid first.

Source: *Credit and Collection: A Practical Guide* by Rick Stephan Hayes, CBI Publishing Co., Boston.

Using The Phone To Boost Bill Collection

Super-tough telephone collections, never pleasant, can be more effective than letters—if properly planned.

How one company does it: Person-to-person call to the individual responsible for paying bills. The caller gives own name only, not company's. (Frequently, he gets through to the right person where an ordinary collection call would not.) He insists on finalizing the terms of payment during the phone call and follows up immediately with a letter "confirming" arrangement. This approach is limited to cases where cost of call doesn't exceed 1% of overdue amount.

If the debtor keeps ducking call, the caller leaves a full message—reason for call, amount owed and for how long, all other facts—no matter who's on the other end of the line. The "message" usually embarrasses debtor into paying, calling back, or accepting future call to work out terms of payment.

This is a high-pressure tactic. Misused, it can raise legal problems if caller isn't careful. Callers should be briefed in advance to avoid personal slurs on debtor, any other statements that could lead to legal liability. It's a good idea to check with attorney and work out a standard "script."

When The Check Is "In The Mail"

Follow up with a telegram saying, "Thorough search shows no record of payment. Stop payment on previous check and send new check for $_____ at once."

Chapter 16
Cash Flow Management

Six Ways To Improve Cash Flow

■Prevent bookkeeping from following the comfortable routine of paying all suppliers on one day.

■Negotiate with suppliers for an installment-payment plan.

■Send stamped, self-addressed envelopes with customers' bills.

■Be sure cash is invested quickly in a money-market fund rather than left sitting in a checking account.

■Take precautions against check bouncing. Common ploys are no date, the figure amount varies from the written amount, no signature.

Copier forgeries of checks are a growing problem. They can be recognized by no indentations on the back from writing or typing.

Source: *The Sales Executive*, New York.

How To Increase Cash Availability

For most companies, accelerating receipts to make cash available quickly may be far more important financially than earning the maximum interest on a disbursement float. The challenge is to get all checks and payments processed and consolidated as soon as possible in the company's main bank account.

The first order of business is to sensitize employees to know the difference between big or important checks requiring special treatment and routine receipts. All checks represent cash and should be taken care of promptly.

Rather than holding checks received after 3 P.M. until the next morning, for example, it may be worth keeping employees overtime or hiring extra help to get checks deposited that day. Also, if mail arrives as early as 7 A.M. and the office staff doesn't normally arrive until 9 A.M., it might be smart to add an early shift. Getting checks to the bank by 8:30 A.M. instead of in the afternoon may save a day.

Become familiar with the bank's clearing procedures and work around those schedules. (It is valuable information to know that the bank has a 9 P.M. clearing or a late Friday pickup.) Never let receipts lie around when they could be deposited and earning interest or defraying expenses. Most banks will accommodate a company's needs once they have been communicated.

For distant customers, bypass the postal system altogether and ask the customer to deposit funds directly into a local bank, preferably one that has a relationship with the company's main hometown bank. Then the funds can be wired directly bank-to-bank with maximum speed.

Plan ahead for special or very large receipts expected from, say, the sale of a piece of property. Alert mailroom employees and leave instructions that the manager should be notified immediately on receipt of this or any unusually large check.

Even if solid check-handling procedures are supposed to be in effect, make sure they are actually working.

Source: John Carroll, partner, Peat, KPMG Peat Marwick, New York.

How To Deposit An Unsigned Check

Write or type the word "over" on the line where the signature would normally appear. On the back, type *lack of signature guaranteed*...and add your company's name, and your name and title. Then sign. This guarantees your bank that you'll take back the check as a charge against your account if it isn't honored. Most banks will then process the check and remit the funds. This saves you the trouble of returning the check to your customer for signature.

Source: *Credit & Financial Management*, 475 Park Ave. S., New York 10016.

Spotting Fake Checks

Fake checks can often be spotted by the first two digits of the account number printed on the bottom left of the check. That's the Federal Reserve Bank code for the state in which the bank named on the check is located. Forgers often use an incorrect code to slow down processing of the check. Example: A criminal prints phony checks for a New Jersey bank and uses a code from Wyoming. That way it takes twice as long for the check to reach the bank and gives the crook extra time to cover his tracks. Code lists are available from any Federal Reserve Bank.

Source: *Security Management*, 1655 N. Fort Myer Dr., Arlington, VA 22209.

Spotting Bad Checks

■Accept only checks with the correct local Federal Reserve number printed in small numbers in the upper right-hand corner. Example: The New York area number is 1-xx/210. (The xx digits vary by bank.) Counterfeiters rarely print the correct number.

■Comparing signatures to detect bad checks. Slants, *i*'s and *e*'s are almost always the same in signatures by the same person. Instruct clerks to ask customers to write their name again and compare these three features if in doubt.

■About 90% of cleared bad checks are numbered 101 to 150, indicating a new account. Spotting forged checks. Legitimate checks have at least one perforated edge. Most forgeries are cutouts. Another difference: Hold a suspicious check up to the light. If the print is shiny, the check is a forgery.

Source: *Lincoln Sees v. Morgan Guarantee Trust Co.*, 8 UCC Rep. 215.

Checks And The Law

■Stale checks. A bank need not pay a check that is more than six months old. Exceptions are certified checks which must be paid at any time. Note that a bank can pay a check that is more than six months old, but it must exercise due care to be sure that the check is still good.

Source: *Advanced Alloys vs Sergeant Steel Corp.*, 12 UCC Rep 1173, 360 NYS2d 142.

■The statute of limitations on a demand note begins to run on the date the note is due. If the limitation period runs out under local law, the holder of the note cannot collect. For example, a note payable 30 days after demand for payment was made on or after September 20, 1967. The statute of limitations provided for by local law was six years. So the holder of the note could not collect on it in 1974.

Source: *Environics, Inc., vs Pratt*, 18 UCC Rep. 143, 376 NYS 2d 510.

■Letters or telegrams may serve as checks. To serve as a check the letter must be addressed to a bank. And it must state that a specific amount is to be paid on demand either to the bearer of the letter or to the order of a named person. If any one of these requirements is not met, the letter will not be valid as a check. And, of course, the bank will make its usual effort to verify that the "check" is valid.

Source: *United Milk Prods. Co. vs Lawndale Nat'l. Bank*, 392 F. 2d 876, 5 UCC Rep. 143.

■Words control figures. When the words and the numbers on a check disagree, the words determine how much the check is worth.

Source: Uniform Commercial Code Sec. 3-118(c).

Chapter 17
Special Tax-Cutting Strategies

Tax Tactics To Increase Cash Flow

Tough-minded managers who focus on tighter financial controls to loosen up the flow of company cash often overlook one area: tax payments. These, too, can be managed to ease the cash pinch.

It is possible to underpay legally. Make payments that total less than the current year's tax liability. In a good year, base payments on the prior year's earnings. This can be done by small corporations (less than $1 million of income) if tax was owed for the prior year. In a bad year, base them on the current year's expected earnings. The company is safe if by the end of the year it has made estimated payments totaling 90% of its actual tax liability.

In a year that starts slowly, base payments on actual quarterly earnings. The result will be small payments at the beginning of the year, and larger payments later in the year when money is coming in.

If the company had taxable income of $1 million in any one of the prior three years, it must make estimated payments totaling at least 97% of the current year's actual tax liability. Companies that fall into this category and are currently basing their estimated payments on last year's earnings must be careful if last year's earnings were exceptionally bad.

Request a quick refund of overpaid estimated taxes. File Form 4466 before filing the firm's tax return. The Internal Revenue Service will refund the excess payments within 45 days.

Another opportunity is to pay taxes on the exact due date. Keep the money in an interest-bearing account until then. If the company invests in commercial paper or Treasury bills, time maturity dates to coincide with the dates tax payments come due.

State and local governments are often slow to cash company checks. Delays of three weeks are not uncommon. So pay taxes with checks drawn on a money-market fund. The money in the fund will continue to earn high interest until the check is cashed.

And the company should withhold at the lowest possible rate for executive bonuses. This may be as low as 20%. If near the end of the year it appears that the withholding has been insufficient to avoid a penalty, the executive may give the company a check for the amount of the shortage. This counts as withholding for the full year. In the meantime, the executive has had use of the money.

Examine the company's accounting methods, and make use of the more beneficial option. Service companies usually have an option to report income on either the cash or accrual basis. The advantage of using the cash basis is that accounts receivable that are outstanding at the end of the year are not included in the company's income.

Manufacturing firms should strongly consider adopting the LIFO (last-in, first-out) accounting method. LIFO will almost certainly cut the taxable income of a firm that holds inventories during an inflationary period.

Also keep tabs on payments to employee benefit plans:
■Medical plans. Form a trust to pay the premiums. Make payments to the trust a year in advance. That way, the company gets a deduction now for premiums that will actually be paid a year from now. And in the meantime, money in the trust earns tax-free interest that can be used to pay part of the premium cost, thus cutting the real cost to the company. The combination may yield more to the company than having the use of the money for that period of time.
■Pension plans. If the company does not have enough cash on hand to make a pension plan contribution, borrow it. Interest paid on the borrowed amount is deductible by the company. And the funds put in the plan earn interest tax-free until it is distributed. This can be a great advantage to company owners who are major beneficiaries of the plan.
Source: Daniel J. O'Kane, vice-president and financial administrator, MMT Sales, Inc., Edward Mendlowitz, partner, Mendlowitz Weitsen, CPAs, New York.

Paying The Least Possible Estimated Taxes

Many people, especially those who get large windfalls during the year, become concerned about paying sufficient estimated tax. Such people are unaware that there's an ironclad exemption from paying full estimated taxes on the windfall if the amount of withholding tax or regular quarterly estimated tax payments is equal to or greater than the previous year's total federal income tax, including self-employment tax. This exemption does not apply if your Adjusted Gross Income is more than $75,000, increased by more than $40,000 over the previous year, and you paid estimated taxes in any of the three previous years. If these conditions apply, your estimated payments must equal 90% of the current year's tax liability.

If you find that you've underestimated your quarterly payments or underwithheld your taxes, give your employer a check to cover the underpayment before the end of the year. This amount will be added by your employer to your withholding and will appear on your W–2. In this way, you'll avoid the IRS's penalty for underpayment of taxes.
Source: *New Tax Traps/New Opportunities* by Edward Mendlowitz, Boardroom Special Report, Springfield, NJ 07081.

Tax Planning That Boosts Cash Flow

Thoughtful tax planning boosts the company's cash flow by reducing taxes and/or deferring the time when tax payments are due.

Estimated Taxes

Estimated taxes affect the cash flow of all profitable businesses. And, the Deficit Reduction Act increases the cost of underpaying estimated taxes by adding an extra two percentage points to the IRS interest rate that applies to underpayments (the normal IRS interest rate is set quarterly).

Small corporations generally must pay 93% of their final tax bill for the year through equal quarterly estimated tax payments (25% of the final tax bill each quarter). However, there are ways to reduce the size of quarterly payments and defer the tax bill.

"Small" businesses (those which have not had more than $1 million of taxable income in any one of the last three years) can base estimated payments on the previous year's tax liability. Thus, each quarterly payment need be no larger than 25% of the prior year's final tax bill, even if this year's bill will be much larger.

Catch: Payments can be based on the prior year's tax bill only if the company owed some tax for the prior year. If no tax was owed, estimated payments must total 93% of the current year's tax bill.

Strategy: A company that sees it may owe no tax for the current year should consider taking steps to generate a small tax bill just before the current year's end to slash the following year's estimated tax liability.

Example: The company could sell a piece of equipment for which an investment credit was claimed in an earlier year, and thus incur a small recapture tax on part of the credit's value.

The few dollars of tax incurred right away by the company could produce big-dollar deferrals of estimated payments the following year.

Benefit From Slow Season

A company which expects to derive most of its income during the last half of the year may defer a large portion of its estimated tax obligations by reporting income on an annualized basis.

Under this method, the company takes income-to-date at the end of each quarter, projects a year-end tax bill on the basis of income coming in at the same rate for the rest of the year, and computes estimated taxes accordingly.

Result: Tax payments due for the early, low-income quarters in the year are reduced.

This method is particularly valuable for growing businesses, seasonal businesses which earn most of their income near year-end (such as many retailers), and firms which expect management changes or improving markets to have a positive financial impact near year-end.

Annualizing income provides an extra benefit by allowing flexibility in choosing the period on which annualized income may be based…

■The second quarter's payment may be based on income received during the first three or five months of the year.

■The third quarter payment may be based on the first six or eight months.

■The fourth quarter payment may be based on the first nine or 11 months.

Tactic: A company which receives most of its income during one part of the year and wishes to minimize the cost of estimated taxes may adopt a fiscal year that ends just after the busy season. For example, many retailers have fiscal years ending on January 31, just after the Christmas shopping season.

The Uniform Capitalization Trap

New opportunities for cutting the cost of Tax Reform's uniform capitalization (unicap) rules are the hot tax topic of the moment.

Background: Tax Reform required that inventory-related overhead costs of manufacturers, wholesalers and retailers be capitalized (added to the value of inventory) rather than deducted immediately. Such costs include storage rent, insurance, repairs, maintenance, utilities, a portion of salaries and other items related to storage of inventories. The bottom-line impact is that the deductions for these items are deferred—they can *not* be deducted until the inventory items are sold…so the current tax bill is increased.

Snag: While Tax Reform required companies to adopt unicap rules on their 1987 tax returns, the IRS did not provide guidelines as to how the new rules were to be applied. Companies were left on their own to figure out the complicated new rules.

Unicap Problems And Opportunities

The IRS has issued a series of announcements which companies can use to simplify unicap accounting and reduce their tax bills.

Problem: Many companies are not in compliance with the new IRS procedures. They set up their accounting methods before the more favorable procedures were announced by the IRS.

Opportunity: By coming into compliance with the new procedures, many companies may simplify their accounting methods and regain large deductions which previously were lost.

Unicap should be seriously looked into by...

■Manufacturers with large amounts of raw materials in inventory.

■Companies with temporarily idled property, plants or equipment.

■Retailers with handling costs at facilities where goods are sold on site.

■Wholesalers and retailers with repackaging costs.

■Companies using LIFO (last-in, first out) accounting and electing LIFO's simplified capitalization method.

We recommend that all companies using unicap accounting review their current accounting procedures...almost all will find tax-saving opportunities.

Unicap accounting procedures can be extremely complex, however, so be sure to consult with a capital cost accounting specialist.

More Cash Flow Boosters

Accounting methods can have a major impact on the company's cash flow...

■Cash-basis accounting provides greater flexibility than accrual-basis accounting. An accrual-basis firm must report income when it is earned (for example, when goods are shipped) whether or not it has received payment. Similarly, it must deduct expenses when they become due, regardless of whether they have been paid. Cash-basis firms, however, report income and expenditures only as cash is exchanged, giving them greater leeway to time income and deduction items by accelerating or delaying payments and billings.

Caution: Not all firms qualify to use cash-basis accounting, so consult a tax adviser for details.

■LIFO (last-in, first-out) accounting can generate a large tax deferral for an indefinite period of time when both inventory costs and inventory levels are rising. LIFO accounting treats the last, and most expensive, item added to inventory as the first one sold, thus increasing the company's deduction for cost of goods sold.

Still More Ideas

■Real estate. A company about to take a large gain on the sale of real estate may be able to postpone the tax due indefinitely by trading the property in a like-kind exchange, instead of selling it for cash. Requirements: Within 45 days of disposing of the old property, the company must designate a specific replacement property to be received. And it must actually take possession of the replacement property within 180 days.

If the company can't find another firm with which it wants to make a straight swap of properties, a commercial real estate broker may be able to arrange a three-way exchange or other multi-party transaction.

At the future date when the company finally wants to dispose of the replacement property, it may be able to defer tax again with another like-kind exchange.

■Bonus payments. The salary base subject to the Medicare portion of Social Security taxes is $135,000 in 1993. This tax is imposed at a 1.45% rate on both the employer and the employee. Result: An extra 2.9% of tax is imposed on income earned in this range.

■Depreciation. Companies should time the acquisition of depreciable equipment for the best tax impact. Normally, a "mid-year convention" applies so that the company gets a half-year's worth of depreciation deductions for new equipment no matter when it is placed in service during the year. This can be costly for property acquired at the beginning of the year, and favorable for property acquired toward year-end.

If more than 40% of all property is placed in service during the last three months of the year, a mid-quarter convention applies—depreciation deductions are allowed from the middle of the quarter in which property is placed in service.

The company's tax adviser should consider how tax benefits will be affected by the simple timing of equipment acquisitions, and plan accordingly.

Source: David W. Jessen, partner and director of entrepreneurial services, Ernst & Young, 3600 Glenwood Ave., Raleigh, NC 27612.

The Best Way To Cut Taxes Is To Plan Ahead

Now is the time to review the company's tax strategies for the coming year. Make sure the company is poised to take advantage of every recent change in the tax law.

The greatest change in the new tax law for business is the reform of depreciation rules. Under the new Accelerated Cost Recovery System (ACRS), first-year deductions are larger than ever before.

Timing is the key to best utilizing the ACRS rules. Deductions are worth more when the company is in a high tax bracket. And the first-year deductions must be taken in the year the equipment is placed in service (regardless of when it was acquired). If the company is in:

■Top tax bracket. Be sure the equipment is in service before year-end. That way the company can reduce estimated tax payments now in anticipation of its lower final tax bill. So it gets year-round cash-flow relief.

■Low tax bracket, but expecting to be in a high bracket next year. The company may benefit by not putting new equipment into service until after year-end. The first-year deductions can then be saved to shelter income that would be taxed at a higher rate.

■No tax is owed this year, but heavy taxes were paid in past years. Consider putting the equipment in service just before year-end. Then use the related tax benefits to file for a quick refund of prior years' taxes (file Form 1139). The refund may more than cover the down payment on the equipment.

Commercial real estate is a special case. ACRS rules allow it to be depreciated over 18 years, with larger deductions in the early years. But if commercial real estate is sold before the 18-year period is up, all the previously taken deductions are recaptured and taxed back to the company in one year at top rates. If there is a possibility the building will be sold in less than 18 years, consider electing the alternative straight-line depreciation method authorized under the ACRS. Deductions will be smaller in the early years. But there will be no recapture on the building's resale.

If expansion is on the horizon, be aware of a recent Supreme Court decision that enables growing companies to cut their tax bills. Instead of expanding the business through the formation of a new operating division, form a new corporation. The old owners retain all the stock of the original corporation, but transfer more than 20% of the stock of the new company to a third party (such as a key executive or outside investor). The two companies are taxed as independent enterprises. Each is taxed initially at the lowest (15%) tax bracket. (Under the old law, their incomes were added together. So the totaled amount could reach into higher brackets.)

At the same time, review qualified retirement-plan programs in light of the heavy cash contributions the company might be required to make to the plan. Two possible situations:

■If the company is suffering a poor business year, it may be able to obtain a waiver of its retirement-plan contributions. Required: The company must show that it is facing genuine financial hardship and that the waiver saving will help the company through its difficulties, so that the employees will benefit from the waiver over the long run.

■If there are excess assets in the plan that are not required to fund plan liabilities, the company may be able to terminate the plan and recover the excess assets. One major corporation is currently recouping $200 million by replacing its defined benefit pension plan with a profit-sharing plan, the contributions to which will depend on company profitability. Caution: Plan termination is a very complicated procedure. Be sure to discuss it with the company's advisers before deciding to act.

Also be aware that many companies that now charge off bad debts on a current basis should adopt the reserve method of doing so. Under normal rules, a company can claim a bad-debt deduction only after it has evidence that a specific debt is uncollectible. But under the reserve method, the company can claim a deduction for the percentage of its accounts that it expects will go bad. So it gets the deduction in advance. If company sales consistently grow, it will be able to claim further deductions for additions to its bad-debt reserve each year.

The company should operate with the tax or fiscal year that yields the most benefits. Typically, the year should end during the middle of the business's slow season. This way executives have more time for end-of-the-year bookkeeping and beginning-of-the-year planning. The company's outside tax advisers may be more readily available as well, since they will not be called on during their busy season.

It is now possible for some companies to change their tax year without IRS permission. The company should consult with its tax advisers about this.

Source: Irving Blackman, partner, Blackman Kallick Bartelstein, *The Book of Tax Knowledge*, Boardroom Books, Springfield, NJ 07081.

Choosing The Best Tax Year

Every business has the option of reporting its income on the basis of either a fiscal or a calendar year.

A fiscal year, which ends on the last day of any month other than December, is best suited for a seasonal business. Its advantages include the reduced cost of taking inventory because of lowered stocks, and the ease in comparing the operating results of successive seasons. In addition, more time is available to attend to tax and accounting matters because of the low level of business activity, and tax advisers are able to give more attention to quarterly returns.

A calendar year makes sense for a firm with a steady stream of business. It simplifies bookkeeping by corresponding with employment tax periods, which always follow the calendar year. As a result, there are fewer calculations to make at year-end.

A firm cannot change its tax year without permission from the Internal Revenue Service. Permission is normally granted if the firm can demonstrate a valid business reason for the change, and if the change won't distort income to provide a significant tax break.

How To Cut Payroll Taxes

Federal, state, and local payroll taxes, covering the costs of Social Security, unemployment insurance, and disability payments often exceed 20% of the company's total payroll cost before voluntary company benefits are counted in. And these costs are scheduled to rise in future years. There are strategies that can be used to cut this growing tax burden.

Federal payroll taxes are imposed on the wages of employees. So the company may be able to cut its federal tax bill by using workers who qualify as independent contractors instead of employees. This usually cuts the state payroll tax bill as well (though rules vary from state to state). The company does not have to withhold income tax on amounts paid to contractors, so tax and administrative costs are saved.

Candidates for contractor status include salespeople, executives who establish themselves as consultants, car and truck drivers, those with talents qualifying them for special tasks (such as artists and computer programmers). Whether or not a worker qualifies as an independent contractor depends on the facts of each case. That status is supported when workers:

■Are trusted to do the job without close company supervision.

■Provide their own work equipment instead of having the equipment supplied by the company.

■Are paid on a per-job basis instead of a time basis.

■Hire their own assistants.

■Are free to perform similar work for other companies.

■Can perform work off the company's premises.

No single one of these factors determines the worker's status. All the circumstances must be considered. For example, workers who perform on the company premises under close supervision may still be contractors if they perform similar work for other companies.

Drawbacks of using independent contractors:

■These workers usually are not covered by workers compensation insurance. If an accident happens and a contractor is injured on the job, he can sue the company for more than the standard workers compensation award.

■If the IRS determines that workers treated as contractors are really employees, the company may become retroactively liable for employment taxes and penalties.

Be sure to review the company's position with a tax expert.

Another area to examine is whether the business is run through a number of affiliated corporations. When the corporations share employees, they can fall into a tax trap: each pays the employees for services rendered to it, so payroll taxes are duplicated. And while employees can file for a refund of overpaid taxes, the company can never get its excess payroll tax payments returned to it.

Consider having one corporation handle the payroll for all the companies in the group. This will allow for flexibility:

■The paymaster can pay all or some of the group's employees.

■It can pay each employee with one check or issue different checks on behalf of the different companies, whichever method best facilitates the company's book-keeping.

■A separate company can be set up to serve solely as paymaster, or there can be more than one paymaster.

The only requirement is that each employee paid by the common paymaster must work for more than one corporation.

Also consider paying employees with tax-favored benefits instead of fully taxed salary. Benefits not subject to Social Security taxes:

■Interest-free loans to employees.

■Group term life insurance that is paid for by the company.

■Personal-problem counseling.

■The right to purchase personal items at discount prices.

■Legal-insurance plans.

■Medical-insurance and medical-expense reimbursements.

■Widow's death benefits.

■Reimbursements for moving and relocation expenses.

■Pension and profit-sharing plans.

■Tuition paid for employees under a company plan.

But while all these items are exempt from Social Security taxes, only some are free from income taxation. And some of these items (such as pension plans) are subject to nontax restrictions. Consult the company's advisers to make sure that any benefit plan is custom-tailored to meet the circumstances of the company.

Source: Edward Mendlowitz, partner, Mendlowitz Weitsen, *Successful Tax Planning*, Board-room Books, Springfield, NJ 07081.

Minimizing State Income Taxes

States have been very aggressive in taxing the income of corporations that do business across state lines. To defend themselves, companies must focus on how income is apportioned to particular states and on managing their interstate activities.

Most states measure a company's in-state income on the basis of a three-factor formula keyed to the percentages of the firm's payroll, property, and receipts in the state. In a typical case, ABC Industries has 20% of its property and 40% of its payroll in state Z, and derives 45% of its receipts from the state. The average of 35% is the percentage of ABC's income that state Z taxes.

The formula applies to a corporation's business income. In certain states, invest-ment income—and any other passive income—may be allocated to the state where the investment asset is located or to the company's home state—technically its com-mercial domicile.

Companies can use various techniques to shift payroll from one place to another. It is worth reviewing the impact on state tax allocations before deciding whether to subcontract work out or hire temporary help.

If the company is planning a major property purchase around the end of the year, time the closing to minimize the tax impact. Generally, consider postponing a year-end purchase in a state with high tax rates and accelerating the purchase in a low-tax or no-tax state.

The destination of goods sold is usually the key factor for states in setting a value on receipts in the formula. Receipts are more heavily weighted in some states than others.

To exclude sales from receipts in a high-tax state, deliver the goods out of the state by mail or by common carrier. If the seller is in a low-tax state, in certain situations it may pay to negotiate the shipping costs and have the buyer accept delivery in the seller's home state.

Generally, goods shipped out of state must be added back into receipts in the origin state if the buyer is either the U.S. government or in a state where the selling company is not subject to income tax.

Sales shipped to a state that has no income tax are usually not recapturable. The destination state must have jurisdiction to tax the corporation's income if it imposed an income tax.

Overseas sales are a gray area. A firm might meet the jurisdiction requirements for taxation in the foreign country but be exempt under a treaty provision. New Hampshire recently took a rigid stand on this issue and is adding back receipts from foreign sales made by companies located in that state. But other states may not.

Companies that overlap in ownership, management, and business operations may be considered a unitary business and be taxed as a single entity under state laws. This can help or hurt.

Say a subsidiary has 10% of its assets, payroll, and receipts in state X and has $1 million of taxable income. Its taxable income in the state would be $100,000. The parent has no income, assets, or receipts in state X, but it has $25 million of taxable income. If the parent and the subsidiary are taxed as a unitary business, the apportionment factor might drop to around $1/2\%$. But applying this factor to the combined income ($1/2\% \times \$26$ million) yields a taxable income of $130,000 (instead of $100,000) in the state.

In a contrary situation, Brother and Sister corporations are both located in state Y, which, like certain states, does not allow loss carryovers. Sister is prospering, but Brother has substantial losses. By qualifying to be taxed as a unitary business, Brother's losses can be offset against Sister's income.

There is no precise standard to define a unitary business. Factors include: overlap in ownership, management, and operation, and how much each business depends on, or contributes to, the other. No consistent formula determines the weight given to each factor. Neither the taxing authority nor the taxpayer may know what the outcome will be without a court decision.

The issue usually comes up when a firm is audited. The auditor's questions generally reveal when unitary taxation is being considered, usually because such treatment will produce more revenue.

If it seems the auditor considered and rejected unitary taxation, the company should review the situation. It is likely that unitary taxation will mean less state taxes. On the other hand, such short-term tax savings should be weighed against long-term consequences.

Most states have a discretionary provision in their rules for apportionment and unitary reporting. Tax officials may disregard or modify an apportionment formula if it does not fairly represent the company's business in the state. It pays to consult a specialist in interstate taxation who is most competent to review the state rules if any planning is to be done in this area or, alternatively, after a state has exercised its discretion.

Source: Richard Krol, director of state and local taxes, and Richard Genetelli, manager of state and local taxes, Coopers & Lybrand, New York.

Year-End Tax Write-Off Opportunities

Be careful when taking last-minute tax write-offs. Make sure that the company can justify them to the Internal Revenue Service. There must be proof that the write-off was duly planned, such as prior approval by the board of directors. And the action must be taken before December 31, such as an entry on the company books, or the scrapping of a machine.

Follow through within the organization. For example, if a debt has been written off as bad, salespeople shouldn't continue to solicit the debtor. Fire insurance should be discontinued on property written off as abandoned.

There are specific IRS requirements for different types of write-offs:

■Bad debts. The IRS insists on an identifiable event for deeming the account uncollectible at year-end. Examples are bankruptcy of the debtor, statements by credit agencies, authoritative reports or analyses of other creditors not being paid. Be prepared to demonstrate that the debt wasn't bad at the beginning of the year.

■Casualty loss. Have proof not only of when it occurred, but also how. (Was it really a casualty, or was it the result of nondeductible gross negligence?) Show that there is no possibility at year-end of recovery from insurance, etc. Settle claims with the insurance company by December 31 to establish the loss.

■Inventory. This is possible only when the inventory is carried on the basis of the lower of cost or market. Have proof of what the year-end market price is for approximately the same number of units. (Examples of proof are quotations, actual sales, offers by other parties.) Also permitted are write-downs of damaged, shopworn, or obsolete goods. The write-down is for the estimated actual realization, less the additional costs of advertising and selling these wares. This does not apply to overstocks of normal inventory.

Remember that any inventory write-down must be brought to the attention of the IRS for verification. The corporate income tax return will ask whether there was any substantial change in determining quantities, cost, or valuations between opening and closing inventory.

■Abandonments. Show the steps that were taken before year-end to dispose of the property or to withdraw it permanently from use. Was it scrapped? Sold for salvage value? Dismantled? Consider deeding abandoned land to the county or city for public use. For patents or other intangibles, surrender the use. Notify the Patent Office that the firm is conveying its rights to public use. Show that costs of investigating and analyzing a business or investment are deductible and not capital expenditures because the attempted acquisition failed or was otherwise abandoned.

■Demolition loss. Have proof that when the company acquired the property, the firm had intended to use it. Show that for reasons then unknown the firm could not do so. (The structure may have turned out to be structurally unsound for the business use the company had in mind.)

■Abnormal obsolescence. Show that business assets have to be replaced before the end of their estimated useful life because of economic, prohibitory law, urban renewal, other causes beyond the company's control, or because another firm has come up with a better, less expensive process for making a product the company sells, and the company can't compete.

How To Save Money On Last Year's Corporate Return

Even when a particular tax year is over, it is not too late to cut the tax liability that will be shown on the corporate tax return that is due March 15. A corporate income tax return is due $2^{1}/_{2}$ months after the close of the company's tax year. That is March 15 for a calendar-year business. If the company uses a different fiscal year, compute the due date and substitute it where March 15 appears in this article. Example: If the company's year ends on March 31, the due date is June 15.

Many deadlines are tied to the date the company's income tax return is filed—the time to make pension plan contributions, the time to make a last-in, first-out (LIFO) election.

When it is useful to stretch out the filing date, the company can get an automatic six-month extension of the time to file its tax return by filing Form 7004.

But a filing extension does not extend the time for paying the company's tax bill. The firm must estimate the tax it will finally owe and pay 100% of that amount two and a half months after its tax year's end. The company may be able to get a payment extension by filing Form 1127. To do that, it must show that payment of the tax on the regular due date will result in undue hardship, for example: The company would be forced to sell assets at a giveaway price to raise funds to pay the tax.

If the company had an unexpectedly poor year, it can obtain a quick refund of estimated taxes that were overpaid by filing Form 4466. The IRS must pay the refund within 45 days. This refund request must be made before the company files its tax return.

When loss carry-backs entitle the company to a refund of taxes paid in prior years, the company can get a quick refund by filing Form 1139. This must be answered by the IRS within 90 days.

It is also possible to extend the deadline for making pension plan contributions for six months by obtaining filing extensions. The company can also amend its pension plan for a particular year (say, to expand coverage or change payment formulas), even though that is over, if it does so before filing the return for that year.

A company that had a poor business year may find that it is difficult to make a big pension plan payment. If so, ask for both a quick refund of estimated taxes and a filing extension. Then use the refund to make the pension payment.

Under the law, the S corporation form of organization is more attractive than ever before. It can be used to eliminate problems resulting from an excess accumulation of corporate earnings; and sidestep the issue of excess salaries paid to corporate officers.

It is also now easier to elect S status because changes in the law eased restrictions applying to the number and kind of permissible shareholders. But an S corporation election must be made within the first two and a half months of the company's tax year. So be sure to discuss the pros and cons of an election with the company's tax advisers before the deadline.

LIFO accounting methods can cut the company's tax bill by reducing its paper tax profits. And new rules have modified the aspects of LIFO that most companies consider to be its major drawbacks (reduced earnings show on nontax financial statements and inventory valuation adjustments that must be made in the year of a LIFO switch).

The company's LIFO election for a particular year need not be made until the return for the year is filed. So the company can get the extra time it needs to reconsider LIFO by asking for a filing extension.

There is now also a credit for research and experimentation costs. Since many firms now expense research costs under various accounting categories, cull through the company's accounts to be sure that all research and experimental costs are segregated and identified, so that no item qualifying for the credit is overlooked.

The credit is keyed to increases in the company's research expenditures. So now is the time to plan how such expenditures will be handled in future years.

A reduction in a particular year's taxable income (through, say, a LIFO election) may result in cash-flow savings in the next year by cutting estimated taxes. This is because in many cases, estimated tax payments can be based on the taxable income the company reported in the prior year. So a reduction of last year's income will result in smaller estimated payments this year. Also, a company with income of over $1 million during any one of the prior three years may have its estimated payments increased. A company that can reduce its income to less than $1 million may avoid higher payments the following year.

Salaries, bonuses, expenses, and interest payments owed by the company to a shareholder owning 50% of the company's stock, and accrued by the company during a particular year, may not be deducted until they are actually paid.

One problem area is that the company may have declared a large bonus for shareholder executives at the end of a profitable year. The IRS may rule that the bonus was really a disguised dividend payout of corporate profits. So the company will lose its deduction for it.

So set salaries for shareholder executives at a level equaling the total of the previous salaries and bonuses. This will show the IRS that the company genuinely intended to raise executive compensation at the end of the previous year. If, in fact, a particular year proves to be less profitable, salaries can be reduced later in the year.

Any loan made between the company and a shareholder should be formalized now with a note, loan agreement, and the terms for repayment, if this has not been done already. Otherwise an undocumented loan's proceeds may be treated as taxable dividend income to a shareholder or as a contribution to the capital of the company.

Keep in mind that adequate records are the key to resolving many tax disputes. So be sure that minutes are complete for board meetings held. Make sure they explain:

■The business reason for accumulating any earnings surplus.
■The reason for a loan arranged between the company and a shareholder.
■The company's salary policy.

Source: Edward Mendlowitz, partner, Mendlowitz Weitsen, New York.

The Power Of Tax Credits

A tax credit is worth more to the company than a tax deduction of equal dollar amount. That is because a credit cuts the company's tax bill on a dollar-for-dollar basis. So if the company is in the top 34% tax bracket, a $1 tax credit is worth $2.94 in deductions.

And the value of the credit goes up, vis-a-vis an equal-sized deduction, as the company's tax bracket goes down. If the company is in only the 15% tax bracket, a $1 credit is worth fully $6.66 in deductions.

Best Tax Shelter In America Is A Business Of Your Own

■ *Living quarters* may be provided on a tax-deductible basis for the corporation and tax-free to the shareholder-employee if the corporation requires him to live on the premises for a good business reason.

This might apply for a shareholder serving as a hotel, motel, farm or ranch manager. It might also apply to the manager of a nursing home, hospital or funeral home and other occupations requiring close and more or less continuous availability in connection with the business.

■ *Use of deductible company car:* The use of a company car can be a valuable fringe benefit. The expenses of the car, including depreciation, are deductible by the corporation and not taxable to the shareholder-employee if it is used exclusively on company business.

If a shareholder-executive is given the use of two cars, and it is clear that one of them is being used by his wife for nonbusiness purposes, he will be taxed on the value of the use of the car. But his tax liability will be less than the cost of renting a car, and most likely less than it would cost him to buy, finance and maintain the car on his own.

If the extra car is treated as extra compensation, the attending expenses are deductible by the corporation as compensation, subject to the overall limitation of reasonableness. If treated as dividend income to the shareholder, it would not be deductible by the corporation.

■ *Deductible chauffeur:* The cost of a chauffeur may be deductible by the corporation and not taxable to the shareholder-employee if deemed an "ordinary and necessary expense," sometimes translated as "appropriate and helpful."

■ *Company dining rooms,* employee cafeterias, and other "eating facilities" operated by an employer for employees are not subject to the 80% limit on business meal deductions if the facility...

1. Is located on the business premises of the employer, and

2. Brings in revenue that normally equals or exceeds its direct operating costs, and

3. Does not discriminate in favor of highly compensated employees.

(New IRC Section 274 (n)(2): Amended IRC Section 132(e) (2).)

■ *Bail-out loophole for family members:* Income and estate tax considerations generally make it desirable for family members to hold stock in a close corporation. The family head may wish to give them money to buy stock from the corporation, or they may already have their own money to buy in.

There are two good reasons why it may be desirable for family members to acquire their stock directly from the corporation as soon as the corporation is set up:

1. The stock will be cheaper at that time than later, assuming that the corporation succeeds; and

2. The rules governing corporate redemptions are less restrictive when the stock is acquired directly from the corporation rather than by a transfer from a family head or other family member.

■*Leasing assets to your own corporation:* The fact that the corporate form is selected as the basic means of conducting a business enterprise does not mean that all of the physical components of the enterprise need be owned by the corporation. Indeed, there may be legal, tax and personal financial planning reasons for not having the corporation own all the assets to be used in the business.

Whether the corporation is to be the continuation of a sole proprietorship or partnership or a wholly new enterprise, decisions can be made about which assets owned by the predecessor or acquired for use in the corporation are to be owned by the corporation and which assets are to be made available to the corporation through a leasing or other contractual arrangement.

For the assets that go to the corporation, decisions must be made about how they are to be held and on what terms they are to be made available to the corporation.

There are several possible choices. The assets may be owned by:

1. An individual shareholder or some member of his family;

2. A partnership, limited or general, in which family members participate; or

3. A trust for the benefit of family members.

A separate corporation is still another possibility, but the risk of being considered a personal holding company and incurring penalties due to passive income (including rent and royalties) may make this impractical.

Normally, a leasing arrangement is used for the assets to be made available for corporate use. Assuming that the rental is fair, it would be deductible by the corporation and taxable to the lessor. Against the rental income, the lessor would have possible deductions for interest paid on loans financing the acquisition of the asset, depreciation, maintenance and repairs, insurance and administrative costs.

These deductions might produce a tax-free cash flow for the lessor. When depreciation and interest deductions begin to run out, a high-tax-bracket lessor might find that he is being taxed at too high a rate on the rental income. At this point, he may transfer the leased property to a lower-tax-bracket family member.

He might also consider a sale of the property to his corporation, possibly on installment terms to reduce the impact of tax liability. This sale would serve to extract earnings and profits from the corporation at favorable tax rates. At the same time, it would give the corporation a higher tax-basis for the asset than it had in the hands of the lessor, thus increasing the corporation's depreciation deductions. This, of course, would reduce the corporation's tax liabilities and benefit the shareholders—the lessor included, if he is a shareholder.

■*Profits reported by low-bracket children. Losses deducted by high-bracket parents:* A business can be organized as a corporation, a proprietorship or a partnership, or even a trust. Use combined forms of ownership to cut taxes.

Example:

1. Use a corporation to operate the business.

2. Have an individual, as sole proprietor, or a partnership own the machinery and equipment and rent it to the corporation.

3. Have an individual or partnership hold title to the real estate and rent it to the corporation.

4. Use a trust (for the benefit of the children of the owners) as a partner in the partnership (in either the equipment partnership or the real estate partnership, or in both).

This arrangement accomplishes these tax benefits:

1. Tax losses are passed through to the owners. When partnerships begin producing income, transfer title to the children for income-splitting purposes.

2. Income from the rental goes to the owners without dilution for corporate taxes.

3. Income to children aged 14 or over benefits from income splitting.

The possibilities for combining the above are endless. Consider such additional entities as S corporations, multiple corporations and multiple trusts.

A diagram of the above example:

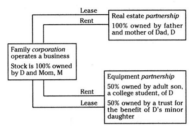

This is a three-generation family business combination:

First generation—Father and mother
Second generation—Dad, D, and Mom, M
Third generation—Adult son and minor daughter

■*Deduct medical expenses without subtracting percentage of income:* One of the healthiest tax benefits you can provide for yourself or your key employees is a corporate medical reimbursement plan under Section 105(b).

You get full reimbursement of medical expenses without reduction for the 7.5% of adjusted gross income limitation on medical expenses. For example, if you are currently earning $40,000, the first 7.5% or $3,000 you spend on medical expenses is lost forever as a deduction.

Medical expenses that are reimbursed to you or are paid directly for your benefit are fully deductible by the corporation as compensation.

The amounts reimbursed to you or paid for your benefit are not included in your gross income.

Simply put, all medical expenses for you and all your dependents can be paid by your corporation and are fully deductible by the corporation without your having to pay one penny of income tax on the benefits.

Uninsured (self-insured) medical expense reimbursement (pay) plans have to meet the breadth-of-coverage requirements applicable to qualified pension plans. In order for medical expense reimbursements to be excluded from the employee's income, the plan must not discriminate in favor of key employees (highly compensated individuals and certain stockholders).

When A Spouse's Expenses Are Deductible

Usually, if a spouse is taken along on a business trip, his or her expenses are not deductible. They're regarded as personal expenses, even if the spouse performs incidental business services, such as answering the phone. However, if the spouse's presence is essential to the business purpose of the trip, the expenses may be deductible. Examples:

■A wife accompanies her husband on a business trip abroad; she knows the language and customs of the country, and he does not.

■A wife serves as secretary on a business trip. She formerly worked for the company and is familiar with technical details.

■An important customer has told an executive to bring "your charming wife" to any business meetings.

In one case, a deduction was allowed for a taxpayer who was a diabetic and whose wife went along to take care of possible medical emergencies, with which she was trained to deal. In such cases, it helps if the taxpayer can prove that he would have had to hire a nurse if his wife did not accompany him.

One taxpayer-husband won by proving that his wife "was not enthusiastic about accompanying her husband on his trips." Another winner showed that his wife had not gone shopping or swimming on a trip to Hawaii.

Even when the spouse's expenses are held to be nondeductible, the taxpayer can still deduct whatever it would have cost him to travel alone. Example: Taxpayer and spouse take a double room at a hotel. The taxpayer can deduct the cost of a single room.

Source: Robert S. Holzman, professor emeritus of taxation, New York University.

100% Deductible Business Meals

Company dining rooms, employee cafeterias, and other "eating facilities" operated by an employer for employees are not subject to the 80% limit on business meal deductions if the facility...

■Is located on the business premise of the employer, and

■Brings in revenue that normally equals or exceeds its direct operating costs, and

■Does not discriminate in favor of highly compensated employees.

Source: New IRC Section 274(n)(2): Amended IRC Section 132(e)(2).

How To Avoid Deduction Limit Traps On Company Cars, Business Meals, Entertainment

Tax Reform rules can unexpectedly increase the tax bills that many executives owe when they use a car for business, whether it's their own vehicle or the company's. And—Tax Reform directly cuts back the deduction for business meals and entertainment.

But with smart planning, executives may be able to minimize taxes on their business autos while securing the maximum deduction for meals and entertainment.

Key: Companies review accounting and expense allowance procedures now. How to handle the new problems:

Company Cars

When a company provides an automobile for an executive, it is necessary to keep very detailed records concerning business use of the vehicle in order to keep the car's value from being included in the executive's income. Methods used by some companies in the past to address these recordkeeping requirements don't work as well after Tax Reform. Examples:

■Giving an executive an auto allowance that is included in his income. The executive then deducts the business use of the car on his personal return.

■Providing the executive with a company-owned car, but including its full value in his income. Again the executive deducts business use of the car on his personal return.

Snag: Tax Reform upsets both these alternatives. Under Tax Reform, business expenses can no longer be deducted on a personal return except to the extent that they exceed 2% of Adjusted Gross Income (AGI).

Example: an executive with $60,000 of AGI gets no deduction for his first $1,200 of unreimbursed expenses, including driving costs.

Thus, an executive who receives a car allowance will have to pay tax on some of it even if it is used entirely to pay business costs…And an executive who reports a company car in income will have to pay tax on some of its value even if it's used only for business.

What To Do

With smart planning it is possible to avoid the tax cost to executives of the 2%-of-AGI limit, whether the company is subsidizing an executive's use of his own car or providing a car to him outright. How to do it:

■Convert a car allowance into a reimbursement program. The difference between an allowance and a reimbursement is that a reimbursement is made for specified expenses. The executive must give the company an itemized report of his business driving—including mileage, tolls, parking fees, and the cost of oil and gas—and receive payment either for actual costs or at a rate not exceeding 28¢ per mile.

Benefit: The payment to the executive is neither included in his income nor deducted on his return, so the 2%-of-AGI limit is avoided. Danger: Many companies that say they have reimbursement programs are in fact providing allowances to their executives, because the payments made to them are not based on sufficiently itemized expense reports. Such programs are now subject to IRS scrutiny.

Any company that provides regular payments on a periodic basis without checking current expense reports falls into this category. So does any firm providing a per-day or per-mile travel allowance which lumps together driving costs with estimated amounts for such other expenses as meals and lodging. Important: Establish itemized expense reporting and reimbursement procedures now.

■Include only part of the value of a company-owned car in the executive's income. The key is for the company to make an allocation of auto use for business and personal purposes. Only personal use of the car is included in the executive's income. Since business use of the car is not reported, the executive does not need to take an offsetting deduction, and again the 2%-of-AGI limit is avoided.

Extra benefits: When a company-owned car is provided to an executive, the firm doesn't have to bother making periodic expense reimbursements—so bookkeeping is simplified. And the company can also claim depreciation deductions for the vehicle. But accurate records documenting the amount of auto use allocated to business and personal purposes are a must.

Two Ways To Keep Records

■The company can set up its own recordkeeping system for each car, for example, by requiring that an auto diary be kept for each vehicle.

■The company can require those using company cars to file written statements saying that they are keeping records sufficient to document the cars' business use. The company then avoids these recordkeeping duties—but an executive who signs such a statement but doesn't keep adequate records may be liable to the IRS for negligence penalties.

Caution: A company that follows neither of these procedures to keep adequate records of business use may have its own auto depreciation deductions disallowed.

Business Meals

By now almost everyone knows that Tax Reform limits the deduction for business meals and entertainment to 80% of their actual cost. But here are several points that are frequently overlooked:

■Client pass-throughs. The party that pays a meal expense is subject to the 80% deduction limit. Thus, if a company pays for a meal on behalf of a client, and bills the client for the meal, the client may deduct only 80% of its cost. But if the client paid only a general fee for services, it could deduct the whole fee as a business expense while the company would have to include the whole fee in income and be able to deduct only 80% of the meal costs it incurred. Here, the billing of itemized meal costs to the client is the key, and this item should be considered when drafting client agreements.

■Company parties. Holiday parties, summer outings and other traditional company gatherings that take place primarily for the benefit of the company's employees are not subject to the 80% limit on meal deductions.

■Dining rooms. Meals provided in company eating facilities are not subject to the 80% limit provided that the facility is located on the firm's business premises, produces enough revenue to meet its direct operating costs, and does not discriminate in favor of top executives.

■Reimbursements. When an executive pays for a business meal (or some other business expense) out of his own salary or a general expense allowance, his deduction will be subject to both the 80% of cost limit and the 2%-of-AGI limit.

Corporations are not subject to the 2%-of-AGI limit. Thus, overall tax costs may be reduced by increasing an executive's expense reimbursements rather than his salary or a general expense account to cover these costs. (Though the company's deduction for reimbursed meals is subject to the 80% limit.)

The 80% limit does apply to business meals taken while traveling away from home, though not to lodging or travel costs.

Many firms pay traveling employees the federal per diem travel expense rate for a given locale. The per diem rate serves as tax-free reimbursement to the employee of meal and lodging costs, and use of this rate saves the company from being required to keep itemized records of travel costs.

Trap: That portion of the per diem that is allocated to meal expenses is only 80% deductible by the company. But the IRS hasn't said what portion of the per diem is allocable to meal costs. Rather, it wants the company to make a "reasonable" adjustment on its tax return. The firm's accountant should be alerted to this problem, and should look for future developments.

Source: Pamela Pecarich, partner, and Steven Woolf, Lynn Hogan and Jeffrey Hillier, managers, Coopers & Lybrand, 1800 M Street NW, Washington, DC 20036.

Deduct Transportation Expenses

If you're an employee, you can convert nondeductible personal commuting expenses into tax-deductible local business driving by keeping an office in your home. The tax rule on commuting expenses is this: Your first trip of the day (from home to office) is nondeductible, as is your last trip of the day (from office to home). All business-related driving in between is tax deductible, either at your cost or at the IRS standard mileage rate of 28 cents a mile for 1992.

The trick is to make your first and last business stops of the day in your at-home office. It doesn't matter if the office qualifies for tax deduction purposes or not. Suppose you have a den where you study reports, go through business papers, read business mail, etc., but you can't write off the office expenses because you don't use the room exclusively for business. But if you make the den your first and last business stop of the day, driving to work and back becomes tax-deductible transportation.

Another option: Collect business mail at the closest Post Office to your home, or make business deposits at a nearby bank. That way, your nondeductible beginning and ending driving trips of the day will be short and all other driving that you do will be tax deductible.

Business/Personal Use of Car

I have a fully depreciated car that I've used in my business, which is a proprietorship. I'd now like to convert the car to personal use. Will this be taxable?

No, it won't be taxable until you sell the car. At that time, you'll have a taxable gain to the extent that the sale price exceeds your depreciated basis in the car—that is, the original cost of the car reduced by the depreciation deductions that you've claimed.

Source: *Tax Hotline*, Boardroom Reports, Inc., 330 West 42nd St., New York 10036.

Entertaining Between Jobs

A salesman who was between jobs could deduct the cost of entertaining customers. He was not in the selling business but was actively seeking another base to serve the same customers, the Tax Court held. It was important to retain the customers' goodwill.

Source: *Harold Haft*, 40 TC 2.

Beat The Limit On Employee Business Expenses

Employee business expenses—including the cost of business meals—are deductible only to the extent that their total, when combined with other miscellaneous deductions, exceeds 2% of Adjusted Gross Income (AGI). This eliminates the deduction for many employees. For example, a person with AGI of $60,000 gets no deduction for the first $1,200 of such costs.

Planning strategy: A deduction for these kinds of items can be preserved by having the company pay for them through an expense account or other reimbursement program. That's because a corporation can deduct these kinds of costs as a business expense without reference to the 2%-of-AGI rule. (The company's deduction for business meals and entertainment is, however, limited to 80% of the cost.)

Business meals: Under tax reform, no deduction is allowed for the so-called quiet business meal—one that furthers good business relations but doesn't involve business directly. To get an 80% deduction for a meal, one must prove not only its cost, but also its specific business purpose.

How To Offset Operating Losses

For the past year I have been running an unincorporated start-up business. So far, it's still losing money, and I don't have enough income to offset my losses. Can I carry them into next year? If so, is there any limit on the amount?

Since your business is unincorporated, its losses must first be deducted on your personal return against your income from other sources. If this leaves you with a net operating loss for the year, you can carry it *back three years* (to get a refund of past years' taxes)…or *forward 15 years* (to offset future income). There's no limit on the amount you can carry back or forward.

Figure your carryback or carryforward using IRS Form 3621. If you carry back your losses, you can get an *expedited refund* of previous years' taxes by filing Form 1138.

Big, Big Benefits

Since the drastic changes made by tax reform, the best source of tax breaks is your own business. Business owner's tax advantages:

Fully deductible business expenses. For the self-employed, business expenses are deductible in full directly from gross income. Employees may deduct their business expenses only if they itemize, and the deduction is reduced by 2% of Adjusted Gross Income (AGI).

Full home-office expense write-off. If you run a business from your home, you may deduct not only property taxes and mortgage interest, but also a percentage of depreciation, utilities, insurance, repairs, and any other costs. You get these deductions even if they result in a tax loss. Essential: To take these deductions, you must reserve a part of your home exclusively for business.

Greater tax-deferred retirement savings. Tax reform severely limited IRAs and capped 401(k) contributions at $7,000 a year, indexed for inflation. But Keogh plans for the self-employed were left practically untouched. Business owners may make annual deductible contributions of up to 20% of business income or $30,000 — whichever is less—to a defined-contribution plan and may stash away even more in a defined-benefit plan.

Potential drawback: If you have employees, you must include them in your plan on a nondiscriminatory basis. Exceptions: You may exclude employees under 21, those who have worked for you less than a year and part-timers with fewer than 1,000 work hours in a 12-month period.

Hiring your kids. Their wages are deductible business expenses, and they can earn up to $3,700 a year tax free. If they open an IRA, up to $2,000 more is tax free. If they do make enough to be taxed, it's at minimum rates. And you may still claim them as dependents.

Caution: Kids must perform actual services for reasonable compensation. Phony jobs and inflated wages don't stand up to IRS scrutiny.

Hiring your spouse. Advantages:

■Your spouse may participate in any retirement plans that you have for employees (pension, 401(k), etc.). In some cases he or she may qualify for deductible IRA contributions.

■If your spouse accompanies you on a business trip as an assistant or colleague, you may write off travel expenses for both of you.

Timing income. If you use the cash accounting method, you can easily defer income from one year into the next. You just don't send out bills late in the year—you wait until January.

More deductible transportation expenses. Going to work and coming home are nondeductible commutation expenses. But if you work out of your home, you're already at your place of business when you get up in the morning. So all travel costs are deductible—trips to visit customers, buy supplies, mail correspondence, etc.

Justifying transportation deductions is also easier for business owners. Employees may be asked by IRS auditors why they weren't reimbursed by their company if their travel costs were truly "ordinary and necessary" business expenses.

Fully deductible casualty losses. Business casualty losses (from fire, theft, accident, natural disaster, etc.) may be written off in full against business income. But personal casualty losses are deductible only for itemizers, and the deduction is reduced by 10% of AGI plus a $100 deductible.

Full write-offs for bad debts. A business's bad debts may be deducted in full in the year in which they become uncollectible. But personal bad debts are treated like capital losses—you may deduct only up to $3,000 a year.

Source: Philip Kimmel, late partner, Hertz, Herson & Co., CPAs, New York 10016.

Business Gift Loophole

An advertising company employed an independent salesman. As favors to prospective customers, he gave out $40,000 worth of tickets to shows and sporting events. The company paid for the tickets and deducted their full cost. IRS position:

The company's expense deduction was subject to the limit of $25 per recipient in the tax law. Court's decision: The ticket expenses were deductible by the company. The $25 business gift limitation applied to the independent salesman, not to the company that employed him.

Source: *World Wide Agency, Inc,* TC Memo 1981–419.

Beating The Home-Office Trap

While a home-office deduction can save you money on your tax return, it can also cost you two big breaks when you sell your home. Namely: Tax-deferred treatment of profits that are reinvested in a replacement residence...and the $125,000 tax exclusion for sale proceeds received by home sellers aged 55 or over.

Trap: A home office is treated as business property, not as part of your personal residence. So the portion of house sale proceeds attributable to the office does not qualify for these residential property tax breaks.

What to do: The IRS has ruled that a house does fully qualify for residential property tax breaks if the seller isn't entitled to claim a home-office deduction in the year of sale, even if the deduction was claimed in previous years. So if you have a home office, don't use it exclusively for business or claim a deduction for it in the year in which you want to sell your home.

All About Home Offices

The ration of time spent working and the precise kind of work performed in a given locale are crucial to all tax determinations on home office status by the IRS. Four landmark cases:

■Homework: A home office is normally deductible only if it is your primary place of business. The IRS uses this rule to deny deductions to many persons who are required to bring work home, but who also have business offices. Case: The Court of Appeals has ruled that orchestra musicians could claim home-office deductions for their practice studios, in spite of the IRS' claim that their primary place of business was the concert hall. Key: The musicians spent more time at home practicing than they did performing. Impact: Salespersons, professors, writers and others who in fact spend most of their time working at home can use this case to try to justify deductions for themselves.

Source: *Ernest Drucker,* 715 F2d 67.

■Proportion: Sally Meiers owned and managed a laundromat. Each day she spent an hour at the laundry and two hours in her home office, where she did necessary administrative work. The Tax Court denied Sally's home-office deduction, because the laundromat, not her home, was her principal place of business. Sally appealed. Court of Appeals: Sally spent more time working at home than anywhere else. Thus, the home office was her principal place of business and the deduction was allowed.

Source: *John and Sally Meiers,* CA-7, No. 85–1209.

■Kind of work: A college professor spent 80% of the work week doing research and writing in an office at home. The IRS ruled the home office was not his "principal place of business" (he had an office at the college), nor was it used "for the convenience of the employer." Court of Appeals: The home office was the professor's principal place of business, as his college office wasn't private enough for the scholarly work required by his job. Moreover, the use of the professor's home was for the employer's convenience, as it relieved the college of the necessity of providing a suitable office. Home-office deductions allowed.

Source: *David J. Weissman*, CA-2, 751 F2d 512.

New Business/Home Opportunities

Corporation owners face the problem of taking money out of the business at the least possible tax cost. Dividends and salaries are fully taxable. You can borrow from the company tax-free, but Tax Reform has limited the tax deduction for the interest you pay.

Big exception: Within broad limits, mortgage interest on your residence (or second residence) is deductible in full. If you're planning to buy or build a home, borrow the money from your corporation, not from a bank. Let the corporation hold the mortgage. The interest you pay goes back to your company, but it will be fully deductible on your personal tax return.

Interest is fully deductible on mortgage amounts totaling up to $1 million when the mortgage financing is used to buy, build or improve your home (or second home).

If you already have a home, you can still borrow an additional $100,000 from your company on a second mortgage or home-equity loan and use the money for a purpose other than home improvement. The interest will be fully deductible.

Be sure the corporation charges market-rate interest on the loan, and document it with a promissory note and a properly recorded mortgage. Make all payments on schedule. Carry the loan, the mortgage and the repayments correctly on company books, so you'll have no difficulty proving the transaction is bona fide.

Source: Irving L. Blackman, partner, Blackman Kallick Bartelstein, CPAs, 300 S. Riverside Plaza, Chicago 60606.

Business Use Of Your Home Computer

Do you have a personal computer in your home? In order to deduct accelerated (ACRS) depreciation of a home computer, you must use it at least 50% for business. Calculate the amount of your deduction by multiplying the percent of business use by the ACRS depreciation rate. Or you can use the section 179 write-off, which is $10,000 in the first year, depending on several variables. (Check this out with your tax adviser.)

If you use your personal computer less than 50% for business, you can take only straight-line depreciation. Caution: Business use doesn't include use for investment purposes.

If you claim a deduction for your home computer as a requirement of your employment, you must prove that you maintain it at the request of your employer.

Source: *New Tax Traps/New Opportunities* by Edward Mendlowitz, Boardroom Special Reports, Springfield, NJ 07081.

Summer Office

An executive could deduct maintenance costs and depreciation on a separate office he built near his vacation home and used exclusively to review the company's long-range plans. The IRS said the office was a nondeductible personal expense. But the court allowed the deduction. The alternate office was appropriate and helpful to the executive in performing his duties.

Source: *Ben W. Heineman,* 82 TC 638.

How To Set Up A Hobby As A Business

You can set up a hobby as a business and deduct your losses. However, you must be able to prove that the hobby is a for-profit business. If you realize some profit in at least three out of the most recent five consecutive years, it is presumed that the business is for profit. But even if you don't show a profit, you may be able to prove that the business is intended to make a profit.

To prove you have a profit motive in conducting your business, keep detailed records. Present evidence of your advertising campaigns, attempts to generate new business, and sales analyses. It's not necessary to show that you run a big business, reaping huge profits, but only that you have genuine intentions of running the business in a businesslike way.

Source: *New Tax Traps/New Opportunities* by Edward Mendlowitz, Boardroom Special Reports, Springfield, NJ 07081.

Free-Lancer Smarts

Report income and expenses on Schedule C of Form 1040. There's a big advantage in doing this. Business expenses, such as transportation costs, are deductible in full on Schedule C. They are not subject to the 2%-of-Adjusted-Gross-Income limitation that applies when the same expenses are taken on Schedule A of the 1040.

If you get a commission, report it on Schedule C, even if you have no business expenses to write off against it. Reason: If the income qualifies as self-employment income, you can use some of it to set up a Keogh plan.

Source: Edward Mendlowitz, partner, Mendlowitz Weitsen, CPAs, Two Pennsylvania Plaza, New York 10121. Mr. Mendlowitz is the author of several books, including *Aggressive Tax Strategies,* Macmillan Publishing Co., 866 Third Ave., New York 10022.

Full MBA Deduction

A business manager could deduct costs of a full-time MBA program even though he had resigned from his job to take the course and after graduation took a job with a different company.
Source: Stephen G. Sherman, TC Memo 1977–301.

How To Keep Your Deductions And Exemptions Despite The New Tax Law

The 1990 Tax Act imposed new cutbacks on income tax deductions and personal exemptions. The cutbacks are based on your level of taxable income. The higher your taxable income, the more deductions and exemptions you lose. New limits:
■When your Adjusted Gross Income (AGI) goes above $108,450 for 1993, you must reduce your deductions by 3% of the excess.
■When your AGI goes above $162,700 on a joint return (above $108,450 for singles), (the 1992 figures are $157,900 for marrieds and $105,250 for singles), you begin to lose the benefit of your personal and dependent exemptions. These are reduced at the rate of 2% per $2,500 of AGI in excess of the limits.
Strategy: Keep your Adjusted Gross Income under $108,450 and you'll keep all your deductions and exemptions. One way to do this is to invest in tax exempt municipal bonds, which produce income that is not reflected in AGI. A simple shift to make if you're close to the cut-off point, would be to switch from taxable corporate bonds to tax exempt municipals.
Source: Randy Bruce Blaustein, Esq., partner, Blaustein, Greenberg & Co., New York. Mr. Blaustein is an attorney and former IRS agent. He is author of *How To Do Business with the IRS: The Complete Guide for the Tax Professional*, Prentice-Hall, Englewood Cliffs, NJ.

Deducting S Corporation Losses Against Other Income

One good use of an S corporation is when a new business is started and expects to lose money at first. The S form can be elected at the beginning and can be continued as long as the business loses money. Those losses will be available immediately to those stockholders who are active participants in the business, and will shelter income from other sources. Then, when the business gets rolling and begins to show a profit, the stockholders may decide to abandon S status so that the profits can accumulate in the business and their taxable incomes are not increased by the addition of the profits from the business.
New S corporations must adopt a calendar year. An exception is made only where there is a strong business purpose for the use of a fiscal year. Furthermore, if

there is a more than 50% change in ownership, then a calendar year must be adopted or the S status ceases.

If the stockholders are confident that the period of losses will be brief, they should time the start-up so that the first taxable year will be very short. For example, start the business in September and the first fiscal year will only be three or four months. The stockholders get the benefits of the losses during the brief start-up period. Then they can terminate the S status for the second fiscal year beginning January 1.

This can be most applicable to a service business, such as a window-washing operation or telephone-answering service that started as an unincorporated organization, keeping its books on the accrual basis. In that case, the accounts payable are negligible as most of the expenses are labor.

In a service business on the accrual basis, taxes are paid on profits represented by accounts receivable. As an example, let's say that such profits in the first year's accounts receivable amounted to $50,000; the profit equals that amount, and taxes are paid on it.

At this point, the business is restructured as an S corporation on the cash basis. But the old organization keeps collecting the cash on its existing accounts receivable, while the new S company pays all expenses. Assume that three months' expenses come to approximately $50,000, and that billed but uncollected accounts receivable also come to $50,000. Cash to pay the bills of the S company can be generated by transferring the $50,000 in accounts receivable collections from the old organization as an investment in the new business. Meanwhile, however—at least for the roughly 90-day period during which no cash collections are coming in to the S company from its own new accounts receivable—the new company reports a loss.

Source: Edward Mendlowitz, a partner in Mendlowitz Weitsen, CPAs, New York.

When Kickbacks Are Tax Deductible

Kickbacks—some legal, some illegal—present some difficult dilemmas for business. Let's examine them.

Kickbacks to government employees aren't deductible by the payor. Payments to businesspersons are—if the payor hasn't violated any state law that would subject him to a criminal penalty. In many states, such as New York, there are commercial bribery laws, which forbid the payment of money to an employee of another corporation unless the recipient's employer knows about it.

The tax relevance: The payor will lose the tax deduction if the employer of the purchasing agent, executive, loan officer, etc., doesn't know about the kickback. That should discourage the making of such kickbacks, which, of course, is what the law is trying to do.

But these are unusual times. The payee's employer may be hard put to pay a valuable person what he demands.

The employer doesn't have to increase the salary if the employee is permitted to sweeten his own income satisfactorily in another way. Many employers consider themselves sufficiently familiar with the product (or service) that their employees are buying to know when shoddy merchandise or inflated prices are involved, and they feel that the employee's acceptance of a commercial bribe won't hurt what the company is getting. For his part the employee is hardly likely to let the kickback distort his judgment if it would result in the loss of his job. So we have the bizarre situation of both employee and employer benefiting from a kickback, which the payor is permitted to deduct for tax purposes.

How To Avoid Tax On Dividends

Individuals can avoid paying taxes on dividends earned from stock investments by investing through a tax managed mutual fund.

How it works: The individual buys shares in the fund. The fund invests in stocks. Dividends are not passed through to the investor, so they are not taxed to him. Instead, they are reinvested in further stock purchases. In this way, the fund grows for the investor's benefit.

How to buy: Shares in a tax managed fund can be acquired through a broker. These funds are generally invested in utilities and steady stocks that pay high dividends such as AT&T, IBM and GM. So they tend to rise less than the average stock in a bull and fall less than average in a down market. These funds charge annual management fees averaging about 0.75% plus up-front "load" fees ranging from 6.75% to 8.5% of the investment. So be sure to consult with an investment adviser and pick a fund that suits your particular needs.

Source: Andrew J. Donohue, secretary and counsel, First Investors Corporation, 120 Wall St., New York 10005.

Donate Inventory And Deduct 2X Your Cost

A little-known provision in the tax law* may enable the company to contribute appreciated inventories to charity to get a deduction of up to twice the donated items' cost basis.

Restrictions that apply:

■The deduction may not exceed the donated items' cost basis plus half of the related appreciation. Nor may the deduction be larger than twice the cost basis.

■Such charitable deductions may not exceed 10% of the firm's taxable income.

■The deduction may not exceed the price that similar items are actually sold for. Impact: This may reduce the deduction available to retail outlets that commonly cut prices to move stock. It may increase the deductions available to industrial distributors who make occasional high-price sales from excess stock.

Also: The receipt organization must be tax-exempt and must actually use the donated items to care for the ill, the needy or infants. Point: This may sound like a tough condition for a contribution of hard goods to meet. But the National Association for Exchange of Industrial Resources, 550 Frontage Rd., Northfield, IL 60093, has 200 members who qualify as donees under this provision of the law.

*IRC Code Section 170(e)(3).

Source: Alan Silver, principal, Alan Silver & Associates, Highland Park, NJ.

Buying Out A Shareholder And Deducting It

One of the worst things that can happen to a closely held company is trouble among the shareholders. Buying out the dissenting shareholders can be very costly.

Some companies have tried to minimize the cost of a buyout by deducting it as a business expense. Problem: Company stock is a capital asset. And the cost of a capital asset is generally not deductible. Opportunity: Show that there is a compelling business reason for the buyout. The elimination of friction between shareholders is not enough. The company must show that without the buyout its business will be in jeopardy.

How the rule works:

■Winner. A company produced a patented product under license. But the conduct of one of the shareholders upset the patent owner, who threatened to cancel the license agreement if the shareholder was not removed from the company. So the company bought the shareholder out and deducted the cost. Court of Appeals decision: Without the license, the company would have been out of business. So there was an overriding business motive for the deal, and the deduction was ruled okay.

■Loser. A company wanted to close an unprofitable subsidiary. But it was contractually committed to buy out interest of the subsidiary's manager first. IRS objection: The company business was healthy on the whole. The fact that the company had made a bad investment in the subsidiary did not entitle it to specially favored tax treatment. The Court's decision: The fact that there was some business motive for the deal did not outweigh the fact that it was a purchase of capital stock. The deduction was disallowed.

Source: *Winner: Five Star Mfg.*, USCA-5, 355 F. 2d724. *Loser: Harder Services*, 67 TC 585.

Personal Deduction For Corporate Donation

There is a way for owners of closely held companies to use company funds to get a charitable deduction on their personal income tax returns. The owner gives the charity stock in his company. Subsequently, the company redeems the stock from the charity. Advantage: A 100% owner would not give up any ownership interest in the company, since his interest in the company after the charity is redeemed would still be 100%. How a bailout works: The owner makes an informal agreement with the charity to offer the stock for redemption shortly after the charity receives it. The owner gives the stock to the charity. He takes a deduction on his personal return for the fair market value of the stock. Later, the company redeems the stock from the charity. If the transaction is properly handled, the stock's redemption will not be taxed as a dividend to the owner. Caution: The agreement with the charity must be informal. The charity must not be under a binding obligation to let the company redeem the stock or to sell it to an outsider. Tax rule: Normally, if a 100% shareholder in a closely held company has some of his stock redeemed, income from the redemption will be taxed to him as a dividend. But the IRS has agreed that a redemption will not be considered a dividend if it is handled by an informal prearranged plan with a charity. Such a transaction must be structured properly to ensure the desired tax results. Check with your accountant or attorney.

Source: Tom C. Klein, CPA, 231 W. 29 St., New York.

Tax Reform and Real Estate Tax Opportunities

Real estate is a major asset in most businesses, whether they buy or lease their premises. The good news is that real estate continues to provide some of the most attractive tax breaks available to companies and their owners, even under the toughened-up rules of Tax Reform.

Tax Shelters

Tax Reform's passive loss rules sharply cut back the availability of tax shelters in general. But real estate investments can still provide old-style tax shelter benefits, especially to companies...

■Corporate shelters. Tax Reform's passive loss rules do not apply to regular corporations (as opposed to S corporations). So, a corporation with operating profits can still shelter the profits from tax by investing in traditional tax-advantaged investments (such as operating oil wells, shopping centers, etc). Tactic: If a company owner finds that Tax Reform prevents him from claiming loss deductions from a shelter that he owns personally, he may be able to salvage deductions by transferring the shelter to the corporation. Caution: Recapture taxes may result on previously claimed deductions, so consider any transfer carefully.

■Passive loss loophole. A major planning opportunity exists in Tax Reform's passive loss rules for owners of closely held corporations, though it is often overlooked. When real estate is owned by a company shareholder personally and is leased to the corporation at a profit for use in the business, the shareholder's real estate profit generally can still be sheltered from tax with passive losses generated by the types of tax shelter investments that were restricted by Tax Reform.

■Tax credits. Most business tax credits, such as the investment tax credit, were repealed by Tax Reform. But real estate tax credits still exist to help offset the cost of renovating certain old or historic buildings.

A 20% credit is available for the cost of rehabilitating a certified historic structure, and a 10% credit can be claimed for the cost of rehabilitating a building placed in service before 1936. Benefit: A tax credit is better than a tax deduction of an equal dollar amount because a credit reduces tax on a dollar-for-dollar basis.

Lease Or Buy

Any corporation that needs to acquire real estate for use in the business must ask a fundamental question: *Should it lease or buy?*

Tax, investment and business factors each must be considered to come to the best bottom line decision...

■Balance sheet. Leasing may keep real estate and related financing off of the company's balance sheet. Thus, mortgage debt that would be used to finance a purchase does not appear as a liability on the company's financial statements if it leases.

■Cash flow. If a company leases, it must, of course, make rent payments. While rent is deductible as a business expense, cash flow may be better if the company buys real estate. That's because an owner gets to deduct both mortgage interest and depreciation expense. And depreciation provides a no-cash-cost deduction which can be used to shelter other income.

■Investment opportunity. If a company can buy in a depressed market and wait for real estate values to rise, a purchase may double as an investment as well as productive property. If real estate values are high, it may make more investment sense to lease.

■Business valuation. Ownership of real estate may lead a business to be undervalued by outsiders, for two reasons...

■Often real estate appreciates in value while being carried on the books at cost (or an even lower depreciated value). Thus, the true value of the property may not be apparent to those outside the company.

■If a company is very good at operating a business, outside analysts may value it more highly if capital invested in real estate was invested in operations instead.

Special Tax Aspects Of Leasing

■Improvements. When structural improvements are made to leased space, their cost must be depreciated at rates specified by Tax Reform, usually over a period of $31^1/_2$ years.

Trap: Tenants often make improvements themselves, receiving some reimbursement from the landlord. This lets the tenant supervise and control construction. But in this case, the reimbursement received from the landlord usually is taxable as income immediately, while the offsetting deduction must be spread over many years. Better way: For tax purposes, it makes more sense for the landlord to make and pay for the improvements.

■Rent leveling. Tenants often receive discounts or "rent holidays" at the beginning of a lease as an incentive for taking space. Unexpected tax impact: When rent rates rise sharply during the course of a lease, the IRS may reallocate rents for tax purposes at a proportional rate over the lease term.

Example: If a tenant pays zero rent in year one through five, and $100,000 rent in each of the next five years of a 10-year lease, the IRS may treat the parties as if the rent was accruing at an intermediate amount annually. Impact: The tenant gets a rent expense deduction in years one through ten, based on a discounted payment stream while paying no rent in the early years. And the landlord owes tax on an equal amount of rental income, even though he has received no cash. This possibility should always be considered when negotiating lease terms.

■Subleases. A special trap confronts partnerships and professional service corporations (such as law firms, accounting firms and medical practices) which sublease substantial space out to other parties.

Example: A firm leases more space than it currently needs in a building, either because it is securing room for future expansion or because it no longer needs space it formerly used. It subleases out the extra space but is forced to do so at a loss. Under Tax Reform rules, the loss on the sublease generally is a passive loss that is not deductible against ordinary business income. Opportunity: Under IRS regulations, a business deduction for the loss will be allowed if no more than 20% of the firm's leased space is subleased out.

Source: Steven M. Friedman, partner and director of Florida real estate tax services, Ernst & Young, 2700 One Biscayne Tower, Miami 33131. Mr. Friedman is principal author of *Acquiring Business Real Estate, Tax and Business Considerations for the International Investor*.

Why IRAs For Kids Make So Much Sense

For a child to make a direct tax-free contribution to an IRA and enjoy the benefits of compound interest, the money must come from earned income or wages.

That's why any entrepreneurial venture that yields income (paper routes, gardening, baby-sitting, etc.) is so prized. Even earnings from chores can be treated as earned income for the purpose of making IRA contributions.

By socking away $2,000 into an IRA early, kids can see the money multiply. The earlier it starts compounding, the bigger the payoff.

Example 1: A 15-year-old who puts away $2,000 a year into an IRA for just 10 years and makes no further contributions but lets the fund sit at an 8% annual rate, will have accumulated $659,756 by age 65. On the other hand, a 35-year-old who contributes $2,000 a year for the same 10 years and at the same 8% rate will have earned only $125,838 by age 65.

Example 2: A 15-year-old who starts saving just $2,000 at 8% every year will have $1.45 *million* pre-tax when it really counts—at retirement.

Source: Jay Goldinger, co-founder, Capital Insight, Inc., 190 N. Canon Dr., Beverly Hills 90210.

Chapter 18
Fighting The IRS

Corporate Self Defense And The IRS

A company that knows its rights needn't feel helpless when dealing with the IRS.

Here are some of the key taxpayer rights as stated in the Taxpayer Bill of Rights, the Tax Code and the IRS's own rules and regulations...

Audit Rights

Right to representation. IRS examining agents in the past have often insisted on talking to taxpayers personally, including the top executives and shareholders of corporations.

The Taxpayer Bill of Rights, however, clearly states that taxpayers have the right to representation. Top company personnel generally need not deal with IRS auditors personally if the company designates a tax professional to deal with the IRS, and the professional is able to supply the information required by the IRS to conduct the examination.

Advantage: Company managers inexperienced in tax matters are spared the inconvenience and anxiety that result from confronting an examiner personally. A professional representative can be of great assistance to the examination process, obtaining the pertinent information needed to assist the examiner.

If a company manager or owner happens to be personally involved in a tax matter that is under examination, he may be required to meet with the auditor. However, he retains the right to have professional representation at the meeting and, therefore, need not deal with the IRS without having expert advice at hand.

Convenient time and place. The IRS's Internal Revenue Manual instructs auditors to schedule an examination at a time and place convenient for the taxpayer, after allowing ample time for the taxpayer to collect necessary books and records. The company has the right to negotiate with the IRS about the time and place of an audit upon receiving the initial audit notice.

Strategy: Negotiate a site for the examination that will be expedient for both the corporation and the IRS. Items to be considered in making the decision include access to the individual who will represent the corporation, accessibility of books and records, and limiting disruption to the corporation.

The IRS does have the right to dictate the time and place of an audit if it concludes that the company is intentionally trying to stall or obstruct the examination. Important: Make reasonable requests and maintain a businesslike attitude.

Audit blueprint. If the examination is a large-company audit conducted under the IRS's Coordinated Examination Program (CEP), IRS manual instructions require that a written audit plan be prepared at the beginning of the audit. The audit plan covers such topics as where the audit takes place, procedures the IRS will follow to obtain records, progress dates and a projected completion date.

Written audit plans are not required of the IRS in non-CEP audits, but IRS agents are supposed to consult with the company being examined about the same planning subjects, and to agree to an informal audit plan, providing the company with much the same benefit. Again, the company should make its planning suggestions on the basis of expediting the audit and avoiding business interruptions.

Many taxpayers fail to avail themselves of this communication tool, even though it can provide significant benefits.

Document requests. The company has the right to have the IRS place its requests for company records in writing, by filing Information Document Requests (IDRs). Benefits...

■It creates a record of information requested.

■It allows for better understanding of information actually needed.

■Requests are more easily understood when made in writing.

■It facilitates the information-gathering process through the representative.

If the company feels that an examiner's IDRs are unreasonable (because they are vague, too broad or irrelevant), it can refuse to provide the requested documents. The IRS may then issue a summons for them, but to enforce the summons, it will have to go to court. There, a judge will provide an independent review of the legitimacy of the IRS's request.

See the auditor's boss. If the company is unhappy with the manner in which an agent is conducting an examination, it not only has the right to contact the auditor's superior (the group manager), but IRS policy actually encourages the company to do so.

Caution: The company may be reluctant to go to the auditor's boss for fear of personally antagonizing the auditor, thereby making the company's situation even worse.

To avoid this danger, don't approach the auditor's superior with general complaints about the auditor's personality or behavior. Instead, talk to the superior about specific decisions the auditor has made concerning the conduct of the examination, and explain how you disagree with them. By expressing your opinions in an impersonal, business-like manner, you give the superior the chance to correct the auditor's conduct without personalizing the dispute.

Point: Further dissatisfaction can be discussed with a second-level manager, the branch chief.

Getting the auditor's workpapers. If an examination results in a recommended tax assessment with which the company does not agree, the company has the right to obtain the workpapers prepared by the auditor to compute and explain the adjustments to the tax return as filed.

Of course, knowing how the IRS has computed a tax bill is a great advantage to the company—the examiner may not have understood how the company's business works and just made a mistake—yet many companies simply neglect to ask for the examiner's workpapers.

Most IRS districts follow the policy of making workpapers available to a taxpayer upon request. In the event that the IRS refuses to release them, perhaps claiming that they contain some sort of confidential information, the company can file a Freedom of Information Act request to obtain them. The request should result in the release of the relevant tax information with any confidential matter deleted.

Right to appeal. The company has a right to appeal any proposed tax assessment that results from audit, before going to court or paying a tax.

Resource: IRS Publication 5, *Appeal Rights and Preparation of Protests for Unagreed Cases*, available free from the IRS. It explains procedures for going to the IRS Appeals Division.

Certain figures show that about 88% of cases that go to the IRS Appeals Division end in a voluntary settlement between the taxpayer and the IRS. Unlike auditors, Appeals Officers consider not only the facts as they pertain to the law but also the hazards of litigation and the high cost of going to court when they review a case. Thus, they may present the company with its best chance for a negotiated settlement.

Heading Off Trouble

Of course, the best way to handle a tax problem is to prevent it from arising in the first place. One method, available to companies with assets over $10 million is to ask the IRS to come in and conduct a record-retention evaluation for the company.

This evaluation is not an audit. Rather, it is a cost-saving step.

How it works: IRS computer audit specialists (not tax examiners) will look at the company's computerized recordkeeping system, describe the records which might be required in a future examination, and also tell the company what records it need not keep.

Benefits: By cooperating with the IRS's computer audit specialists, the company may be able to develop a computerized record-keeping system that greatly reduces both the effort and cost involved in its record keeping system. For large companies, the savings can be impressive. At the same time, if the IRS says a company need not keep certain computer records as a result of its review, IRS examiners will be precluded from requesting those records in future tax examinations.

Although executives are naturally reluctant to invite the IRS onto their premises, the benefits of a machine-sensible record retention evaluation are so great that every large company should consider one. The company's tax adviser can get further details by referring to Revenue Procedure 86–19 which explains procedures to request an evaluation.

Source: Ronald Friedman, tax partner, and Donald H. Anderson, senior tax manager, national tax department, Ernst & Young, 1200 19 St. NW, Washington, DC 20036.

Audit Survival Tactics

Knowing how the system at the IRS works gives an experienced practitioner an advantage when it comes to representing a client at an audit. Here are some of the truly "inside" things that go on:

■Postponing Appointments: It is possible, though not likely, that the IRS will actually change its mind about auditing you if you have postponed the appointment enough times. The IRS is constantly under pressure to start and finish tax examinations. If the return selected for an audit becomes "old" (i.e., more than two years have passed since the return was filed), the IRS may not want to start the audit. This situation may develop if you are notified of an audit about 15 to 16 months after filing. By the time you have cancelled one or two appointments, the 24-month cut-off period may have been reached.

When is the best time to cancel? The day before the appointment. By that time, the next available appointment will probably not be for 6 to 8 weeks.

■Best Time to Schedule an Audit: To someone uninitiated, it may seem ridiculous that one time of the day or month is better than another to have your tax return audited. However, a real advantage can be gained by following some simple tips. Try to schedule an audit before a three-day weekend. The auditor may be less interested in the audit and more interested in the holiday. Another excellent time to schedule an appointment is at the end of the month. If an auditor has not "closed" enough cases that month, he or she may be inclined to go easy on you to gain a quick agreement and another closed case. As for the best time of the day, most pros like to start an audit at about 10 o'clock in the morning. By the time it comes to discussing adjustments with the auditor, it will be close to lunch time. If you are persistent, the auditor may be willing to make concessions just to get rid of you so as not to interfere with lunch plans.

Source: *How to Beat the IRS*, Ms. X, Esq., a former IRS agent, Boardroom Books, Springfield, NJ 07081.

What IRS Computers Look For

Tax returns are selected for examination by a combination of computer and human factors. It is possible to improve the odds slightly against having your tax return selected by doing what the tax pros do for their own clients. Be aware, though, that there is nobody around (at least nobody who is talking) who knows the IRS computer program used to determine whose tax return is a candidate for audit.

What is public knowledge about the computer side of the selection process is that the computer determines the likelihood of a particular tax return generating additional tax dollars, if it is examined, by using a scoring system known as the Discriminant Income Function (DIF). Each tax return processed by the computer is assigned a DIF score. The higher the score, the more likely the return will be audited. The formula used to arrive at the DIF score is updated on a regular basis with information gathered by IRS examiners. Data is compiled from the thousands of tax returns actually audited, and the highly guarded and secret DIF formula is then modified. No public information is available on the factors that go into the DIF scoring.

Another scoring factor used by the IRS computers is known as Total Positive Income (TPI). TPI is the sum of all positive income values appearing on a return, with losses treated as zero. The purpose of this system is to eliminate or minimize the use of Adjusted Gross Income as a factor in deciding the potential for additional tax dollars if a return is audited.

The IRS found that it was not getting a true reading of tax returns when it relied on Adjusted Gross Income. An Adjusted Gross Income of, say, $15,000 can represent either a salary of $15,000 or a salary of $150,000 with tax write-offs that bring the Adjusted Gross Income down to $15,000. High-income taxpayers are less likely to escape audit now that the IRS computers have a second method to check for high audit potential.

The human process of tax return selection is much less scientific but just as important. After a tax return has been identified by the computer as having audit potential, it is shipped to the district office and manually screened by the classification division. An IRS examiner assigned to the classification division gives most tax returns a quick "once over" to determine if the computer has made an obvious error in selecting it or if there is a special item to be brought to the attention of the examining agent ultimately assigned to the return.

If at this initial human level of contact there is adequate explanation or proof of a particular deduction attached to your return, the classifier may decide that an audit is not in order. For example, receipts attached to your tax return that prove property was donated to a charity may satisfy the classifier and eliminate the need for an audit to document the claims.

If your return reaches the classifier at the end of the day, he or she may be bleary-eyed and less concerned about what you reported, and the special attention that might have been given to a particular issue will not be given. When your return actually reaches the classifier is, of course, out of your control.

Know Average Deductions

Some tax professionals attach great importance to the latest statistics correlating deductions claimed with Adjusted Gross Income, in an effort to determine the degree of risk of an audit their clients face. The latest numbers released by the IRS concerning personal income tax returns reflect only average amounts. An assumption is made that the computers use average numbers to determine if your particular tax deductions are likely to be disallowed if they are higher than average.

Reduce Your Chances Of Being Audited

You may have the impression at this point in the discussion that the IRS computers are quite sophisticated and that it is virtually impossible to do anything legally to divert their eagle eye from your tax return. By and large this is true, but there are at least two things that may help minimize the effect of the IRS's high-tech capabilities.

First, how income is reported on the return may make a difference. Suppose you have freelance income. If it is merely reported as "Other Income" with an appropriate description as to its source, chances of having the return selected for audit may be smaller than if the same income is reported as business income on Schedule C (Income from a Sole Proprietorship).

Second, you can minimize your chances of being audited by filing as late as legally permissible. A tax return filed around April 15 generally has a greater chance of being audited than one filed on October 15 (the latest possible date). This is because the IRS schedules audits more than a year in advance. As returns are filed and scored by the computer, local IRS districts submit their forecasted requirements for returns with audit potential. The fulfillment is made from returns already on hand. If your return is filed on October 15, there is less risk that it will be among the returns shipped out to the district office in the first batch. As a result of scheduling and budget problems that are likely to develop in the two years after your return has been filed, it may never find its way into the second batch slated for examination.

Although the IRS is wise to this ploy and has taken steps to make sure that the selection process is as fair as possible, inequities invariably result. Why not try to be part of the group that has the smallest chance of being audited?

The best way to reduce your chances of being audited is to avoid certain items universally thought to trigger special IRS scrutiny. There are also some common-sense considerations that should be thought about before you mail in your return. They are often overlooked by the very people who can least afford to be the subject of an audit. Here are a few examples:

Some people who are in cash businesses are not content with merely skimming some of their income. They also want to get every possible tax deduction—which is where the potential for audit comes in. When a business owner reports only a modest income, the IRS naturally becomes suspicious if that person also claims many business expenses and has high interest expense deductions. Two immediate questions are raised in the mind of the IRS examiner: Where does this person get money for personal living expenses and how is he or she able to make the principal repayments to justify the interest expense? When you are preparing your return, step back and think like an IRS auditor. If you can spot questions, so can the IRS.

What else can be done to minimize the chances of being audited? The following items should be reviewed carefully:

■Choose your return preparer carefully. When the IRS suspects return preparers of incompetence or misconduct, it can force them to produce a list of all their clients—all of whom may face further IRS examination, regardless of their personal honesty.

■Avoid formal membership in barter clubs. Members of these clubs trade goods and services on a cashless basis. The club keeps track of all transactions between members. Although no cash changes hands, these trades are taxable like any other profitable deal. Very often, however, they are not reported to the IRS. The IRS can force such clubs to produce membership lists, so that the returns of all club members can be examined.

■Answer all questions on the return. IRS computers generally flag returns with unanswered questions. For example, there is a question asking if you maintain funds in a foreign bank account. Even if you do not, you should answer no to the question.

■Fill in the return carefully. A sloppy return may indicate a careless taxpayer. The IRS may examine the return to be sure the carelessness did not lead to any mistakes.

■Categorize each deduction. Don't place deductions under headings such as miscellaneous or sundry. If you can't categorize a deduction, the IRS may decide you can't prove it.

■Avoid round numbers. A deduction that's rounded off to the nearest hundred or thousand dollars will raise IRS suspicions. The IRS will think the taxpayer is guessing at the deduction's size rather than determining it from accurate records.

Source: *How to Beat the IRS* by Ms. X, Esq., a former IRS agent, Boardroom Classics, Springfield, NJ 07081.

The IRS Hit List

Doctors and dentists are high-priority targets for tax audit. Items IRS agents look for: Dubious promotional expenses. If the same four people take turns having lunch together once a week and take turns picking up the tab, a close examination of diaries and logbooks will show this. Agents also take a close look at limited partnership investments, seeking signs of abusive tax shelters. And they take a dim view of fellowship exclusions claimed by medical residents. Other target occupations:

■Salespeople: Outside and auto salespeople are particular favorites. Agents look for, and often find, poorly documented travel expenses and padded promotional figures.

■Airline pilots: High incomes, a propensity to invest in questionable tax shelters, and commuting expenses claimed as business travel make them inviting prospects.

■Flight attendants: Travel expenses are usually a high percentage of their total income and often aren't well documented. Some persist in trying to deduct pantyhose, permanents, cosmetics, and similar items that the courts have repeatedly ruled are personal rather than business expenses.

■Executives: As a group they are not usually singled out. But if the return includes a Form 2106, showing a sizable sum for unreimbursed employee business expenses, an audit is more likely. Of course, anyone whose income is over $50,000 a year is a high-priority target just because of the sums involved.

■Teachers and college professors: Agents pounce on returns claiming office-at-home deductions. They are also wary of educational expense deductions because they may turn out to be vacations in disguise.

■Clergymen: Bona fide priests, ministers, and rabbis aren't considered a problem group. But if W-2s show income from nonchurch employers, the IRS will be on the alert for mail-order ministry scams.

■Waitresses, cabdrivers, etc.: Anyone in an occupation where tips are a significant factor is likely to get a closer look from the IRS nowadays.

Many people, aware their profession subjects them to IRS scrutiny, use nebulous terms to describe what they do. Professionals in private practice may list themselves as simply "self-employed." Waitresses become "culinary employees," pilots list themselves as "transportation executives." But there's a fine line here. Truly deceptive descriptions could trigger penalties. And if the return is chosen for audit, an unorthodox job title for a mundane profession could convince the agent you have something to hide. Then he'll dig all the deeper.

Source: Ralph J. Pribble, a former IRS field agent, president of Tax Corporation of California, 5420 Geary Blvd., San Francisco 94121.

What Are Your Chances Of An IRS Audit?

The IRS audits far fewer returns than most people suspect. The percentage of personal returns subject to audit has been declining for years. And the percentage of audited business returns has decreased more dramatically. The latest audit facts and figures:

■Individual returns. An individual's audit risk depends on the total positive income reported on his tax return—that's the amount of income reported before deductions and losses are subtracted. Latest audit-risk figures:

Total positive income	% audited	
$10,000 to $25,000 (with itemized deductions)	1.30%	
$10,000 to $25,000 (without itemized deductions)	.64	
$25,000 to $50,000	1.40	
Over $50,000	2.24	

■Business returns. For business owners, incorporation helps. Small and medium-sized businesses that are run as corporations are audited less frequently than similar-sized businesses that are operated as proprietorships or partnerships. Comparisons:

Noncorporate business income—Schedule C	% audited	
	1987	1986
Under $25,000	1.41%	1.34%
$25,000 to $100,000	2.01	2.27
Over $100,000	3.86	4.47
Corporations (assets)	% audited	
	1987	1986
Under $100,000	.67%	1.07%

$100,000 to $1 million	1.16	1.74
$1 million to $10 million	4.10	6.19
$10 million to $100 million	22.92	29.99
Over $100 million	69.08	74.51

Source: Irving L. Blackman is a partner with Blackman, Kallick Bartelstein, 300 South River-side Plaza, Chicago 60606.

A Winning Presentation

A winning presentation goes a long way toward convincing an IRS agent that your position has merit even though the facts are weak. Example: You took a deduction for home entertainment, but you don't have any receipts to prove it. Your presentation at the audit might include the following: A guest list showing the business relationship of each guest. Affidavits from guests stating what you served at the party and how many people were present. A caterer's written estimate of the cost of serving that number of people. Photographs taken of the affair.

Source: Ms. X, a former IRS agent, who is still well connected.

Accountant-Client Conversations

Be careful what you say to your accountant…if you have something to hide. Suppose that for years you consistently neglected to tell your accountant about a certain source of income. If you now tell the accountant about it, he can be called on by the government to testify against you in court, since accountant-client communications aren't privileged. But conversations you have with an attorney are privileged. An attorney can't be compelled to testify against a client who has admitted that he committed a crime. Best advice for someone in this position: Hire an attorney, who can then hire the accountant and include him under his umbrella of privilege.

Source: Ms. X, a former IRS agent, who is still well connected.

Not-So-Private Returns

New rules enable the IRS to hire outside contractors to process tax return information for it. The new rules state that providing tax return information to the outside companies will not violate taxpayer confidentiality.

Source: *Regulation 301.6103(n)-1, amended.*

Hide Assets From The IRS—Legally

Many people keep assets in a safe-deposit box thinking that no one will ever find out about it. But the name of the renter of a safe-deposit box isn't kept secret. It doesn't help to rent a box in your own name; there's an organization that, for less than $100, will run a search of every bank in the country to see if you are a safe-deposit box customer. And the IRS, if it's looking for assets of yours, will do a bank search for safe-deposit boxes held in your name. (It's especially easy for the IRS to track down boxes that you pay for with a personal check…it simply goes through your canceled checks.)

To conceal the existence of a safe-deposit box:

■Ask your lawyer to set up a nominee corporation—a corporation that has no other function but to stand in your place for the purposes you designate, such as to rent a safe-deposit box.

■Rent a box in the name of the corporation and pay for it in cash. Your name and signature will be on the bank signature card, but the corporation, not you, will be listed as the box's owner on the bank's records. And because you paid cash, there will be nothing in your records to connect the box with you.

■You can, if you want, name another person as signatory in addition to yourself. Then, if something happens to you, that person will be able to get into the box.

Additional protection: Having a safe-deposit box in a corporation's name permits the box to be opened by your survivors without the state's or the bank's being notified of your death and having the box sealed. Otherwise, the survivor must get to the box before the funeral to look for a will and to find whatever else may be there.

Source: Edward Mendlowitz, partner, Mendlowitz Weitsen, CPAs, New York 10001.

Negligence Or Tax Fraud?

Failure to report income deposited in a bank could be considered careless. Carelessness is punishable, generally, by a 5% negligence penalty. But when the omitted income represented deposits made in a bank in a different state, one court regarded the omission as a fraudulent, willful attempt to conceal income.

Source: *Candella et al. v. United States*, USDC, E. Dist. WI.

Your Company Vs. The IRS

If the IRS says your company owes more taxes, don't despair. Smart planning can get the company extra chances to settle or win its tax dispute outright—without going to court. An IRS field agent, for example, has come to the company's office, finished an examination of the books and decided that a large extra tax bill is due.

The next move depends on how strong your case is.

If the company's position is clearly correct and that the agent was incompetent, unreasonable or unfair, ask for a second opinion from the agent's supervisor.

An IRS field agent is required to provide the name and phone number of his supervisor upon a taxpayer's request. The supervisor will meet with the taxpayer and field agent to review an agent's decisions.

Trap: Since supervisors are more experienced than field agents, they're also likely to catch taxpayer mistakes that the field agent missed. So don't use this tactic unless you're sure that the company has filed a clean return.

If there's a genuine disagreement as to how the law should apply and your opinion differs from the agent's, ask the agent to write to the IRS National Office for technical advice.

The procedure is fairly simple. You prepare a letter explaining the facts and the law as you think it should apply—and prepare a statement of the ruling you desire. The field agent does the same. The experts in the National Office will then examine the matter and issue a ruling, which will be binding on the agent but which you can still appeal.

If a field agent refuses to ask for technical advice, you can go over his head to the chief of the examination division for your IRS district and ask him to request technical advice.

If the chief doesn't think technical advice is warranted, he can refuse to ask for it, but he must refer your request to the National Office anyway. The IRS National Office reviews all such requests on its own, and the record clearly shows that, when appropriate, it will issue pro-taxpayer technical advice even when IRS field-level and district-level personnel have recommended against it.

Useful strategies if you don't get the desired result from the above...

■Let someone else fight the case. If you think some other company is likely to fight the IRS on the matter, it might be smart to wait and let the other company pay all the relevant legal costs. If the other firm wins, you can file for a refund using its case as a precedent. If it loses, you'll see that you'd probably have lost, too. Either way, you save on legal bills.

How to do it: At the end of the examination the IRS auditor will inform you of the tax adjustment that he is proposing. Instead of appealing his decision, agree to pay the tax and sign Form 870, Waiver of Restrictions on Assessments and Collection of Deficiency, or the "consent" at the bottom of Form 4549. Don't let the way the IRS describes this form fool you—by signing, you are not agreeing that you owe the tax, even though the IRS and some practitioners call it an agreement.

After signing this form you have two years in which to file a claim to cover the tax paid on the assessment, and after filing the claim you have another two years to file a refund suit in District Court. So you effectively get four years in which another taxpayer can win your case for you.

Advantages and disadvantages of the strategy: You have to pay the disputed tax up front. But if you ultimately win a refund, you will get the tax back plus interest. By contrast, if you avoided paying tax by going to Tax Court but then lost, you would wind up paying the tax, plus interest and lawyers' fees.

■Delay the tax. If you want to fight your own fight and delay the payment of tax, the next step is to get an appellate conference with an IRS appeals officer. At the end of the audit process, the IRS will send you a 30-day letter explaining the auditor's proposed adjustment to your tax bill. If you want to appeal the results of the audit, you must answer this letter within 30 days, protesting the proposed adjustment.

Appeals are good: The IRS will then schedule a meeting for you with an appeals officer—probably in about six months' time. Benefit: Appeals officers have a different attitude than auditors. Their job is to resolve cases quickly; they have the authority to compromise on issues where auditors can't.

When an appeals officer considers your case, he thinks not only of its merits but also of the cost in terms of a bad precedent for the IRS of losing the case in court, the likelihood of your winning, and the relative importance of your case to other cases that the IRS is pursuing. For example, appeals have an objective of securing an 85% agreement rate in cases involving less than $100,000. The officer may be willing to "split the difference" on an unclear issue, or to trade a concession on one issue for a concession from you on another.

Source: Interview with Walter T. Coppinger, partner and special consultant in tax practice and procedure, Ernst & Young, 2121 San Jacinto St., Dallas 75201.

Loopholes In Dealing With IRS Collectors

The collection of unpaid taxes is handled by the IRS's collection division, which has broad powers—including the power to seize property for non-payment of taxes.

Best strategy: Pay your tax bill voluntarily before the IRS threatens you…but for those who can't pay in full, here's useful advice…

There are two main categories of IRS collection personnel—revenue reps and revenue officers.

Revenue reps: Handle correspondence and phone calls. Revenue reps are the people who make the first contact on delinquent tax bills. They are usually very inexperienced. They have no power to modify a bill. Their primary function is to locate a source of funds that can be impounded for payment of taxes.

Revenue officers: Professionals in the collection division. They have a considerable amount of authority. They can recommend abatement of penalties and negotiate installment payments of a tax bill.

Strategy: If you're planning to do any negotiating about your tax bill, you're best off dealing with a revenue officer. Don't say anything to a revenue rep about your finances. Request that your case be transferred to a revenue officer. This isn't easily accomplished, but if you're completely uncooperative with the revenue rep, your case ultimately will be transferred to a revenue officer.

If the revenue rep refuses to transfer the case, ask to speak to his supervisor or manager.

Loophole: Always ask that the revenue officer recommend the abatement of penalties that have been assessed against you. In cases where the delinquency in taxes is a single isolated instance, and not a pattern of behavior, and the taxpayer comes up with a good excuse for falling behind, penalties are usually abated.

Telephone tactic: An IRS notice demanding payment may give you a telephone number to call if you have any questions. When you call, you'll be asked to give your name, Social Security number, and an explanation of the problem you're having. If the person you're talking to is uncooperative or unsympathetic, terminate the call and try again. Excuse yourself politely by saying, for example, "I've got to speak to my accountant." Then call back.

Loophole: You'll get a different person each time you call. Calls are assigned to a group of IRS employees in sequence. Keep trying until you find an employee who seems sympathetic to your problem.

The collection people will not speak to a representative of yours unless that person has a power of attorney—IRS Form 2848. The minute you get a notice of delinquent taxes, write to the IRS saying you are in the process of granting power of attorney to your representative and ask if they will hold off on taking any action for 30 days. This generally is effective.

Caution: Don't assume the IRS has received your letter. Follow up with a phone call. Get the name of the person handling your case and send a copy of your letter directly to that person.

Once you've given a power of attorney to your representative, don't talk to anyone in the collection division. Refer all calls and letters to your representative. Keep copies of the power of attorney so that you have one to send in if someone from the collection division contacts you directly.

If you owe back taxes that you genuinely can't pay, the IRS will usually work out an installment arrangement with you. This generally requires taxes to be paid within six months.

A payment period of longer than six months can be granted only by a revenue officer. To get it, you are required to submit financial statements showing that you will have the ability to pay within the stated period.

Caution: If a revenue officer feels you're not being cooperative and are withholding financial information, he will attempt to seize assets, levy your bank accounts, or garnish your salary. So, don't withhold information.

If you have assets of value, they'll want you to borrow against them or show that you tried to borrow, but couldn't.

If you owe payroll taxes from a business, the collection personnel's instructions are to use any methods to stop the continuing accrual of tax liability. What this means, in most cases, is to liquidate the business…and use the proceeds to pay off the back taxes.

Loophole: Pay current payroll taxes first, before back taxes. The collection division will be less inclined to close your business if you keep up to date on current payroll taxes.

Source: Edward Mendlowitz, partner, Mendlowitz Weitsen, CPAs, Two Pennsylvania Plaza, New York 10121. Mr. Mendlowitz is the author of several books, including *New Tax Traps/New Opportunities*, Boardroom Books, Springfield, New Jersey 07081. Another one of his books is *Aggressive Tax Strategies*, Macmillan, 866 Third Ave., New York 10022.

Tax Laws And Avoidance Strategies

Here's what companies need to know to plan ahead…

Good News And Opportunities

■The 1990 Tax Act renewed for 1991 several business tax credits and benefits that had expired under old law. Credits:

■Targeted jobs credit. Up to $2,400 (40% of the first $6,000 of wages) for each employee hired from one of a number of designated economically disadvantaged groups.

■The research and experimentation credit. This generally amounts to a percentage of a company's increase in its expenditures for technological research related to product development or improvement. Benefits:

■Educational benefits for employees. The company may provide up to $5,250 per year tax-free to an employee to cover the cost of tuition, books, fees and similar items. And support can now be provided for graduate study. (Old law allowed support only for undergraduate students.)

■Group legal plans for employees. The exclusion from employees' income for this benefit expired on October 1, 1990, but has been extended through tax years beginning in 1991.

Note: The above tax breaks are currently on hold, waiting for Congress to extend them.

■Filing break. Affiliated companies often can benefit by filing a tax return as a consolidated group—for example, the losses of one company can then be used to offset the taxable income of another.

Catch: The companies in a consolidated group must have 80% common ownership. If the common-ownership level of a company falls below 80%, that company ceases to be a member of the group and can't rejoin it for five years without receiving IRS permission.

The IRS has just announced new procedures under which it will automatically grant a company permission to rejoin a consolidated group within the five-year period. This can provide a great benefit to companies that were forced out of a group in recent years. For details, see IRS Revenue Procedure 90-53.

■Private company break. The 1990 Tax Act gives owners of private companies more freedom in planning for estate taxes that will be due on the value of the business when they die.

Background: Company owners for many years practiced "estate freezes." In a typical freeze, an owner would recapitalize the company so it would have both common and preferred stock. The common stock would be given to the owner's children. It would have little value, but all future growth in the company's value would accrue to it. The owner would keep the preferred stock, which would have a high, but fixed, value and pay cash dividends. Thus, the owner would secure income while shifting future value in the business to his children, free of estate tax.

In 1987, Congress passed tough anti-estate freeze rules, effectively eliminating them as a tax-planning device. But in the 1990 Tax Act, it repealed the rules and established new guidelines which, if followed, allow estate freezes to be accomplished.

Business owners should consult with their tax advisers on how to use the new rules to eliminate the threat to the business which estate taxes may pose.

Dangers

■Consumer packaging costs. A new trap faces companies with consumer products for which they have incurred the cost of developing and modifying packaging designs. Almost all companies deducted the cost of developing packaging as a normal business expense. But the IRS now says that the cost of developing a package design for a product cannot be deducted at once. It must be deducted at an even rate over the period during which the product will be in use, or, if certain conditions are met, over a period of four or five years. The new rule applies retroactively to tax years beginning after 1986.

Impact: All businesses which have deducted consumer packaging costs in the past must file IRS Form 3115, Change of Accounting Method, to come into compliance with the new rules. Any costs that were previously deducted and related to package designs still on-hand at the beginning of the year of change must be added back into income for that year. Danger: Many firms may be completely unaware of this requirement.

For details concerning the new packaging design accounting rules, see IRS Revenue Procedure 90-63.

■S corporation trap. A requirement imposed on all S corporations is that they have only one class of stock. Danger: Newly proposed IRS regulations threaten the tax status of many S corporations by treating them as if they had more than one class of stock, even when only one class of stock has been formally issued. Under the rules, shareholders who are treated differently by the company may be deemed to own different types of stock. Examples:

■A shareholder/executive receives excess salary from the company. The excess compensation is treated as an extra dividend, creating a second class of stock.

■A shareholder takes a loan from the company at below-market rates. Again, the financial benefit is an extra dividend creating a second class of stock.

■Shareholders take the same cash distribution from the company, but at different times of the year.

Danger: A company may inadvertently find its status as an S corporation endangered. Have the firm's tax adviser review its situation in light of the proposed regulations to avert this risk.

■The AMT. Companies not alerted to changes in the way the Alternative Minimum Tax (AMT) is computed may be surprised with a higher tax bill than they expected.

Why: The AMT is an extra tax computation designed to keep firms with high operating profits from eliminating their tax bills through the use of tax credits, accounting methods such as accelerated depreciation, and similar devices.

A company must separately compute its tax under both regular income tax rules and AMT rules, and pay the higher tax that results. Trap: If the company falls under the AMT, many of its normal tax-planning strategies will lose their value.

Before 1990, companies had to add back into income for AMT purposes an amount equal to 50% of the difference between alternative minimum taxable income (taxable income increased by adjustments and tax preference items)…and book income (as reported on financial statements).

For 1990 and later, the adjustment is based on 75% of the difference between alternative minimum taxable income and Adjusted Current Earnings (ACE).

ACE is not based on financial statement income, but on complicated accounting concepts of "earnings and profits" and statutory adjustments. The rules are complex, but ACE is likely to be incurred when a company has large amounts of depreciation deductions relative to income…and/or income from long-term contracts…and/or net operating losses…and/or intangible drilling or percentage depletion costs…and/or a large amount of proceeds from life insurance (perhaps from a key man policy).

Key: Companies planning ahead should project their AMT position for the full year ahead and take steps to avoid an unexpected tax bill.

■Customer lists. Through a Coordinated Issue Paper, the IRS has instructed its agents to closely examine company deductions for intangible assets—especially customer lists.

Danger: IRS auditors often argue that a business (such as a magazine, cable television system or mail order firm) would not exist without its customer list, so the cost of acquiring the list must be a nondeductible cost of being in business.

Defense: Show that the company's list has both a clearly defined cost and a limited useful life. Appraisals should be done to determine how much it costs to gain new customers, and how often the customer list turns over. The courts have repeatedly held that companies can deduct the cost of a customer list over its demonstrated useful life.

■Interest rate trap. The 1990 Tax Act increases by two percentage points the interest rate that corporations must pay on tax deficiencies exceeding $100,000. The object is to raise revenue and put extra pressure on companies to settle tax disputes with the IRS, by increasing the amount of interest a company has to pay if it contests a tax assessment and loses its case at the IRS Appeals division or in Tax Court.

Companies should consider the potentially higher cost of prolonging a dispute with the IRS.

Source: James M. Ward, tax partner, KPMG Peat Marwick, 345 Park Ave., New York 10154.

Advertising Expenses Aren't Always Deductible

Advertising is such an ordinary and necessary business expense, it's easy to believe that all such spending is tax-deductible. Not always the case. When the deduction can be denied:

■Costs are excessive in terms of expected benefit.

■The advertiser isn't actually soliciting orders, because he has nothing to sell. Examples: 1. All of the company's capacity is committed to government contracts. 2. No inventory is available because of strikes, lack of raw materials, etc.

■The advertiser isn't yet in the business that he is advertising. Deduction for pre-business expenses must be spread out over the first five years a firm is in business.

■The advertising is in the nature of a penalty. Example: A governmental regulatory agency orders a manufacturer to run advertisements that correct misstatements in previous advertising.

■Advertising that attempts to influence legislation.

■Advertising expenditures of another corporation. Example: The parent company pays for ads of products that actually are sold only by subsidiary companies.

Source: *The Book of Business Knowledge*, Boardroom Books, Springfield, NJ 07081.

Justifying Tax Deductions For Executive Salaries

A successful IRS challenge to the reasonableness of executive compensation hurts both the corporation (which loses the tax deduction) and the executives (who probably then have a hard time justifying any further increases).

■Each executive should be responsible for proving the extent and value of his services to the company. Keep track of little-publicized improvements, cost-cutting, salary offers from other companies.

■When an individual serves as an executive of two or more related companies, how much any one corporation can deduct as reasonable compensation for such a person must be established by credible records. Otherwise the Internal Revenue Service will decide how much each company can deduct.

If the companies are all 80% subsidiaries of a common parent, under most circumstances a consolidated federal income tax return may be filed. Then it doesn't matter how much each company deducts as long as the total for all companies is reasonable.

But consolidated returns can't be filed by brother-sister corporations (where the same individuals own substantially the same proportion of each related company).

■Good strategy is an agreement that requires the executive to repay any amount disallowed the corporation as a tax deduction because it was excessive. He can then be paid a very generous salary without fear of tax loss to the corporation.

Justifying High Salaries When Company Is Losing Money

An executive is paid to make money for his company. If the corporation loses money, is he really worth his princely salary?

The Internal Revenue Service used that logic to throw out part of a president's salary as unreasonable in a year when a company experienced the loss that resulted from shutting down its manufacturing operations during an essential relocation of the plant. (Poor plant layout and inadequate space had resulted in costly and cumbersome operations.) The move, for which the president was largely responsible, laid a foundation for the highly profitable years which had been logged by the time the case reached court. Verdict: Deduction of the full salary was allowed in that loss year.

Source: *Roux Laboratories v. U.S.*, D.C., M.D., FL.

When Supper Money Is Taxable Income

Supper money paid in cash to late-working employees is not taxable to employees. But it is taxable to business proprietors, partners, and officers who are major stockholders of corporations. (No tax, though, to either employees or owners, if meals are served at work premises and are paid for directly by the company. That's different from making cash payments so that employees can eat elsewhere.)

Source: *Antos v. Comm'r.*, TC Memo 1976–89, affd. CA-9, 2/24/78.

Tax Rules On Deferred Compensation

■Compensation can be deferred to retirement, to any specified year, or spread over a number of years.

■It will be taxed as income (and deductible by the company) only when actually paid.

■Agreement can provide for payment sooner under specified conditions. Examples: It can be payable immediately if the executive becomes disabled, or to his beneficiaries on death.

■Deferred tax treatment does not depend on pay being subject to conditions, such as being forfeited or reduced if the executive leaves the company. But such a provision is okay if the company asks for it and the executive agrees.

■Compensation can't be put into escrow or a special account subject to control of the executive. The company can establish a reserve or buy insurance, but funds must remain part of general company assets.

■Deferred compensation arrangements are allowed for owner-officers of closely held companies. But they are still subject to IRS scrutiny as to whether total compensation for the year (including both paid and deferred) is excessive.

The executive cannot say to the company, "Don't pay me now, I'll let you know when I want it." That's called constructive receipt and makes the amount taxable immediately.

Important to consider:

■Money paid in later years will probably be worth less because of inflation.

■Do not assume that your income tax bracket will be lower after retirement. Executives now in the top tax bracket could be in the same bracket then if they have substantial income from investments.

How Deducting Bad Debts Can Misfire

Seven mistakes the IRS is waiting for you to make:

1. A bad debt is not deductible if there was no reasonable prospect of payment when it was contracted—for instance if sale was made to an insolvent party.

2. The bad debt must be legally enforceable. No tax deduction is allowed, for instance, if interest is charged in excess of state's maximum rates.

3. No tax deduction is allowed for unpaid bills unless the taxpayer is on an accrual basis and the debt was reported as income in the same year or the previous year.

4. It is not enough that the debt has not been paid. The account must also be uncollectable because of the debtor's financial inability to make the payment.

5. There is no deduction unless creditor can cite an "identifiable event" that made the debt worthless. Some examples: Debtor's bankruptcy; his balance sheet showing no possibility of equity for credits; destruction of debtor's plant by uninsured casualty; newspaper report that debtor has lost a government contract accounting for 80% of revenues; death or permanent incapacity of debtor's one truly indispensable presiding officer.

6. Debt is deductible only in the taxable year when the identifiable event took place. A company that does not hound its debtors mercilessly may not discover the worthlessness of the debt until it's too late for the company to get a tax deduction.

7. Only business bad debts are fully deductible. Nonbusiness bad debts are considered to be short-term capital losses. Business bad debt must be connected with either the taxpayer's trade or business, but not with the taxpayer's outside investments.

Here is how taxpayers can deduct partial bad debts:

Most taxpayers don't seem to know this privilege exists. An example of when you can use it: A credit agency or certified public accountant with particular expertise in the matter concludes that chances of collecting on this debt are only 60%. If properly documented for a particular debt (not total receivables), this could justify deducting 40% of the account as a partial bad debt. But no tax deduction is allowed if the credit was extended to the debtor after the debt became partially worthless.

Even Faster Depreciation For Some Companies

The accelerated cost recovery system (ACRS) allows most businesses to claim generous depreciation deductions according to fixed schedules. But capital-intensive companies that must replace assets frequently may be able to obtain even larger deductions by using the unit-of-production depreciation method. Promising candidates: forest-product companies, mines, oil producers.

How it works: Take the cost of the new productive asset and subtract the salvage value that the asset will have at the end of its useful life. Divide this net cost by the number of units the asset is expected to produce. This simple calculation results in the depreciation cost of each unit of production. The annual depreciation deduction is computed by multiplying this unit cost by the number of units produced during the year.

Advantages: The unit-of-production method provides even faster depreciation deductions than are available under ACRS when the company uses up its productive assets quickly. It also matches deductions more closely to operating profits that result from use of the assets.

Alternative: Consider the operating-day depreciation method. The net cost of the asset divided by the number of days it will be in use. The annual deduction is determined by multiplying the per-day cost by the number of days the asset was used during the year.

Source: Dr. Robert Holzman professor emeritus of taxation at New York University and the author of *Encyclopedia of Estate Planning*, Boardroom Books, Springfield, NJ 07081.

Deducting For Premature Obsolescence

Extra depreciation deductions are possible when assets become obsolete before the end of their normal lives. Write off all the remaining cost in one year by proving that the assets are out of date and continuing to use them would put the company at a competitive disadvantage. But it isn't enough to show that there's something newer, better, or cheaper on the market. The company must prove that the facility was abandoned because continuing use would hurt its competitive position.

Source: *Fort Howard Paper v. Comm'r.*, TC Memo, 1977-422, 12/14/77.

When Local Taxes Are Not Deductible

With the passage of California's Proposition 13, and fears of taxpayer revolts elsewhere, some cities are increasing revenues by imposing new taxes but calling them something else. For example: To pay for a new water system, one city hit taxpayers with a "front door benefit charge," covering the cost of building the new water system, plus interest on money borrowed for construction, plus the cost of maintaining the new system.

The problem: "Local benefit taxes" are not deductible on IRS returns, because the revenues raised to pay for new water lines or curbs or other local improvements increase the value of taxpayer's property. One exception: Local benefits taxes assessed to pay for more than physical improvements. In the case of the city's "front door benefit charge," the portion of that local tax covering interest payments and maintenance costs was deductible on IRS returns.

What taxpayers should do: Insist that cities furnish them with a breakdown on exactly how all local benefits tax revenues are used.

Source: Revenue Ruling 79-201.

When A Minor Child Works For A Family Business

A favorite tax-planning tactic is to have a minor child work for the family-owned business. The first $3,000 earned by the child is tax-free, and further income is taxed at very low rates. In addition, the company gets a deduction for the child's salary. Now, a dramatic taxpayer victory shows just how effective this tactic can be.

The facts: The taxpayers owned a mobile home park and hired their three children, aged 7, 11 and 12, to work there. The children cleaned the grounds, did landscaping work, maintained the swimming pool, answered phones, and did minor repair work. The taxpayers deducted over $17,000 that they paid to the children during a three-year period. But the IRS objected, and the case went to trial. Court's decision: Over $15,000 of the deductions were approved. Most of the deductions that were disallowed were attributable to the 7-year-old. But even $4,000 of his earnings were approved by the court.

Key: The children actually performed the work for which they were paid. And the work was necessary for the business. The taxpayers demonstrated that if their children had not done the work, they would have had to hire someone else to do it.

The case: *Walt. Eller,* 77 T.C. No. 66.

Source: Irving Blackman, a partner, Blackman Kallick Bartelstein, CPAs, Chicago 60601.

Tax Traps When Buying Or Selling A Business

Watch out for the tax consequences of good will (the part of the price paid for a going business that exceeds the net fair market value of the tangible business assets).

Problem: The Internal Revenue Service does not recognize good will as a deductible expense.

Solution: If the excess can be termed part of "a covenant not to compete," it's completely deductible (to be amortized over the period of the agreement).

Seller's interest is the reverse. Adjust the purchase price to even out net after-tax effects. And don't forget that an installment deal reduces the seller's tax burden by spreading it over several years.

Avoid IRS problems by specifying exactly what both sides want in the sale contract. IRS generally will go along. Such contracts normally provide some form of noncompetitive covenant.

Make sure the contract also spells out allocation of other components of the price. Don't allocate more to depreciable property (trucks, machinery, etc.) than fair market value. That part of transaction may require payment of sales taxes. Allocation to the covenant is probably the simplest, clearest, and quickest way to get maximum deduction.

Alternative: Where customer service contracts are transferred, good will can apply on a per-item basis to the individual contracts. As contracts are terminated, this cost can be deducted. It can take longer than a covenant to get deductions, but still provides a way to write off the good will cost.

Another cost: Leasehold purchase. Used when a specific site, such as a retail store, carries the good will. Purchase price should allocate good will cost to purchase of leasehold. Then cost can be amortized over the life of the lease, since the asset's value falls to nothing at termination.

Important: Unnecessary inclusion of covenant not to compete, as when seller is retiring, can transform part of the proceeds of sale from capital gains into ordinary income. IRS reasoning: The covenant is deemed to be worth something to the seller, but what he's selling (i.e., his right to compete with the buyer) isn't a capital asset. So whatever portion of the sales price is allocable to the covenant isn't a capital gain. The Court of Claims agreed.

Source: *Proulx v. U.S.*, 594 F.2d 832, Ct. Cl. 2/21/79.

Selling A Company For Cash Without A Big Tax

There comes a time in the life of many closely held corporations, and even some publicly held ones, when the controlling shareholders begin to feel locked into their investments. They would like to cash in without having to pay to the tax collector on the appreciated value of the company they built up. Here is a tax-wise way to achieve this goal.

What kind of company would be a candidate for this tax-saving idea? It must be:
■A healthy one with good earning prospects.
■One that is controlled by a few shareholders.
■One whose stock is undervalued in the marketplace.

The procedure: The corporation agrees to sell all the assets (factory, machinery, customer lists, good will, etc.) and the liabilities of the company for cash. The sale price for the assets must be lower than their tax basis (original cost minus depreciation). That produces a tax loss for the sellers, which is guaranteed by the buyers. With the tax loss in hand, the sellers will give the buyer some price concession.

Note that the stock hasn't changed hands. The shareholders have sold only the assets. They keep their stock in a corporation that has no assets except cash.

Now, with that hard cash, the corporation converts into an investment firm. It buys a diversified portfolio with the cash—anything from stock or real estate to other companies.

Potential problems: The selling company becomes a personal holding company. It must distribute its earnings at least annually or face a heavy personal holding company penalty tax.

■There is also the problem of double taxation—income taxed once at the corporate level and again when distributed to shareholders as dividends. The personal holding company status makes distributions mandatory, precluding the use of the corporation as a tax shelter.

Ways to minimize the dual taxation problem: Use of the 85% dividends-received exclusion by the corporation, which should invest in tax-free securities, or low-dividend-paying growth stocks.

■The buyer's guarantee of a tax loss also creates a potential problem. The seller could be viewed as increasing the sales price and thus reducing the anticipated loss. And payment of the guarantee would appear to be taxable income.

The model for this technique will be found in the Big Bear Stores Co. proxy statement dated July 24, 1976, on file with Amex and the SEC. The technique has also been used with unlisted, closely held companies, although there is a more difficult problem in determining the value of the company.

Acquisitions: Cash Versus Stock

Cash deals are subject to capital gains tax when the cash is received by the seller. But though cash deals are taxable, they are best when there are doubts about the buyer's solvency—or when the stock doesn't suit seller's investment criteria or estate planning.

Minimize taxes by treating the deal as an installment sale.

■Business risk. Will the buyer be able to pay? In an installment deal, the seller is just as tied to the fortunes of the buyer as if he had taken stock instead of cash.

■Purchasing-power risk. Present value of $1 million is much more than the same amount paid out over 10 years. The seller should keep in mind the net amount he will sell for, discount future dollars, and negotiate from that position. The new original issue discount rules could also apply, making more of the annual payments taxable as ordinary income.

For the buyer, paying cash is more expensive than issuing treasury stock or new preferred, but it can have advantages:

■When companies are nearly equal in size and a stock deal would dilute the buyer's control of company.

■If the buyer wants the tax advantages that stem from being able to take depreciation on a larger sum (the cash payment) than on the seller's tax basis (usually below the selling price). The buyer can do this only when there is an all-cash deal.

The seller should take stock only when the stock of the acquiring company is an attractive investment on its own merits. Advantages of a stock deal:

■Defers tax liability. Can shift it to the next generation if the stock is left to seller's heirs.

Installment-sale strategy in stock deals: Also takes advantage of any future easing of capital gains taxes. Seller has much more flexibility than with a cash deal on what to sell and when. Disadvantage: Vulnerability to vagaries of the stock market.

When buyer should use stock:

■To conserve cash.

■When company stock is selling at a high price/earnings multiple.

■For the seller: Cash is taxable when received if stock makes up at least 50% of total (making the deal a merger). Stock is not taxable until sold.

■For the buyer: A hybrid deal is treated like a stock deal. Buyer loses the advantage of getting stepped-up depreciation of seller's assets. He can't pick up half the advantages for paying half cash. It's not a good choice unless buyer is afraid of diluting his present stock interest.

Source: Robert Willens, KPMG Peat Marwick, 1025 Connecticut Ave. N.W., Washington, DC 20036.

Deducting Acquisition Expenses

A mistake made too often by acquisition-minded companies: Assuming that all expenses incurred in the search for a suitable company are tax deductible. Not so, if these expenses were related to a trade or business in which the firm was not already engaged and no successful acquisition was made.

What can be deducted: Expenses for attorneys to draft purchase agreements and any other costs of an effort to complete the purchase of a specific business or investment.

Source: *Revenue ruling 77-254.*

Corporate Tax Returns

Corporate tax returns are due on March 15—or two-and-a-half months after year-end for companies using a fiscal year. Time is running out for finding smart filing strategies to use to cut the past year's tax bill...and to aid planning to reduce this year's tax liability as well.

Depreciation

Companies that made major acquisitions of depreciable real property and equipment during the year should take care to classify the property in the most advantageous way.

Example: Buildings generally are depreciated over $31^{1}/_{2}$ years, while equipment typically is depreciated over seven years. But many items which might be thought of as building components may qualify for faster depreciation in the equipment category when installed in a building to support or facilitate the use of movable equipment...special wiring, concrete pads, climate control systems, plumbing lines, etc.

Also, while most equipment is depreciated over a period of seven years, some types of equipment (such as computers and research and experimental equipment) qualify for shorter three-year or five-year depreciation. So be sure the company's newly acquired equipment is allocated to the most advantageous category.

Businesses that placed up to $200,000 worth of depreciable property in service during the year can elect to claim an immediate expense deduction of up to $10,000 for such property. The full $10,000 deduction is taken in one year, instead of being spread out over the depreciable life.

Inventories

One of the most dramatic changes imposed by the 1986 Tax Reform Act is the requirement that, like manufacturers, wholesalers and retailers capitalize overhead costs related to inventory.

Meaning: Many costs that previously were deducted as a current expense have to be carried as part of the cost of inventory and can be deducted by the company only as inventory is sold.

Examples: Insurance, repairs, maintenance, handling, packaging, rent, utilities, salaries and benefits of warehouse workers, and even a portion of compensation paid to managers who make decisions affecting inventory.

Companies subject to this provision of Tax Reform should have adopted capital-cost accounting methods on their 1987 returns. But many firms have not yet properly done so, because the required accounting methods are so complicated and unfamiliar to firms that were not previously required to use them. Trap: There have been so many rule changes concerning this part of the law since it was enacted in 1986, that even companies that have adopted the new rules should review their compliance with the law.

Other companies are becoming subject to the new rules for the first time, due to the growth of their businesses. (The rules apply only to those wholesalers and retailers who have had average annual gross receipts exceeding $10 million over the past three years.)

In either case, the company should get the advice of an expert in capital-cost accounting and comply with the new rules to avoid potential penalties.

Elections

Installment method reporting. A company may elect on its tax return not to use installment sale reporting methods for a transaction to which they would otherwise automatically apply.

Installment reporting provides the benefit of deferring tax. But it can make sense to have the full gain on an installment sale taxed immediately if the company has other tax deductions, credits or losses that will shelter the gain from tax.

It also makes sense if the company thinks its tax rate is likely to go up in the near future, either because increasing income will push it into a higher tax bracket or because it anticipates a future increase in tax rates.

LIFO. As companies begin to feel an increase in the inflation rate, the last-in, first-out (LIFO) inventory accounting method is attracting renewed attention. LIFO can be a big money-saver for firms experiencing both rising inventory levels and rising inventory costs. LIFO is elected for the year just past by filing IRS Form 970 with the company's tax return. Have the firm's accountant check out the impact of LIFO before the tax return's due date to see if an election makes sense.

Writedowns. Claim a writeoff for any reduction in the value of inventories that occurred during the past year. Key: The company must have evidence (such as market sale prices) supporting the new value assigned to inventories. Important: Make sure the company talks with its tax adviser and pulls together all needed data by the time the tax return is filed.

52–53-week tax year. A company can elect a tax year that always ends on a particular day of the week, rather than the last day of the year.

Example: The last Tuesday in December, or the Tuesday closest to December 31, rather than December 31 itself.

Benefit: Many businesses (especially retailers) find it a valuable convenience to be able to close the books, and perhaps conduct an inventory, on a particular day of the week.

First-year elections. A regular corporation filing its first tax return has the option to choose a fiscal year that ends in a month other than December.

Advantage: The company may end its year during a period when business is slow, making it easier to close the books. Or it may choose a time when income is cyclically low, minimizing its tax liability.

New corporations should also make the election to amortize organizational and start-up costs over a five-year period even if they think the election will have little value.

Reason: During an audit conducted in a later year, the IRS may disallow the company's deduction for first-year costs that were treated as business expenses and recategorize them as start-up costs.

Trap: If the company hasn't made the election on its first-year tax return, its deduction for such items will be lost forever. But if it has made the election, it can still claim the five-year write-off for the recategorized items.

Reporting

Recent tax law changes have toughened tax-compliance rules and created new reporting requirements…

■A company that bought a business during the past year must file IRS Form 8594, reporting how the purchase price has been allocated to the business's various assets for tax purposes.

■A company that is more than 25% foreign-owned must file IRS Form 5472, reporting the payments of sales proceeds, rents, lease payments and interest between the company and the foreign owner. Trap: The foreign ownership limit has been reduced from over 50% to over 25% by the 1989 Tax Act, effective tax years beginning after July 10, 1989, so some businesses will be required to file this report for the first time.

■A corporation with a net operating loss must file an information statement with its tax return every year that it is a loss corporation. It must also report any change in ownership that occurs while it is utilizing a loss carryforward. See IRS Regulation 1.382-2T(a)(2)(ii) for a description of the information that must be provided.

■The 1989 Tax Act will require any corporation that experienced more than a 50% change of ownership during the year to report the change on its tax return. The IRS will be interested in seeing that costs related to the purchase of the business are properly treated as capital costs rather than deducted as business expenses.

Refunds

The company can get extra time to devise tax strategies by requesting an automatic six-month filing extension by filing IRS Form 7004.

But if expecting a refund, the company should act to get the refund as quickly as possible…

■A firm that overpaid its estimated taxes can get a quick refund by filing Form 4466 before the regular unextended due date of its tax return. The IRS is required to respond within 45 days.

■A company that has suffered losses and intends to use a carryback to get a refund of a prior year's taxes can get a quick refund by filing IRS Form 1139. The IRS is required to act within 90 days.

■If losses are expected in the current year, the company can get an extension of the time to pay last year's tax by filing IRS Form 1138. The coming loss can then be carried back to cut last year's tax, eliminating the need to pay last year's tax at all. Trap: Penalties will result if the projected loss doesn't actually occur.

Filing

When sending in the tax return to the IRS, be sure to send it by certified mail—return receipt requested.

There seems to be an increasing incidence of cases where returns are lost—and the IRS denies ever receiving them. Non-filing penalties may result. However, the Tax Code specifically states that a certified mail return receipt constitutes proof of delivery to the IRS.

Source: Tom Sherman, tax partner, and John Morris, senior tax manager, Coopers & Lybrand, 1000 TCF Tower, Minneapolis 55402.

When IRS Will Accept Less Than You Owe

People who have old tax debts outstanding often don't realize that it's possible to work out a compromise payout with the IRS.

How it works: The tax debtor files an "Offer in Compromise" on IRS Form 656. This is simply an offer of terms the taxpayer can live with. There is a question on the form asking why the taxpayer wishes to compromise. Best answer: "I am unable to pay the total tax liability in full."

A financial statement listing all assets and liabilities must accompany Form 656. It is signed under penalty of perjury.

Danger: If the offer is rejected, the IRS may move quickly to seize assets listed on the statement.

Solution: The offer should always be made through a tax specialist who is familiar with the local IRS procedures and able to judge whether an offer is likely to be acceptable.

How much must be offered: There is no set percentage. But it must be clear that the taxpayer is making a sincere effort in the light of his financial situation. And that situation must be fully revealed. It isn't necessary to tender payment.

Sample offer: I agree to pay $1,000 upon the acceptance of this offer and an additional $500 per month for the next 12 months.

Future income. In most cases the IRS won't accept less than 100% of the tax due unless the taxpayer agrees to make additional payments in the event his future income improves. Typical requirement: For the next five years, the taxpayer pledges 10% of anything he makes over and above the first $20,000; 15% of any income beyond $35,000; and 25% of anything beyond $50,000. Unless the taxpayer agrees to this type of pledge, the IRS will usually reject the compromise offer. However, they may accept lower percentages.

When does it pay to make an offer: When the tax debt has been on the books for a number of years and the taxpayer wishes to reestablish his credit by having the IRS withdraw its lien on his property.

Key: The IRS must be convinced that conventional collection procedures won't work. That's why a relatively recent tax obligation won't be compromised. But if the IRS has had a chance to collect and hasn't succeeded, they'll be more reasonable.

Source: Randy Bruce Blaustein, Esq. M.R. Weiser & Co., 535 Fifth Ave., New York 10017.

Delayed Bonus

A executive retired knowing that he had earned a $20,000 bonus under a company incentive plan. But under the plan's terms, the bonus wouldn't be paid until January of the year following his retirement. IRS ruling: The bonus will be treated as earned income in the year the executive receives it, even though he'll be retired in that year. Thus, the executive can use the bonus to make an IRA contribution for that year, even if he doesn't work at all during the year.

Source: IRS Letter Ruling 8707051.

Chapter 19
Tax Strategies For Tight Times

Tax-Wise Ways To Prepare For A Bad-Earnings Year

Lagging sales and high costs mean many businesses are bracing themselves for a poor-earnings year.

It is important to devise tax strategies to strengthen the company's cash flow as earnings erode by using the tax code to the company's advantage.

If the company made money in one year but expects to lose money in the next, it can effectively avoid paying any tax that it still owes for earlier, money-making years by filing Form 1138. This extends the time for paying the earlier year's taxes until the date the present return is due. And the loss shown on the return can be carried back to wipe out the earlier year's tax bill.

A company with losses can get a quick refund of prior year's taxes through its loss carry-back by filing Form 1139. The Internal Revenue Service must generally respond to this refund request within about 90 days. It is required that the company must file its regular tax return before the Form 1139 is filed. So file the previous year's tax return as quickly as possible.

Using a Subchapter S. The Subchapter S form of corporate organization presents both an opportunity and a danger for company owners when the company faces a loss. Shareholders of a Subchapter S corporation can deduct the firm's operating losses on their personal tax returns. So they can use the company's losses to cut taxes on their income from other sources.

A company with 25 or fewer shareholders may consider reorganizing under Subchapter S to take advantage of this break. A Subchapter S election must be filed by the 75th day of the company's tax year. For a calendar-year firm, the deadline is March 16.

But there is a limit to the amount of losses that a Subchapter S shareholder may deduct. The limit equals the adjusted basis of the shareholder's stock (basically its cost) plus the amount of any debts owed by the company to the shareholder. Owners frequently overlook this limit. But any losses that exceed it are truly lost. They cannot be deducted by the shareholder or carried forward by the company.

A company that is already organized under Subchapter S should examine its situation closely to be sure its loss limit will not be exceeded during the present years. If the prospect is that the limit will be overrun, the company may do best by ceasing to qualify as a Subchapter S corporation.

When it comes to estimated taxes many firms routinely base one year's payments on the previous year's tax liability. But the resulting tax payments will be too high if this year's income goes down. So be sure the company's accountants base estimated payments on actual earnings as the year progresses. During a stretch when the company is losing money, it need pay no estimated taxes at all.

If business turns good later in the year as the economy picks up, the company may wind up with a large tax liability after all. And the IRS may ask why the company did not make any estimated-tax payments during the course of a profitable year. If this occurs file Form 2220. This shows that the company was actually losing money for most of the year and did not owe the taxes. Make sure the company's bookkeepers examine Form 2220 at the beginning of the year. It will show them what records must be kept to protect the company from tax penalties.

And now the tax law allows loss companies to sell investment credits and depreciation deductions that they cannot use. Technical requirements must be met, and planning is involved. So consider this carefully with a tax specialist.

If the company is locked into making large pension-plan contributions this year and is afraid that it may not be able to afford them, plan now to ask the IRS for a waiver of the contribution requirements.

The company must be able to show that it is suffering from genuine economic hardship to qualify for a waiver. And it must show that the waiver is in the best interest of the pension plan's participants. Show that the waiver will help the company regain economic strength and continue in business.

Often businesses are operated through several different corporations. And the swift-changing economic conditions may affect the separate companies differently. Some profit while others lose. Look at the effects of filing a consolidated tax return. The profits of one company may then be offset by the losses of another. And the net tax bill may be reduced. A consolidated return does not have to be decided upon until the normal time for filing the tax return. At that point, with all the good and bad news in, the results of consolidated and separate filings can be compared to see which one produces the best outcome for the company as a whole.

There are two things a company should not do when confronted by financial difficulties. Never ignore an IRS communication about a tax problem. The IRS takes the worst actions when companies are silent. Instead, have the company's tax adviser answer the IRS in a businesslike manner. And never use taxes withheld from employee wages to meet a cash need of the business. That use of withholding is a crime, involving a possible fine and/or jail term.

Source: Henry A. Garris, tax manager, Richard Eisner & Co., New York.

Corporate Charity

Even if taxable profits are low because of a slow economy, high depreciation deductions or an investment credit, the company may still want to make a charitable contribution to establish goodwill with influential business and community leaders. But a corporation cannot claim charitable deductions exceeding 10% of its taxable income.

To avoid the 10% limitation, find a business reason for the donation. Business expense deductions have been allowed for donations to:

■Local charities, when lobbying for a favorable community vote on a business license.

■An organization planning a convention that would generate extra business for the company.

■A community group that is engaged in rehabilitating the neighborhood in which the company offices were located.

■A hospital that agreed to provide medical services for the company.

Be sure that corporate records document two things: The business reason for the donation, and the fact that the company expects a return on the expenditure.

Bad-Debt Write-Offs

A debt can be written off for tax purposes as bad only where there is reason to believe that it won't be collected. Slow payments don't in themselves imply uncollectability. Nor does the simple fact that a debt isn't being paid. A tax write-off is limited to accounts that are not paid because the debtor is financially unable to do so. And a loss that results from compromising a debt is not deductible if the debtor is solvent.

The test of reasonable expectation of payment when the obligation was incurred usually rules out deductions on loans to friends or relatives. Money owed by a close relative can be deducted as a bad debt if there was a provable business transaction with reasonable expectation of payment. There must be proof that every effort had been made to enforce the obligation.

If the debt did not arise from a business transaction, it is treated as a short-term capital loss. That's only a limited tax usefulness.

There can be no bad debt if there was no genuine debt in the first place. Examples are gambling debts (in most states) or loans at illegally high interest rates. A cash-basis business cannot deduct a bad debt when its merchandise or services are not paid for, since income had never been reported in the first place.

A bad-debt deduction is allowed only in the taxable year when some identifiable event occurs that indicates the account can't be collected. Such an event might be discharge of the debtor of its obligations by a bankruptcy court. But it needn't go that far. If the debtor's liabilities exceed its assets, there is technical insolvency. If a bank reports that a debtor is defaulting on trade obligations or cancels its own purchase orders, that is an identifiable event.

A bad debt is not deductible at the end of a taxable year unless it can be shown to have been good at the beginning of that year. (The debt actually may have become bad in an earlier year.) Deduct in the year when the debt actually became bad, not in the year when it was discovered to be uncollectable.

If there is real doubt as to whether a debt will be paid, those stuck with it don't have to wait until uncollectability is proven to get a tax deduction. A partial bad-debt deduction can be taken for the portion of the debt that has become uncollectable in that year. If, for example, an experienced attorney advises that there is only a 40% chance of collecting from a certain customer, that justifies a deduction of 60% of the indebtedness as a partial bad debt. (This applies only to business bad debts.)

If a bad debt is written off in one taxable year and subsequently payment is received in whole or in part, the original deduction is not affected. The amount recovered is taxed in the year received, but only if the original deduction created a tax benefit, that is, if the creditor reduced his taxable income by deducting the bad debt. But if the creditor had no income to reduce by the amount of the bad debt, the recovered money isn't taxable.

Recession Tax Planning

Tax planning can ease the cash-flow problems a firm is likely to experience during any recession. Possible steps to take are:

■Extend the payment time for the previous year's taxes by filing Form 1138, if a loss is expected this year.

■Obtain a quick refund of estimated taxes by filing Form 4466 within two and a half months after the close of the tax year.

■Expedite refunds resulting from net operating losses, capital losses, unused job-credit carry-backs, and investment tax credits: File Form 1139.

■Reduce estimated tax payments by basing them on this year's expected income rather than last year's tax.

■Extend the payment time for this year's taxes to avoid undue hardship to the firm by filing Form 1127.

Source: Deloitte & Touche, New York.

Interest Deductible; Principal Too

Employee stock ownership plans are a tax-saving means of corporate financing. The essence: A firm sets up a plan, which borrows money from a bank on a note guaranteed by the corporation. The plan uses this to buy stock from the corporation. The corporation makes contributions annually in cash or stock to the plan, for which it gets tax deductions. The contributions are used to pay off the bank loan. In effect, the corporation raises capital with tax-deductible dollars.

The ESOP can be used as a personal financial planning tool for the shareholder-owners of a close corporation who are otherwise locked into the corporation.

If the corporation redeems part of their shares in an ordinary way, they're almost certain to be taxed at ordinary income rates. And that transaction will be treated as a dividend distribution (which the corporation pays taxes on) rather than a sale or exchange.

The corporation itself faces a major problem on redemptions. It must accumulate the necessary funds. They can be accumulated only out of after-tax dollars.

By interposing an ESOP, the picture changes dramatically. The shareholders have a market for their shares—the ESOP. The plan buys their shares with deductible contributions made with pretax dollars.

If there isn't enough money in the ESOP at the time to effect the purchase, then the plan borrows money from a bank in the procedure outlined above.

The same approach may be used by the shareholder's estate as a means of realizing cash on stock held by the estate without getting dividend treatment.

Insurance angle: The ESOP, as an alternative to borrowing to raise cash to purchase stock from the estate, may, according to current thinking among practitioners, carry life insurance on a key shareholder. If the corporation itself were to carry such insurance to facilitate redemption, the premiums paid wouldn't be tax deductible. By interposing an ESOP, the premiums effectively become tax deductible, since they're paid by the Plan out of tax-deductible dollars contributed to it by the company.

Other Benefits

The shareholder-executive will be able to participate in the plan himself and enjoy its benefits.

■His company will make tax-deductible contributions to the plan.

■He won't be taxed until the benefits are made available to him.

■The payout is required to be made in company stock and he won't be taxed on the unrealized appreciation in the stock over the cost to the plan until he sells the stock.

■On a transfer of his plan benefits to his beneficiaries, other than his estate, upon his death, they won't be includable in his estate and will escape estate taxes.

Chief Problem

Valuation of shares on a sale to the ESOP. Another is the necessary distribution of corporate information to the employee-shareholders. If corporate progress isn't to the liking of employees, expect worker dissatisfaction.

The concepts are new. But the idea is one well worth exploring.

Chapter 20
Tax-Wise Business Strategies

How To 'Cash In' With Minimum Tax Bite

Practical way to transfer a business to the principal's children (or other family members) with a minimum of tax liability: First, arrange to transfer some stock to family. Later, have the corporation redeem the rest of principal's share. But, instead of paying a lump sum of cash, have the money paid as a life-time annuity. In that way, the money is distributed in fixed, annual installments. The advantages:

The business is removed from the owner's estate immediately, without the imposition of gift or inheritance taxes. It becomes the sole property of the remaining shareholder.

The owner gets a lifetime income, which can meet retirement needs just as well as a lump-sum payment.

The estate isn't swollen with cash or notes that would be received in a lump-sum redemption. The annuity lasts only during the principal's lifetime.

Business isn't saddled with a traumatic outflow of working capital. The annuity is paid out of profits and is spaced evenly over the lifetime of the former owner of the business.

How to do it: Calculate the fair market value of the shares. Then use Internal Revenue Service actuarial tables to translate the value of those holdings into a monthly lifetime annuity plus interest.

Taxes are paid only on the income that's received each year, not on the cash value of the annuity in the year received. The annuity payments are divided into three layers: 1. return of capital (not taxed); 2. profit on the sale of stock (capital-gain) tax; 3. interest on the unpaid balance (taxed as ordinary income).

Tax Opportunities In Buying A Business

Record-high interest rates provide an opportunity to buy out the business of a financially shaky supplier, customer, or competitor to broaden the business without the strain of starting a new division or subsidiary from scratch. In some cases, the tax savings can pay the entire cost of the transaction. The tax implications will depend on whether the business has been making money or losing money.

In buying a health company, suggest to the present owner that the company redeem some of the shares he holds, paying him cash directly for those shares. Simultaneously, have the owner transfer the rest of the shares to the purchaser. Section 302 of the Tax Code provides the owner with tax-favored long-term capital gains treatment for his profit on the deal, and the seller avoids paying any funds out of pocket.

The purchaser must not commit itself in writing to purchase all the seller's stock, and then use funds taken from the company to make payment. The used funds are a taxable dividend to the purchaser, who winds up paying both the seller and the government.

In buying an unhealthy company, have the old owner put the company into Chapter 11 bankruptcy proceedings before the sale is announced. The liabilities of the company are declared and defined, so the purchaser avoids buying unknown debts. The business's creditors will probably be ready to negotiate a reasonable reduction of their debts, rather than risk loving everything by having the buyer walk away.

It may take some time to turn around a business that has been losing money. But the purchaser gets immediate tax benefits:

■Continuing losses of the company that is bought can be used on a consolidated return to offset the profits of the purchasing company.

■Capital investments made to turn around the acquired business will result in large investment credits and depreciation deductions. These benefits are now larger than ever.

■When the acquired business turns profitable, its post-acquisition losses may be used to offset future gains. The period during which these losses may be carried forward has been increased to 15 years.

When purchasing a company, it may become necessary to give key managers a stake in the business. These employees should not be given more than 20% of the company's stock. Consolidated returns cannot be filed unless the purchasing company owns 80% of the stock of the other. Without consolidated returns, the tax benefits will be lost.

A key consideration in buying a business is assigning a cash value to the purchased company's assets. A high value for the depreciable assets increases the depreciation deductions available in the future, whereas a high value for a noncomplete agreement signed by the seller increases the business expense deduction available for its cost. The seller may want little value attached to the noncomplete agreement (its price is taxed as ordinary income to him) and as much as possible attached to the goodwill of the business (to qualify for long-term capital gains).

Source: Edward Mendlowitz, Mendlowitz Weitsen, New York.

Dividing Up A Company—Tax-Free

Cutting state and local taxes is often a prod to corporation breakups. A business can profit by incorporating some of its operations in low-tax states. But there are other powerful motivators for dividing up:

■Split liabilities. A retail firm's credit line could be frozen if a large personal-injury lawsuit is filed against one of its several stores. Separate incorporation of each store can help contain the liabilities of each.

■Reduce accumulated earnings. A corporation with $250,000 in retained earnings faces a possible penalty tax. But two corporations with $125,000 each in earnings are both safe, provided there is a business reason (as opposed to a tax reason) for creating them.

■Provide employee incentives. A firm may want to give its branch managers an equity interest in the business, but only in each one's own branch. The solution is to incorporate each branch separately.

■Obtain financing. When a company operates several businesses with different financial needs, the credit rating of one or more might be strengthened by having them separately organized.

■Contain labor disputes. A labor dispute at one plant may result in the entire company being picketed or boycotted. It is easier, legally, to contain a dispute within an operation that is separately incorporated.

■Avoid conflicts of interest. A wholesaler or manufacturer may create a different named subsidiary to begin selling directly to the public without going into direct competition with its retailing customers.

■Settle management disputes. Two groups of shareholders in a mid-size corporation might disagree on management policy and paralyze the company. Dividing the business between two new corporations gives each group control of one.

■Avoid regulation. When one of two businesses is regulated, the entire firm may be subject to restrictions. Similarly, when a firm operates one business in several states, the regulations of one state may affect the entire operation.

The most commonly types of tax-free reorganization is the split-off. The company creates a subsidiary to run part of its business. The parent company's shareholders then exchange some of their stock for that of the subsidiary. The shareholders can vary their interest in the two corporations by varying the amount of stock they exchange. Each can emerge as a shareholder of either company, or of both. Split-offs are used to settle management disputes and to provide employee incentives.

■In the spin-off, the subsidiary's stock is distributed directly to the parent company's shareholders. No stock is exchanged. The shareholders keep the same proportional ownership of the two businesses that they had when there was one company. Spin-offs are frequently used for financing purposes.

The least common type of division is the split-up. The parent company's entire business is transferred to two or more subsidiaries. Stock in the subsidiaries is distributed directly to the parent company's shareholders. The parent then ceases to exist. Split-ups are used only when there is some reason to terminate the parent corporation.

Certain conditions are essential to qualify the breakup as tax-free. There must be a business purpose to the deal, not just the avoidance of federal taxes. The parent company must own at least 80% of the subsidiary's stock just before the division. A controlling amount of the subsidiary's stock must be transferred to the shareholders of the parent. (There must be a good reason not to distribute all of it.) The subsidiary's business must have been actively conducted by the parent for at least five years—unless the business was acquired in a tax-free reorganization. Finally, if stock is exchanged, the value of the stock surrendered must equal that of the stock received. The transaction's purpose must not be to withdraw earnings from the business.

Source: Dr. Robert Holzman, professor emeritus of taxation, New York University, author of *The Encyclopedia of Estate Planning*, Boardroom Books, Springfield, NJ 07081.

Tax Treatment Of Noncompete Agreements

The buyer of a business usually seeks to call part of the purchase price a payment for the seller's promise not to compete for a specified number of years, since he can deduct payments made for that promise. The seller wants as little of the price as possible allocated that way, since money received for such a covenant is taxed as ordinary income. In one case, the seller argued that the amount labeled in a contract as payment for a covenant not to compete should be disregarded as an economic unreality. The seller had terminal illness and couldn't compete. But the court refused to disregard the terms of the contract. It had not been proven that the seller had been too ill to know what he was signing. Since the contract referred to a big slice of the consideration as payment not to compete, that's the way it was taxed.
Source: *Clesceri vs United States*, USDC, N. Dist. IL, 11/21/79.

Recapitalizing For Personal And Tax Advantages

If a corporation has only one class of stock, all shares must be treated identically as to dividends, voting rights, etc. But shareholders have different needs. Older ones may require income; younger ones may want growth; not all may be active in the firm's management. The solution is a tax-free recapitalization that allows different shareholders to acquire different types of stock, according to their needs. The standard choices are preferred stock, which usually pays regular dividends, but does not share in the firm's growth, and common stock, which need not pay dividends but increases in value as the company grows. Both common and preferred stock may be classed as either voting or nonvoting.

A typical candidate for recapitalization is a company with only common stock outstanding whose founder is approaching retirement age. The founder owns most of the stock, but all his children own some. Only one child is active in the business.

All the firm's stock is now exchanged. The founder receives voting preferred stock, which becomes nonvoting on his death; the child in the business receives voting common stock; and the other children receive nonvoting common stock. In this way the founder retains control of the business and gets a regular income for life. The children all profit from any future growth in the company's underlying value. And the child active in management gains control of the company when the founder dies.

Here are other reasons for recapitalizing:

■Estate planning. The chief shareholder's estate may be so large that the company may have to redeem much of the shareholder's stock to pay estate taxes when he dies. This cash drain could hurt the business. Strategy: The shareholder exchanges his common stock for preferred. Result: The value of his interest in the business is frozen. Estate taxes are reduced, since future growth goes to other shareholders who won't be taxed on the major shareholder's death.

Income taxes. A firm's sole owner might not want to receive dividends, because they are taxable at rates up to 50%. But the firm may have to pay dividends because of Internal Revenue Service limitations on accumulated earnings. One solution is to create a new class of preferred stock and place it in trust to benefit the owner's children. Since they are in a lower tax bracket, the family as a unit would receive dividends taxed at a lower rate.

■Employee incentives. Key employees may wish to acquire an interest in the business but the value of the firm's stock may be so high they cannot afford it. Solution: The company exchanges each share of old stock for several new ones (common, preferred or both). Result: The value of individual shares is reduced.

■Shareholder harmony. Passive shareholders may want to receive large dividends from the company while those who are actively managing the business may want to reinvest profits. Worse: Active family members may resent working for the benefit of inactive ones. Solution: Inactive shareholders exchange their common stock for nonvoting preferred. Result: Shareholders who actually manage the company get control and the benefits of future growth. They may choose to forgo dividends on the common and invest earnings as they wish. The passive shareholders get the regular dividends they desire.

Before plunging ahead on a recapitalization plan, consider the company's needs carefully with its business and tax advisers. Mistakes can be expensive. A parent might give all the children voting stock in the business, then decide later that only the children active in the business should have voting stock. But the others won't give up their voting interest. A bitter family fight results. Or a shareholder receives preferred stock in exchange for his common stock, then he sells some of the preferred. Under some circumstances, profit from the sale will be considered ordinary income and be taxed at up to the 31% rate. But if the shareholder had received preferred stock to begin with, the profit would have been a capital gain, taxable at a lower rate.

Questions to ask when recapitalizing the company:

■If the business is successful, will it be sold? If so, it may be best to give family members small blocks of stock. Reason: When the business is sold, gain will be spread among family members in lower tax brackets.

■Who will be the company's ultimate shareholders? Possibilities: Near family, distant family, employees, outsiders. What kind of stock should each own?

■Who will ultimately control the company—all the shareholders, or those who are active in the business? Point: Create voting and nonvoting stock accordingly.

There must be a business purpose for the transaction. Reasons accepted by the Internal Revenue Service are efficient management, shareholder harmony, and estate planning (when the business might be affected by a large redemption). The new stock received by each shareholder must be equal in value to the old stock that was exchanged. And a formal plan of reorganization must be adopted by the company and the shareholders. A copy of it must be filed with the firm's tax return.

The firm's tax adviser might ask the IRS for a private-letter ruling concerning the transaction before it is done. If the ruling is favorable, the company can rely on it should problems later arise. If the IRS raises an objection, the problem area will be known before the deal is completed, and a costly mistake can still be averted.

When To Choose The S Corporation

One of the chief attractions of an S corporation is the fact that losses and profits are passed through to the stockholders, reducing the shareholders' taxable income in the case of losses, and avoiding double taxation of dividends in the case of earnings. An amendment to the tax law has liberalized the treatment of losses on Section 1244 stock, which is frequently used for corporations starting up. Losses on this stock would be allowed up to $50,000 and, in case of a joint return, up to $100,000.

When starting up a new business, discuss with professional advisers the desirability of qualifying as an S corporation as well as under Section 1244. This can be especially important if initial losses are anticipated. Once the corporation starts making money, it can always terminate the Subchapter S election and become a regular corporation later.

The S election is especially good for companies with high start-up costs for equipment as well as expected losses. A new restaurant venture, for example, might require $50,000 of equipment. If the S is made, shareholders would be eligible for the 10% investment credit. But in an ordinary C corporation with operating losses, there would be no income against which to take the credit immediately. Under the S corporation election, the credit would be passed through to the stockholders of record.

Other times when Sub S makes sense:

■When you anticipate accumulating earnings. In a normal C corporation, the earnings would have to be paid out as dividends from after-tax funds, then taxed again in the recipient's income. For S firms, there's no tax on the distribution at the corporate level.

■For speculative ventures. An S corporation election allows immediate tax write-offs of operating losses up to the amount paid into the company for equity or as loans.

■To simplify some intrafamily transfers. In one case, the owner of an executive recruitment agency wanted to shelter substantial income. He incorporated the business as an S corporation and gave stock to his children. Profits from the business were then taxed in the children's lower tax bracket.

The S corporation election should not be used when the corporation will be using internally generated cash for growth. A C corporation is taxed at a lower rate than high-income individuals.

S corporations can now enjoy the same liberal pension benefits enjoyed by regular C corporations.

Companies that used Sub S to recapture heavy start-up losses and wish to convert to regular corporation status can do so, but once converted, a corporation cannot change back to Sub S for five years unless the termination resulted from circumstances beyond the shareholder's control.

Note: The IRS may grant exceptions to the five-year rule in certain cases.

Source: Sidney Kess, retired, KPMG Peat Marwick, 630 Fifth Ave., New York 10111.

Chapter 21
Financing Strategies

Financial Strategy For A Recession

Now is a good time to take protective action.

Aim: To avoid much of the pain that comes with hard times—and even make some profits.

The best preparation: Saving.

Make sure you have a rainy-day fund that can cover three to six months of your total living expenses if you are in danger of losing your job.

Don't take any risks with that money. Keep it in ultrasafe CDs, money market mutual funds, or short-term Treasury bills.

But be more aggressive if your job is secure. No-risk investments will only earn about 2%—after inflation and taxes. For people with good job security...

■Increase your holdings in high-quality corporate bonds. Interest rates usually decline during recessions, and bond prices increase when rates fall. So your corporate bonds could actually increase in value as the economy stumbles.

■Take your profits in the stock market now—and reinvest a fixed amount each month as the economy falters. This way, you'll be buying low as prices fall—and be set to reap profits when the economy recovers.

Better strategy: Since the stock market usually bottoms when a recession is officially announced, start your buying programs a month after the downturn is official. (A recession is generally defined as two quarters of negative economic growth).

■Buy stocks or stock mutual funds that have good recession track records. Avoid economically sensitive issues—autos, aerospace or defense stocks. Stick with companies that produce necessities—food, electricity, etc. And look for mutual funds that have good long-term track records.

■Keep a higher proportion of your money in cash as the recession hits. That way, you'll be able to take advantage of "fire sale" prices when the stock market declines.

■Cut down on debt. When times get tough, paying off debt makes life all that much harder. A good rule of thumb: Keep your total debts under 30% of your pre-tax income. It's not easy, but it will give you peace of mind. Postpone buying high-ticket items, like cars or refrigerators, unless you really need them. That will just increase your debts at a time when you should be saving.

■Strategy for paying off those debts: Take out a home equity loan to cover high interest consumer debts such as car and credit-card debts. The interest rate will probably be lower, and in most cases, you'll be able to deduct the interest from your taxes.

Another advantage to the home-equity route...flexibility. Many home-equity lines have a minimum, interest-only payment. Anyone who gets laid off will find that lower payment handy. Others would pay both interest and principal.

Better strategy: Pay as much on your home equity payment as you did on your old bills. You'll be paying 30% to 40% more than your required payment but you'll pay off the important principal much more quickly.

■Think about dumping that adjustable-rate mortgage. Adjustables are at about the same rate as fixed-rate mortgages now. And when a recession hits, the last thing you need to worry about is high mortgage rates.

■Keep your mind open. Most people resist changing their portfolios or their budgets when a recession hits. But you can turn bad times into winners if you take advantage of the opportunities around you.

Source: Mitchell Keil, financial planner with IDS in Irvine, CA.

Building A Sensitive Reporting System

To design a sensitive financial reporting system, management should ensure that:

■A few (8–10 at most) crucial and sensitive financial measures are generated regularly and appear right on top of the report.

■Key nonfinancial measures of output are included, especially productivity and market penetration.

■Data are subdivided according to managerial lines of responsibility, not simply by legal or accounting guidelines.

■The financial record is broken down by major product lines.

■The regular report immediately identifies the company's weakest and strongest performers. Goal: A weekly, monthly or quarterly profile of the company's operating and financial status.

Strategies For Smart Borrowing

Basic errors in a company's borrowing strategy often do not become apparent until the company needs money fast. By then, it may be too late. For smart corporate financing:

■Maintain contact with several lenders. If possible, do business with more than one. Relying on one lender is dangerous. A company that has used the same lender for 20 years is extremely vulnerable. If that lender refuses a loan or terminates the relationship entirely, the company will have trouble arranging for alternate financing quickly.

■Anticipate financing needs and make arrangements well in advance. Patchwork financing is an expensive and risky way to operate. Put money on standby whenever possible. A standby fee, if necessary, is cheap insurance against the risk of suddenly running out of money.

■Borrow as much as possible. It is better to have too much than to have too little. Lend out excess funds to reduce net borrowing costs. Large companies view money as a resource to be inventoried, like coal or steel. Smaller firms should too.

■Get all commitments in writing. This includes standby agreements, loans, and increases in credit lines. If there is nothing in writing, the company might not really have what it needs. No professional lender objects to written commitments.

■Never assume that silence is tacit approval of a loan request. Some lenders do not like to say no, so they say nothing. Then when the company inquires about its loan application, usually around the time it needs the money, it suddenly learns that it has been turned down. When applying for a loan, ask when the answer will be ready. Call the lender on that date if there has been no response.

■Do not make the interest rate the major consideration in evaluating a credit. No company wants to pay more interest than necessary. But the most important aspect of a financing is the availability of money—how much and how soon. The second most important is how the deal is structured. Interest rate is third.

■Do not limit sources to banks alone. Too many companies rely on a local bank for all financing needs. This is unfair to the bank, and it restricts the company's growth. Even smaller companies can, and should, borrow from insurance companies, pension funds, venture-capital funds, and other institutions.

Source: Russell Hindin, managing director, Hindin/Owen/Engelke, Los Angeles.

How Much Should A Company Borrow?

Total borrowings should not exceed the sum of:
■10% of the net working capital
■Plus 5% of cash and receivables
■Plus 10% of one year's net income.
From this total, deduct 3% of the long-term debt.
Bankers use this formula to make sure they don't lend too much money.

Source: William G. Torrace, management consultant, Troy, MI.

Chapter 22
Dealing With Banks

How To Find The Right Banks
For The Company's Money

There are two parts to good corporate banking...
■Finding the most financially healthy banks to do business with.
■Finding the banks with the right services for the company at acceptable prices.
Challenge: Satisfying both criteria at a time when commercial banks are failing by the hundreds each year, while healthy banks' services become increasingly complex and often overpriced.

Seeking Safety

Though the headlines are full of drama about bank failures, there are still many thousands of well-managed, very profitable banks. To measure the financial condition of the company's bank as well as that of other banks in the company's region, get a recent rating report from Veribanc,* the independent bank-monitoring service. Its reports can rate any of the nation's 13,000 banks. What to look for:

■Equity-to-assets ratio: Healthy banks have ratios of 5% or higher. This usually means the bank is operating profitably. Anything below 5% could mean trouble. Veribanc's rating system gives banks a green rating if the ratio is 5% or more, yellow for ones that are 3%–5% and red for ones below 3%. I recommend considering only green-rated banks.

■Annual income: A key measure of profitability. Any bank with no net loss gets a green from Veribanc. Banks with modest losses get a yellow, while banks with large losses that could erode the bank's equity get a red. In addition, Veribanc shows the actual dollar amount of each bank's income. The bank with the biggest profit isn't necessarily the best. It doesn't need your business as much as a smaller bank does and therefore is less likely to be flexible when it comes to negotiating services and fees.

■Problem loans: The Veribanc rating system includes the amount of loans that are not being paid on time or that are in danger of default, as a percentage of the bank's equity, after deducting the bank's reserves for loan losses. If that ratio exceeds 100%, the bank is in serious trouble. The vast majority of banks aren't in that condition.

And More Probing

In the evaluation process, I also advise studying the quarterly Abbreviated Report of Condition on individual banks from the Federal Deposit Insurance Co. in Washington.** These are financial reports on banks showing details of the bank's performance. Look for...

*Box 461, Wakefield, Massachusetts 01880, 800-44-BANKS. Call for varying fee schedules.

**FDIC, Disclosure Section, 550 17th St. NW, Washington, DC 20006, 800-424-4334. Copy charges are normally minimal or waived.

■Trends in the bank's earnings. Steady profit growth is desirable. Very rapid or negative growth is suspect.

■Trends in loan-loss reserves. Steady increases in loan-loss reserves indicates prudent preparation for possible loan defaults. Big jumps in loss reserves are a danger signal, indicating the likelihood of very large defaults. Decreasing loan-loss reserves means the bank is experiencing substantial, possible dangerous, loan losses.

■Total deposits. Steady growth in deposits is normal and desirable. Rapid jumps in deposits often means the bank is offering high-yields on accounts that could get into trouble. No deposit growth usually reflects a bank unable to compete in its market.

Aim: From Veribanc and the FDIC Call Reports, narrow down the choice of banks to three or four, remembering that smaller banks with top ratings are the ones more likely to go out of their way to get the business of new customers.

Service Deals

There are hundreds of services banks can offer businesses, most of which aren't new...and most of which the average business doesn't need.

To get what the company really needs at the best price, make a list of the needed services before you approach any bank. Then negotiate with the bank, with the aim of getting them for no charge. Examples:

■Freedom to move money between accounts by phone or computer. Many banks will charge you each time this happens.

■Unlimited phone inquiries on balances. Some banks are now charging a fee each time you call for an account balance. Don't let the bank get away with that.

■Controlled disbursement service. This gives you daily reports on outstanding checks that will clear the bank that day. It enables you to keep the absolute minimum balance in the account to cover those checks. Many banks now offer this as a package service, with a set monthly fee. If the bank won't budge on this, fine. But don't let the bank convince you that this is a new high-tech convenience deserving a big fee. The ability to provide the service has been around for years, and really shouldn't cost a good customer anything.

■Payroll processing. Banks charge different amounts for different types and sizes of companies. Compare, compare, compare.

Important: Choose the best bank for the company's specific requirements. Bank A may offer the best payroll service for the best price, while Bank B may offer the best cash management services.

Having more than one, or even several, banks can also be advantageous if one gets into trouble. A switch to a bank the company already does business with is an obvious benefit.

In addition, if the company anticipates the need for bank loans in the future, having several banks familiar with the company's business increases the chances of getting a good deal.

Long-Term Monitoring

Because the U.S. banking system is in such turmoil, I advise companies, much as banks do with their commercial loan customers, to constantly monitor the financial condition of all the banks where they have deposits. The best way to continually monitor banks is to request a new Abbreviated Report of Condition on the company's banks from the FDIC every six months. That way, as soon as a problem arises, management will have reliable first-hand warning.

Source: Edward F. Mrkvicka, Jr., author of *The Bank Book: How to Revoke Your Bank's License to Steal*, HarperCollins, 10 E. 53 St., New York 10022.

Maintaining A Good Bank Relationship

Although the company may not be a borrower at the current time, it pays to stay in touch with the bank's lending officers. Maintain contact with them by:

■Seeing the officers periodically on social occasions. Invite them to lunch and to company functions. Tell them any news about the company that will interest them.

■Sending them the firm's quarterly financial statements updating the bank's records on the company.

■Keeping good balances always is of interest to bankers.

Games Bankers Play With Interest Rates

Banks teach their loan officers a number of strategies to get an extra $1/4\%$ or even $1/2\%$ from borrowers.

Recognize some of their tricks:

■Doing the negotiating at the bank. Familiar territory to the banker, intimidating to the borrower.

■Not mentioning the rate at all, but simply filling it in on the note.

■"Since you need the money today, let's write it up at X%. Then we can talk later about changing it." The banker hopes you'll never bring it up again. He certainly won't.

■Flat Statement: "The rate for this type of loan is X%." (Never true except for small consumer loans. There is always room to negotiate.)

■Postponing the rate discussion as long as possible, hoping borrower will weaken under deadline pressure.

■Ego-building. Bank president stops by during negotiations.

■Talking constantly about how little the interest costs after taxes. And comparing it with finance company rates, second mortgage rates, or the cost of equity capital.

The banker looks at the company's account as a package, including loans, average balances maintained, and fees for services. Borrower options: Trade off higher average balances for a lower interest rate on borrowings, or vice versa.

The borrower is at a disadvantage because he probably negotiates a loan only once a year or less, while the banker spends full time at it. So prepare carefully for negotiations.

Good tactics for the borrower:

■Ask interest rate questions early—in your office, not his. Don't volunteer suggestions.

■Negotiate everything as a package—rate, repayment schedule, collateral, compensating balances. Banker's strategy will be to try to nail down everything else and then negotiate interest rate when the borrower has no more leverage and no room to maneuver.

■Be prepared with an expression of surprise and shock, even rehearse it before a mirror. React that way when the banker mentions the interest rate, no matter what the figure is.

Source: Lawrence T. Jilk, Jr., executive vice president, National Bank of Boyertown, PA, writing in *The Journal of Commercial Bank Lending*.

Best Way To Get A Loan From Your Bank

■Prepare a loan proposal. Include amount of capital needed, type of loan (long- or short-term, revolving credit line), terms (secured, unsecured, endorsed, guaranteed), desired interest rate, and proposed pay-back schedule.

■Clearly explain purpose of loan.

■Show company fundamentals. Include cash flow and operating projections, balance sheets and income statements for past three years, collateral, inventory, fixed assets, life insurance, marketable securities, listing and aging of accounts receivable.

■Provide related nonfinancial information. Show business strategy, data on company's industry and its position. Also: List trade suppliers for references.

Some Banks Are Better Than Others For Getting A Small Business Loan

Try taking your firm's loan request to a bank that is working with the Small Business Administration's secondary market program. The program greatly multiplies the bank's lending ability, increasing the possibility that your company's loan will get considered.

How the secondary market works: Bank gets a line of credit from the SBA. Ninety percent of each loan made to a company under the SBA program is guaranteed by the U.S. government. The bank then sells that 90% portion (or packages several loans and sells them together) to a broker. Result: Bank has that amount of money back again to lend.

The broker, in turn, sells the loan to an insurance company or pension fund, which picks up a 100% government-guaranteed instrument that pays 9% or more.

Details: For names of local banks in SBA program, write Office of Public Information, Small Business Administration, 1441 L. St. NW, Washington, DC 20416.

How To Negotiate For Below-Prime Bank Loans

Now that several recent lawsuits have exposed the common bank practice of making loans to favored customers at interest rates below the prime, all companies should be especially aggressive in getting the best loan deal possible.

Caution: Don't be fooled by new terms that some banks use instead of prime—base rate, index rate, reference rate. They all mean what the prime has come to mean in practice—the lowest rate charged to commercial customers, with the understanding that a few borrowers get even lower rates.

What To Look For

To improve your chance of getting the best rate, figure out how much your account helps the bank's profitability, and then use that information to negotiate loans.

To determine what your business is worth to a bank, look at:

■Idle balances. Many banks have gotten away from the tradition of demanding 10%—15% of loan value in compensating balances. But if the company does maintain big balances, or is willing to, it has a strong negotiating tool for getting a better loan rate. Don't forget to weigh the personal bank accounts of company employees into the equation.

■Fees. If the company uses lots of bank services (payroll, pension program or cash management), which bring the bank big fees, that too can be used for leverage.

Strategy: When a shrewd consumer buys a car, he first determines the price level at which the dealer makes a profit. Then the buyer negotiates as close as possible to that price. In the same way, you can use profitability to bargain with your bank. If you know your business contributes heavily to a bank's profit, it's often worthwhile to bargain. If it doesn't, you may have to swallow a point or more on a loan rate.

There are several useful guidelines that can help you to determine how the bank earns its profits and then to use that information in negotiating.

The Federal Reserve Bank of New York publishes *Functional Cost Analysis*, an annual that breaks down the average cost of various services for banks throughout the Fed's twelve districts. There are figures for banks with deposits up to $50 million, from $50 million to $200 million, and over $200 million. The report is available at Federal Reserve Banks in each district.

How to use the data: Compare the average costs of various services for banks of a similar size with the charges your company is paying. Example: If check clearing costs an average of 8¢, and you're paying 12¢, the bank is probably making a profit.

Most financial officers and CPA firms can interpret the data. There are also several commercial services that collect and publish useful cost and profit data on banks. Sheshunoff & Co., for example, publishes annual reports on profit data for banks in each state. Write: Box 13203, Capitol Station, Austin, TX 78711, and ask for *The Banks of* (name of state) *1985*, $245.

Sheshunoff also publishes *Pricing Bank Services and Loans* ($150), an annual report that covers a cross section of $1,650 banks, broken down by bank size and profitability. The report shows how each bank prices special services, including loan charges and commitment fees.

Source: Dr. Paul S. Nadler, professor of finance at Rutgers University Graduate School of Management. His office is at 14 Friar Tuck Circle, Summit, NJ 07901. Dr. Nadler is also contributing editor to *The American Banker*.

Mistakes Borrowers Make

Desperate as a company may be for money, it's extremely important not to give the lender more security than absolutely necessary.

A loan officer obviously needs some kind of a lien to show his superiors. The less the security interest, the stronger the relationship with the lender will be.

■Key points: 1. The lender is in effect a partner. 2. The more given in security, the greater the commitment the borrower should seek.

■Common mistake borrowers make: Automatically agreeing to the lender's loan request. It isn't always necessary to say yes or no. There is usually something in between. It's to the company's advantage to explore all possibilities.

■Example: Offer a lien on inventory but not receivables; on plant, furniture, fixtures (all requiring time to dispose of); on contract rights; or some combination of these.

■The worst thing to sign over is receivables. They mean quick cash. They are also the easiest thing for the lender to collect. The lender collects—and the business is ruined.

■Inventory, however, is good for a lien. Even though it may turn out to be virtually worthless, it looks good for the loan officer to show his superiors.

On the other hand, resist giving all inventory as security. Some can be rapidly converted into receivables, often by selling to a competitor.

From borrower's standpoint, it is best to offer things that will take months, even years, for lender to collect. That time may mean the life-and-death difference for the company. Even if it is necessary to sign over receivables, try to sign over only a percentage of them, retaining the rest to keep business running.

When lender asks for a personal guarantee, be careful not to sign away everything—and don't have your wife as a co-signer.

Here's where you need a smart lawyer:

Wording: There's a difference between a guarantee of payment and a guarantee of collectibility. If you guarantee payment, the lender is legally entitled to get his money fast. In some cases, one also forfeits the right to countersue the lender when there is a serious misunderstanding. A guarantee of collectibility, on the other hand, requires the lender to take all of the company's assets and liquidate them before coming after you. In a privately owned company, this gives one valuable time and may save personal assets so that the firm can survive and start over.

■Don't overlook the possibility of limited guarantees. Think of the guarantee as basically an indication of good faith. Agree to perhaps $50,000 on a $1 million loan. But don't be deceived by lenders' disclaimers about enforcing personal guarantees. When push comes to shove, they will.

Typically, borrowers are enthusiastic, sometimes over-optimistic. Even if a company avoids serious trouble or bankruptcy, realize that over a five-year period, 40%–50% of companies have a bad year. Maybe a big customer goes sour and it takes time to recoup that loss. Or payments start coming in late and cash flow becomes a problem.

The only defense is a continuing frank, friendly relationship with lenders. The best time to take a banker out to lunch is when things are going well. Always keep lenders informed about business and upcoming problems. The uninformed lender tends to overreact in times of surprise or crisis. The better he understands your business (the fatter his file, etc.), the stronger the case he can make for your company with his superiors. It's harder to say no to someone you know.

Source: Arthur Malman, Brown & Malman, 299 Park Ave., New York 10017.

Recovery From A Bank Loan Turndown

Common mistake: Giving up after the first try. Instead, prepare immediately a new thrust. What works:

■Asking for specifics on why the loan was refused. Two common causes: The bank is overextended or doesn't know the company's type of business.

■Inviting the loan officer and one of the officer's supervisors to visit the plant. This builds confidence by showing off equipment, facilities and personnel.

■Soliciting ideas on how the application can be made more acceptable through financial or accounting changes, tax regulations, government programs or production changes.

■Applying for another type of loan or a different credit basis. Possibilities: Pledging machinery as collateral, using a third-party guarantee or borrowing against seasonal receivables.

■Reapplying when the timing is better. Use an upswing in sales or profits to obtain a line of credit or get close enough to the banker to be informed when the bank has excess funds to loan.

■Changing banks, particularly to one that is newly chartered and looking for customers. Possibility: Splitting a loan between the old and new banks.

The way the loan proposal is presented can be critical. A friendly banker will advise the company on which documents to present and the best ways to compile financial data.

Source: *Finding Money: The Businessman's Guide to Sources of Financing* by J.G. Hellmuth, Boardroom Books, Springfield, NJ 07081.

Alternatives To Borrowing From Bank

A company may be able to borrow more from a commercial finance or factoring company than it can from a bank. Of course, the interest rate will be higher, too.

Here's how such organizations work and how your company can borrow from them:

Commercial finance companies: A company might borrow 75% to 85% of the value of receivables (excluding those that are past due). Or it might borrow 50% to 70% of the value of raw material inventory or work in process. Most commercial finance companies don't like to lend on plant and equipment, but a few specialize in this activity.

They usually take a lien on the assets they lend against. Banks, however, generally make unsecured loans based on the company's general credit and balance-sheet strength. The bank probably won't lend more than 50% or 75% of the company's net worth, but the finance company may lend several times the net worth if sufficient assets are pledged to secure the loan.

Commercial financing is usually done on a revolving basis. That means that the loan is reduced as receivables are collected or other assets liquidated. Then it can be increased again as the pledged assets increase. Some commercial finance companies will consider making three- or five-year term loans secured by plant and equipment if the company is also borrowing on a revolving basis against current assets.

Interest rates usually float—from $3^1/2$ to 6 percentage points above bank prime rates. If the same borrower went to the bank, it would probably pay 1 to 2 points over prime, but the difference is less than it seems. Banks usually ask for compensating balances, so the bank's effective interest rate is higher than its stated rate. And the bank may insist on lending for 60 or 90 days, even though all the money isn't needed for that long. The commercial finance company calculates its interest charges daily.

A possible way to get a lower rate: Ask the commercial finance company to bring in a bank to take half the loan. If the finance company charges four points over prime and the bank two points over prime, the borrower pays a blended rate of three points over prime. Sometimes the entire transaction can be done in the bank's name, so that nobody knows the company is borrowing from a commercial finance company.

Such knowledge can generate problems. If a company uses commercial financing, some people will think it's in financial trouble. This is less true than it used to be. Some very large listed companies use commercial financing for seasonal needs. (Usually a company's customers aren't notified of the commercial financing. But Dun & Bradstreet will pick the information up, and the lien on the assets will probably be entered in public records.)

Factoring: In this approach, a factoring company signs on to perform a package service—for lending, credit management, and protection against credit losses. How it works:

■The factor makes credit investigations of the company's customers.

■The factor takes over all approved receivables and pays the company face value for them a few days after the due date. This is called maturity factoring.

■The factor assumes all collection problems and all credit losses on approved receivables. Thus, the factor, in effect, provides credit insurance to the company.

■The factor charges a fee—usually between $3/4$% and 2%—of receivables collected.

■In addition, the factor is willing to lend money to the company by paying for the receivables in advance of the due date. This is called discount factoring. The factor will discount receivables by subtracting from their value an interest amount (usually an annual rate $2^1/2$–4 percentage points over bank prime rate).

■The company's customer is notified that the factor has acquired his obligation and he is asked to send payment directly to the factor.

Factoring is commonly used in the textile and apparel fields, where there is no stigma attached to it. It is also being used somewhat more in furniture, shoes, plastics, and hardware and by wholesalers and importers.

How to find commercial finance companies and factors: Write to National Commercial Finance Conference, One Penn Plaza, New York 10001, for a free copy of *Roster of Membership*. It includes names and addresses of over 150 commercial finance and factoring firms throughout the country.

Swiss Bank Accounts

It's best to open a Swiss bank account, especially a large one, in person. However, you can easily open an account by mail. Just write to the bank, asking for forms and information. (Type your letter. Swiss bankers complain of illegible mail from America.)

You must have your signature verified at a Swiss consulate or bank or by a notary public. The bank will provide forms.

You should execute a power of attorney over the account (unless it's a joint account). Under Swiss law, the power of attorney remains in force even after the depositor's death. If you have qualms about a power of attorney, you don't have to deliver it to the person. Leave it with your attorney, to be delivered only in case of your death or disability.

Swiss banks offer current accounts (checking), deposit accounts (saving), and custodial accounts (the bank will hold your stock certificates, gold, or other property for a fee).

As in America, there are demand deposits and time deposits. Some accounts require notice to withdraw more than a specified amount. Interest varies with the type of account. The rates are not high, however, compared with those of American banks. The appeals of Swiss banks lies in safety and the soundness of the currency.

Accounts may be in Swiss francs, American dollars, or another stable currency (depending on economic conditions when the account is opened).

Taxes And Regulations

Although there are no US restrictions on Swiss bank accounts, your income tax form asks if you have any foreign bank accounts. If you answer "yes," you must fill out Form 90-22.1 and file it by June 30.

Interest on foreign accounts is taxable like any other income. You can take a credit for foreign taxes paid.

If you have an account in Swiss francs and the franc increases in value relative to the dollar, you may be liable for a capital gains tax when you withdraw money and reconvert it to dollars. Losses arising from decreases in value may not be deductible in regard to personal accounts.

Switzerland imposes a withholding tax on interest, but Americans can get refunded by showing they are not Swiss residents. Your bank will send you the forms. (Note: The bank sends in the tax without disclosing depositors' names. To claim the refund, however, you must, of course, disclose your identity.)

At one time, the Swiss imposed severe restrictions on foreign accounts. Only the first 50,000 francs of an account could draw interest, and accounts above 100,000 francs were charged "negative interest" of 40%—nearly a confiscatory rate. These restrictions, and others, could conceivably be reinstated if economic conditions change.

Even when the restrictions were in force, however, the were not retroactive. They did not apply to existing accounts—only to deposits made after the rules were adopted (another reason you might want to act now).

Source: Stanley C. Ruchelman, tax partner, Deloitte & Touche, New York 10019.

To Keep Your Banking Secrets Secret

The only thing banks can legally tell a third party about your company is whether it has an active account. In practice, banks often give out much more information than that. Though most banks use sound judgment, it makes good business sense to keep a tight rein on data that can get into the hands of customers, creditors and competitors. Best safeguards:

■Send a written order to the bank officer that handles your accounts, instructing him not to release any information without the company's approval. This step seems obvious, but many businesses don't make the demand clear and explicit. Never rely on oral instructions.

■Instruct the bank in writing to refer all requests for information to the company's financial officer.

■Remind the bank, again in writing, of your instructions whenever you suspect that someone might try to get credit data. Send a copy of your instruction to the bank's legal department. Attempts are often made when a new competitor enters the market or when the company is a takeover candidate.

■When the bank lets information slip out, notify the account executive immediately. Waiting makes it appear that the breach of confidentiality isn't important.

The Realities

It's virtually impossible to protect financial information completely. Credit agencies and people interested in your company employ a variety of ruses to get data…and they're usually successful.

Examples: An agency representative calls the bank. He says he's from a fictitious business and asks the bank if a $65,000 check drawn against the company's account is good. Any answer the bank gives (other than saying it can't answer) gives an indication of the company's creditworthiness. Credit agencies also request that their bank make a bank-to-bank inquiry about the company. These questions are usually answered.

If it appears that the bank is giving out information, retain a credit agency to find out how much data it can get on the company itself. This way, you'll find out how much information parties are likely to get and how accurate the information is.

If the bank still doesn't plug the leaks, the company has two options:

1. Change banks. That's a drastic step since most banking relations are built up over several years. But the mere threat of a change will often let your bank know how serious you consider the breach.

2. Threaten to sue the bank for defamation if the information it gave out was false. That's another drastic step, but it may be the best recourse when the company has suffered large damages because of the leaks.

If the company was damaged by accurate information that the bank gave out, it can also sue for damages. For instance, if a bank reveals information that encourages a takeover attempt, the company may be able to recover its costs to fight the takeover from the bank. Caution: Litigation of this type is complex and usually time-consuming.

Source: Dan Brecher, head of the investment banking department at the law firm of Demov, Morris & Hammerling, 40 W. 57 St., New York 10019.

Can't Meet Bank Payment?

Make an appointment to see the company's loan officer at the bank as soon as it is clear that the company will not make the payment on time. The officer can sometimes keep the company off the bank's delinquency list. Benefit: Preserves maneuvering room. Once an account is on the list, it comes to the attention of the bank's top officers. And that reduces the company's negotiating ability.

Tactics:

■Be honest. Withholding information only hurts in the long run.

■Do not wait for the bank to initiate a new payment plan. Bring one to the bank that fits the company's cash-flow projection. This preparation shows the company is sincere in trying to make good on the loan.

Be prepared to give the bank additional collateral if necessary. Caution: Do not strip the company of all collateral. Hold on to as much as possible so that management retains future bargaining power.

If the bank is uncooperative about negotiating new terms, shift the accounts necessary to manage the company's cash flow (everything above compensating balances) to another bank. Banks have the legal right to dip into a company's accounts to satisfy a delinquent loan. (It is called setting-off and can be done without notice.)

Bottom line: If the company's credit history has been good all along, most banks will work with management as long as they believe the delinquency can be cured. They do not want to lose customers any more than the company wants to lose its credit rating.

Source: Malcolm P. Moses, Malcolm P. Moses Associates, financial consultants, Merrick, NY.

Profiting From 'Bank Float'

Most companies underestimate their checking account balances by at least 30%, according to a consultant in cash management. The corporation doesn't estimate the float and doesn't know at any given moment what checks haven't cleared yet. Learning to analyze and monitor the float can mean extra earnings with little effort.

What to do: Make a six-month study of outgoing checks to major suppliers (chances are 80% of dollars paid go to 20% of vendors). Check each one's float pattern, then estimate how long new checks will take to clear, have money on deposit only as needed.

How To Cut Banking Costs

Most companies know how much interest they pay on bank loans, but comparatively few know what they're charged for other banking services.

Examples: Fees for deposits, check clearing, account maintenance, zero-balance accounts, controlled disbursement, lock boxes, inter-account transfers, etc.

Reality: Individually, these banking services are not expensive, but the total can be substantial for a company. As a rule, these fees are paid through maintaining balances with the bank at a level sufficient to compensate the bank for these services.

Trap: By not looking closely at these non-credit banking charges, companies might wind up paying for services they don't need...or they overlook less-expensive services they could be getting if they negotiated or shopped around.

Depending on the kinds of services and number of transactions, medium-size companies can spend up to $100,000 a year on banking services. And doing without services they could be getting can cost a company far more than that.

Tighter Control

Companies don't always have a handle on bank charges because banks aren't required to provide all the information...and company financial officers generally don't take time to review the data that are provided.

The first step toward getting control is to ask the company's financial officer to get a periodic account analysis from banks the company uses. The analysis is a statement of services being used in all active accounts, the costs of the services, the customer's balances and available funds, and the earnings credit rate the company will receive for its available balances. Banks usually prepare analyses on all accounts, but furnish them only on request.

If the company hasn't been receiving regular account analyses, chances are good that it has bigger idle balances than necessary.

Opportunities: Always request and review account analyses. And, if balances are substantially higher than necessary to compensate for bank services, shift excess cash to other accounts or into non-bank vehicles such as Treasury bonds, where it can be put to more profitable use.

Shopping For Services

If the company uses more than one bank, compare the different account analyses closely.

Examples: In a recent survey of eight banks whose assets ran from $500 million to more than $44 billion, we found that deposit fees varied from 25¢ to $1.10, monthly account maintenance from $5 to $15 and daily balance reports from $16 to $213. Surprisingly, there's not always a correlation between the size of a bank and what it charges for services.

Next, ask other banks in your area for their standard price lists. As the name implies, this is a catalog of services and their cost, often depending on how much business a company does with the bank. The object, of course, is to find the lowest prices, but also to find out about services that can mean an even greater saving.

Example: Banks in any one area rarely clear checks at the same speed. Shaving a day—or even a half-day—off the clearing time can mean huge savings for a company with high cash flow.

Negotiating Strategy

It's rare to find services so much cheaper at another institution that it makes sense to pull out of a long-term banking relationship. But specific services may make it worthwhile to move some of the company's business. And, in some cases, the offer of inexpensive service from one bank can be used to persuade the company's existing bank to lower its rate for the same service.

The Error Factor

When a company looks at its account analyses, it is not uncommon to find mistakes. Example: Fees based on a standard price list, rather than the prices quoted or negotiated.

Don't hesitate to ask for a correction. Then, where applicable, go one step further...if the volume of business the company does with the bank has increased, ask for a reduction of fees.

Possibility: When negotiating a loan, the company may want to agree to a half-percentage point higher interest in exchange for a cut in other banking fees (or conversely, tolerate the high fees in exchange for a slightly better interest rate).

Myth: That a company will jeopardize its banking relationship if it complains about fees. As long as customers are diplomatic, good banks respect those who keep track of what they're being charged. In the long run, that type of customer is more likely to get loans when it needs them.

Source: Benjamin Arvizu, Arvizu Financial Group, banking and corporate cash management consultants, 3860 W. Northwest Highway, Dallas 75220.

Chapter 23
Acquisitions, Mergers, And Start-Ups

Guide To A Successful Acquisition

Before looking for an acquisition, a company should set realistic goals for what it expects from the venture. These goals will vary substantially in each situation. But a buyer should not expect a perfect match between the acquisition's value and present objectives.

The first step is to do careful homework on the acquisition target. Know where it stands in the market and whether it's an innovator. Find out as much as possible about its strengths and weaknesses before negotiations.

Use book value in relation to market purchase prices to determine whether the deal is attractive. A healthy return on equity and a good growth curve will usually ensure profits from an acquisition for at least a couple of years.

Keep in mind that acquisitions tend to progress more favorably with the use of a professional intermediary or investment banker, one with a proven track record and good references. Make sure the actual professional, not just the firm, has the right experience and credentials.

Next, set up an acquisition team to work with the intermediary. The chief executive officer should be part of that team. The final decision should be the CEO's alone.

Don't pursue a company that wouldn't survive a merger. Entrepreneurial companies that rely on a highly personalized management style fall into this category.

Keep negotiations moving at a steady, but not necessarily fast, pace. Lagging negotiations may be taken for lack of interest. Conducting them too quickly, however, creates an impression of overeagerness and can lead to errors of judgment.

If either side has serious problems, see that they're discussed at the outset. When a company discovers a problem just before the close, it can't help but question the wisdom of the entire deal. Examples are a buyer who doesn't reveal immediately that action can't be taken on the deal for several months, or a seller who delays mentioning that a lease may not be renewed.

Use due diligence in checking on the target company, but don't go to extremes. The term due diligence refers to the acquirer's legal responsibility for performing a full audit, a review of minutes, leases, contracts, etc., and an inspection of plant and inventory. Due diligence can be overdone and mess up the deal. If the target of an acquisition really wants to hide something, it will probably succeed.

Understand the seller's motivation for wanting to be acquired.

Unless the buyer plans sweeping changes in policy and management, it should prepare both teams of executives for the aftershock of acquisition. Except in cases where the company was bought for its plant or inventory, its management should be one of its strongest assets.

Source: Gilbert W. Harrison, chairman, Financo, Philadelphia.

Sizing Up A Possible Acquisition

While a potential buyer should leave full analysis of an acquisition candidate's financial statements to experts, the buyer can sharpen his instincts by looking at those statements for potential danger signals:

■Look at the average age of accounts receivable. If the average is lengthening, find out why. There may be more doubtful accounts than raw figures suggest.

■Check the method by which the company ages its receivables. If that method has changed recently to improve the numbers, beware.

■Are the receivables from related parties significant? Did the deals with related parties take place on terms equal to arm's length?

■Study the company's inventories. If inventories listed as work in process have risen relative to inventories listed as raw materials and finished goods, this suggests a possible slow-down in sales.

■See how labor and overhead have been allocated to inventories. This is one way inventories get padded.

■Closely held companies with unaudited financial statements often reduce their inventory through "reserves." Personally inspect them. Often, they're dumping grounds for unsalable finished goods.

■Scrutinize all contingent liabilities. If the company is a defendant in litigation, or has been threatened with litigation, find out how much a settlement could cost.

■Are the intangible assets overvalued?

■A surplus that the Internal Revenue Service decides is unreasonably retained earnings can sour a bargain acquisition.

If the IRS decides that salaries paid to top management in recent years are disguised dividends, the new owner may face a sizable tax liability.

■Analyze the standard ratios determining the level of the company's profitability. Look for any recent change, then investigate the reasons for it.

■Find out what percentage of sales comes from major customers. Consider including a clause in the acquisition agreement voiding the sale if the sellers don't disclose the number of customers accounting for more than 10% of sales volume.

■Find out what percentage of transactions are with related parties. This includes leases, loans, purchases of property, guarantees of indebtedness, capital transfers, and sales. Beware if the terms of these transactions are hidden or not clear.

■Check maintenance and repair costs to see if they've risen in proportion to sales volume. If they haven't, management may have been running down the capital plant.

Additional points to study:

■Reasons for auditors' qualifications on financial statements.

■Reasons for any significant transactions entered into the last year and their impact on earnings.

■Reasons for large legal bills.

■The number of years for which the IRS has yet to close the books on the company's tax returns.

Source: Samuel P. Gunther, partner, Richard A. Eisner & Co., New York.

Before Okaying Acquisition

The failure rate of acquisitions is very high. About 50% do not reach expectations, according to informed estimates. There are certain obvious mistakes that should be avoided. If they are, the chance of the merger or acquisition being successful goes up significantly. Questions to ask:

■Is the decision to acquire chiefly a response to the fact that the competition is doing it? Every decision to acquire should be based only on the company's own growth needs and capabilities.

■Is the acquisition being considered simply as a reaction to an idea? Intermediaries (brokers, investment bankers, lawyers, etc.) who frequently present interesting acquisition candidates to chief executives are often unfamiliar with the specific technical and management needs and capabilities of the acquiring company. Management time and energy spent in reacting to proposals is probably better spent clarifying business strategy for growth, including the question of acquisitions.

Is there a member of management, or an outside adviser, who understands the operations of the prospective acquisition well enough to identify less obvious problems? It is very important to eliminate poor candidates quickly.

■Who will competitors be? The share of market projections will depend on what competitors the acquisition faces. The larger the combined company's market share, the more of a leader it can be in setting prices, market strategies, etc. Best opportunity to consider: Buy into a market that is fragmented, if possible, not one with one or two strong market leaders.

Special acquisition strategy for a smaller company: Management capabilities are usually narrower and more specialized, thus less able to provide expertise in a number of different industry areas. Acquisitions should not stray far from home.

Source: William Kirschenbaum, Neuberger & Berman, 522 Fifth Ave., New York 10036.

Eight Ways For Buyers To Evaluate A Business

Emotion and other less than pragmatic considerations often play major roles in deciding how much a business is worth. For buyers who want to rely on more logical techniques, there are eight basic methods for evaluating a closely held business with no publicly traded stock and owners who are near retirement:

1. Capitalized earnings. The value is judged according to the previous year's earnings, income over the last few years, or projected earnings.

2. Corporate and shareholder earnings. Both of these are capitalized. This amount is paid out over a period that is usually two to four times the capitalization period. If earnings were capitalized for the previous two years, for example, payment could be over the next four to eight years.

3. Percentage of future profits. The definition of profit can include any items that management determines. Payments can be spread over a number of years and arranged in diminishing stages.

4. Book value. The sum of assets as they appear on the books (excluding goodwill) less liabilities.

5. Adjusted book value. Current values are applied to the balance sheet. For example, fixed assets are valued at either their replacement or their knockdown value rather than as they appear on the books.

6. Book value plus pensions. Consideration is given to retirement plans currently in effect at similar companies and an equitable compensation program for the retiring sellers.

7. Start-up cost. A buyer who wants to enter an industry will often pay more than a business is actually worth, since the price may still be less than the cost of entering the field from scratch.

8. Industry custom. Some types of businesses are valued on the basis of historic formulas. Dental practices may sell for the previous year's gross income. Insurance brokerages can sell for a price equal to the first year's retained renewals.

Source: Edward Mendlowitz, partner, Mendlowitz Weitsen, New York.

Before Buying A Small Business

Questions to ask in assessing the potential of a business you are thinking about purchasing:

■Was the initial planning effective? To evaluate this, look at lease terms, fixtures and equipment, recordkeeping, advertising, marketing, and site selection.

■What were the start-up costs? Some sellers try to include these in the selling price. A basic rule is that all one-time costs should be absorbed by the owner. Exception: The sale price should reflect the current market value of fixtures and equipment.

■What mistakes did the founder make? Could they eventually kill the business?

■How solid is the current customer base? Avoid any business that depends on strong customer loyalty to the current owner.

■Will the current owner stay on for a few months to ease the transition? This helps transfer supplier and customer trust to the new owner and gives immediate assistance on unforeseen problems.

Source: Kenneth J. Albert, *Straight Talk About Small Business*, McGraw-Hill, New York.

Buying A Business Without Down Payment

For many, the idea is just a fantasy, but for a growing number of entrepreneurial managers, it's a practical solution to a long-held wish: Buying the division or business department from the parent company.

The idea: Buying the business operation with little or no down payment. The method is called leveraged buy-out—and it's gaining increased attention from financial people and would-be entrepreneurs. Here's how it works:

A new corporation is created that purchases the division by borrowing up to the hilt against the divisions' assets. It might borrow 80% of the value of receivables,

60% of inventory, and 60%–75% of land, buildings, and equipment. If it isn't possible to borrow the full purchase price (plus working capital that the new company may need), the selling company may take back a subordinated note for part of the purchase price.

Many lenders are willing to finance leveraged buy-outs, even where the new owner-managers don't have much cash to invest, if the division had a good track record and if they believe management is strong. Their reasoning: If execs did a good job working on salary, they'll probably do even better as owners.

The best sources for this kind of borrowing are the selling companies themselves. Some banks are becoming active, too. And equity capital or subordinated loans may be obtained from venture companies (their terms are tough, though).

It's a way for good managers, now on salary, to build a personal fortune. If the new company does well, their stock holdings should become very valuable in a few years.

Managers of divisions who are thinking about going on their own should consider these points:

■Lenders will want ironclad assurance that the management team will stay. They'll probably ask for five-year employment contracts and expensive life insurance on top officers.

■Lenders will insist on a pledge of all assets and will supervise operations very closely. Management may find itself restricted, may have to go to finance company for permission to do anything new. (One disappointed owner said, "All I did was change bosses.")

■Because the load of debt is so heavy, lenders may insist on personal guarantees of loans by owner-managers and their wives. That means the house, the bank account, and all personal assets are on the line.

■Risks are high, too. Managers are so dazzled by the chance to be independent that they sometimes fail to analyze the company's future dispassionately. It's a good idea to review the company and industry outlook with an experienced adviser whose thinking isn't colored by personal involvement.

Source: Dan Brecher, attorney, 230 Park Avenue, New York 10017.

People Problems In Corporate Mergers

Many potentially successful mergers fail because of inadequate assessment by both parties of the human factors.

The most common error made by the buying company is overreliance on gut feelings about the seller's management and organization, and on the seller's past financial performance. People who work effectively in one environment may not do so in another.

High-risk merger candidates are companies in which the entrepreneur/owner is to function as a manager within the merged structure, or companies with a unique image. An example is a small high-technology company, proud of its creativity and independence.

Before making an acquisition, the buyer should know the quality of the seller's management and work force. Look for a diversity of skills and the ability to accept authority.

The seller should ask himself if he will be comfortable operating under the system of the buying company. Before the deal closes, he should clearly determine with the buyer details about reporting, managerial and financial autonomy.

Sellers who often become unhappy are those in the so-called creative businesses. They frequently get frustrated adjusting to the discipline of the new system. The ideal seller is one who views the sale as an opportunity to turn illiquid wealth into cash, and to grow through the additional resources of the acquiring company.

Source: Arthur A. Rosenbloom, Standard Research Consultants, and Abraham K. Korman, BFS Psychological Associates, New York.

Incorporation Dangers

When incorporating a business, be sure that everyone knows about it. Case: A retailer incorporated without telling anyone. When it fell behind in paying its bills, the shareholders were ruled to be personally liable to the unpaid suppliers, just as if there were no corporation.

Source: *Detroit Pure Milk Co. v. Farnsworth,* 319 NW2d 557.

The Secrets Of Successful Joint Ventures

Companies are learning to stretch their own resources of money, people and innovation by forming strategic alliances with other companies.

Such alliances have been growing at well over 20% a year in the U.S.

While there have been some successful examples of joint ventures that have lasted 35 years or more, the average life span of the alliances I've studied is only $3^{1}/_{2}$ years.

Companies go into these alliances expecting them to be temporary, but most think they'll last about seven to 10 years as entrepreneurial ventures typically do.

Unfortunately, most companies find they aren't getting what they want out of the alliances. Worse, a company may find that it has given away precious know-how or technology to a potential foreign competitor.

Such mistakes can be avoided only by very carefully selecting partners and relying on a tightly drawn contract that specifies exactly what each of the companies will give and get out of the deal, including specific remedies if things don't work out as planned.

Alliances Supplanting Companies

My notion of strategic alliances includes everything from equity joint ventures (in which each company contributes cash to form a separate entity) to cross-licensing, cross-manufacturing, cross-marketing and/or distribution agreements, to research and development consortia, to "Texas Handshake" deals where companies simply agree to work together to accomplish some objective. (It's understood in Texas that if you don't live up to the terms of an agreement, no one will do business with you in the future.)

With so many strategic alliances taking place, the boundaries between one firm and another—and between supplying industry and consuming industry—are beginning to blur. Sometimes it's hard to determine exactly who invents, makes and sells a particular product or service.

Example: Pharmaceutical companies, strapped by the high cost of developing new drugs, are spreading these costs by forging co-marketing and co-promotional relationships with other firms at an increasing rate.

Hoffmann-La Roche recently made a deal with Glaxo, which created and owns the patent for *Zantac*, an ulcer medication, which gives Hoffmann the right to market the product in the U.S. for 10 years, after which Glaxo itself will also market the product in the U.S.

Prediction: Instead of trying to do and be everything unto themselves, more companies will combine in networks, shoring up their own weak spots.

Reasons To Form Alliances

We used to see joint ventures formed only for projects that were very expensive or risky, such as offshore oil drilling. Now, however, they're being formed to help projects move faster. The rush to take on partners is often an effort to quickly capitalize on what little competitive advantage a company has.

Alliances are sometimes required for certain kinds of defense contracts. Occasionally, they're the only way to get technology out of a country where currency blocks prohibit an outright sale.

Certainly alliances offer companies a way to explore synergies of scale and scope that they couldn't do alone. Finally, alliances are becoming a way of getting venture capital when traditional sources of financing dry up.

It's now a joke that Japanese partners are so popular because they can provide so much financing. What's not so funny, however, is that they want in return right of first refusal or right of first information on any new technology created. Often, Japanese partners manage to learn much more about the operations of U.S. partners than the companies intended.

Example: In one case, the Japanese sent representatives around to follow a U.S. company's salespeople. When they found out who the customers were, they wined and dined them—planning to woo them away. Then they backed out of the alliance because they didn't need it any more. The U.S. company sued and won damages because the Japanese had clearly gone beyond the terms of the agreement.

Right now, there's a danger that U.S. companies will rush to make hasty alliances with European partners in advance of 1992. Problem: Europeans are much more familiar with alliances than are U.S. executives, who are often naive in setting up these deals.

Advice: Don't hurry. It won't be a seamless move to a unified European market. It may take years to work out. Meanwhile, if the company has something to offer a European company in the U.S., that may be the best approach now, with the proviso that your company will get European rights later on.

Picking A Partner

The way most companies get into alliances is a hit-and-miss process of dancing with a lot of different partners, and eventually finding out which ones they like best.

But before taking up with any partner, the company owes it to itself to find out if the partner is trustworthy. Check references carefully. If there's no track record of previous joint ventures or alliances, interrogate suppliers, bankers and customers to see if the company has a reputation for reliability and integrity. If anybody has anything bad to say about the company, check it out carefully.

When in doubt about a partner, start with very limited small projects to test the waters.

Always try to verify that the partner actually has the technology it claims to have and that it can deliver on the promises it is making. (Whether it will deliver is another question.) To get a reliable assessment, there's no substitute for trusted eyes and ears. Be prepared to send your own people over, if necessary.

The biggest mistake U.S. companies make in forming alliances with foreign partners is relying too much on lawyers. There comes a time to review any deal with counsel, but most foreign companies entrust negotiations to operating people who know what is doable. Too often in the U.S., management negotiates in secret and, by the time operating people are involved, they're handed something totally unrealistic. There's no easy answer to this problem because secrecy is important. But management must get input from operating managers before an alliance is finalized.

Traps To Watch Out For

Companies should avoid alliances in countries that don't adhere to our copyright convention, especially those that have a well-educated population. These include India, Russia, China, Taiwan, Eastern European countries like Hungary, and even Italy and Israel.

Danger: They will simply take your intellectual property and reverse-engineer your products.

Never give a joint venture every piece of information needed to understand your proprietary technology. Just sell pieces of it in a turnkey form as you would to another third party. Also avoid giving the alliance any power to change your proprietary information. If you can't control the knowledge, lay down very strict terms governing its use or walk away from the deal.

To protect a famous brand name, structure the alliance as a franchisee with a very tight contract that can be rescinded if there are any infringements.

Companies that become dependent on strategic alliances for technological development and innovation risk losing their in-house ability to innovate. Then they're in real trouble.

Source: Dr. Kathryn Rudie Harrigan, professor of strategic management, Columbia Business School, 716 Uris Hall, New York 10027. Director of the Strategy Research Center, professor Harrigan is a well-known consultant and worldwide authority on industrial survival strategies, mergers and acquisitions and joint ventures. She has authored seven books and many articles on the subject.

Start Your Own Business With Accrued Pension

Employee Getum has "had it" working for his present boss. He wants out now. He has $100,000 coming from his employer's qualified plan, and he is entitled to and qualifies for lump-sum treatment. Getum finds out the tax bite on the $100,000, if distributed this year, would be $35,000; he needs $50,000 to finance his new business. What to do?

The steps would be as follows:

1. Getum forms a new corporation, Go-Getum Co.
2. Go-Getum Co. adopts a qualified profit-sharing plan.

3. The distribution—the full $100,000—from Getum's former employer's qualified plan is rolled over to the new Go-Getum plan.

4. The new plan would have a provision to allow loans to be made to participants in an amount not to exceed 50% of the participant's vested interest, or $50,000.

5. The new profit-sharing plan would loan $50,000 to Getum to be repaid over five years at 11% interest per annum.

Obviously, the documentation from the new plan itself, the plan administrator's minutes describing and approving the loan, and the note payable by Getum to the profit-sharing trust must be impeccable in every detail.

Source: Irving L. Blackman, partner, Blackman, Kallick, Bartelstein, 300 S. Riverside Plaza, Chicago 60606.

How To Start A Business On A Shoestring

Shoestring businesses aren't limited to small ventures tucked away in the dusty corner of someone's garage. Many are capitalized at hundreds of thousands of dollars. They're called "shoestring" because the owner has invested little—if any—of his own cash.

Shoestring businesses are more a state of mind than a modus operandi. They work only if the owner is willing to adhere to the One-tenth Principle. Starting a business with one-tenth of the required capital demands that you exert 10 times the effort.

Planning Comes First

Don't fall into the trap of thinking that the smaller a business, the less risk involved. Starting too small is actually more of a risk than starting too big. If you're starting a service business, microscopic beginnings might work. But new retail and manufacturing ventures require some more to begin—and enough to internally generate profits.

Careful planning and well-researched start-up costs are the keys to attracting financing. Helpful: Get a copy of the Small Business Administration's cost worksheet. It's been invaluable to me in pinpointing frequently overlooked cost items.

Once you've identified costs, the next crucial step is figuring out how to slash them. Don't emulate the small journal publisher who struggled in his plush $66,000/yr. offices when a $10,000 facility would have sufficed...and would have produced profits instead of red ink.

If your shoestring business does require extensive quarters, however, look for retail basement space or space in a large, older home. Both are usually priced well below conventional commercial property.

Retail businesses must focus on location. These businesses need immediate cash flow, and that means a high-traffic, high-rent location. Bad alternative: Low-rent space that will force you to plow rent savings into advertising to attract customers.

Better: Negotiate with the landlord to pay partial rent early in the lease and a higher rent later when cash flow is likely to be more substantial. Or, negotiate to pass renovation costs on to the landlord. Keep in mind that a landlord who pays for your new ceilings, carpets and air-conditioning is going to charge a higher rent. But this can save you as much as $100,000 in initial costs.

Equipment bargains are next on the shoestringer's cost-slashing list. In fact, it should be part of every entrepreneur's game plan to scour auctions, chain stores, equipment supply houses, classified ads, bankruptcy sales, and trade journals for secondhand equipment and fixtures.

Nothing Down...The Smart Way

One-hundred-percent financing abounds if you know where to look. Although banks and finance companies aren't prime lending sources for shoestring businesses, they'll usually consider full financing on bargain-priced equipment with established collateral value. And equipment sellers are often more interested in unloading unneeded equipment than in getting immediate cash.

Manufacturer financing can also be arranged. Trade-off: Manufacturers' lending standards are more lenient than banks'...but you'll have to pay two or three percentage points more.

Leasing is often a wiser choice than buying, especially for motor vehicles, computers, carpets and cash registers. Rule of thumb: If it will last more than five years, buy. If it will wear out or become obsolete within five years, lease when possible.

Inside idea: Whether buying or leasing, negotiate with the equipment manufacturer for a 30- to 60-day trial run. If you've planned well, your business should be generating enough cash flow to complete the buy or lease agreement by the end of the trial. If it isn't, return the equipment...and you've spent nothing.

Look to suppliers for financial support. Big suppliers can usually afford to let you defer payment for a while if they see the possibility of more and more business from you down the road. And, if your business looks like it will do well in the future, small suppliers might offer price breaks or better terms.

Example: A small enterprising baked-goods manufacturer convinced his flour supplier to buy him $40,000 of baking equipment against $800,000 in flour purchases over four years. The deal amounted to nothing-down for the baker, and a long-term customer for the supplier.

If you can't offer good collateral to a traditional lender, you'll have to look to nontraditional financing sources. Best bets: Friends, relatives, high-tax-bracket investors, and the SBA.

The Shoestring Corporation

Incorporating your venture is essential. But don't buy shares with all of your investment funds. Instead: Use a small portion for share-buying and loan the balance to a friend or relative who, in turn, loans the money to the new corporation in exchange for a mortgage. In the event of a failure, your friend or relative will be a preferred creditor...when he gets his money back, so will you. By contrast, if you loan directly to the corporation as a shareholder, repayment may be disallowed by a bankruptcy decision.

Should a loss occur, you can pass some of it to the IRS by taking advantage of Section 1244 of the Tax Code. That allows losses of a small business to be deducted in full against ordinary income. Limit: $100,000 a year on a joint return ($50,000 a year if you are single). All it takes is a clause in the corporate bylaws stating that shares are sold to you under this section of the Internal Revenue Code. To qualify under Section 1244, the corporation must have capital of $1 million or less. It must operate as a business. And the stock must have been issued for money or property.

Source: Arnold S. Goldstein, Meyer, Goldstein, Chyten and Kosberg, Chestnut Hill, MA.

Sole Proprietors Win Big

Sole proprietorships win a big one. The Supreme Court has granted extra protection to individuals who run their businesses through proprietorships. When the business's records contain evidence of criminal wrongdoing, the owner may claim the Fifth Amendment right against self-incrimination, and refuse to deliver them to the IRS. The same protection does not extend to corporate records because corporations aren't persons and so can't claim the Fifth Amendment privilege.

Source: *U.S. v. John Doe*, S. Ct. Docket 82–786.

Selling The Company Upon Retirement

Despite the temptation to sell out and forget the aggravations of stagflation (especially if a bidder comes along with an attractive offer), many owners of privately held companies will benefit most by staying private and devising a plan that allows them to sell out on good terms when they are actually ready to retire.

Unless an owner wants to make a life or career change, or believes the business is going bad, the attractions of selling out are usually less than meet the eye:

■Taxes may take up a large percentage of the profit from selling out.

■Selling out via an exchange of stock with a public corporation is risky in an uncertain market.

■Continued ownership of a privately held company guarantees unique financial flexibility.

An alternative for continuation is to offer selected managers a minority, noncontrolling equity interest in the company. This makes managers into ready buyers whenever the owner wants to sell out, since it gives managers the borrowing power to come up with the necessary cash for a buyout. As a bonus, equity participation will inevitably improve the manager's performance, which is crucial in the increasingly tough business environment.

If the principal wants to pass on the company to his heirs, the equity participation plan should be structured so that when the time comes to sell out, the owner gets a sizable lump sum with which to retire but keeps enough stock for the family to retain control of the company.

But making managers minority partners changes their relationship with the owners. The change is not necessarily perceived by the principal as for the better. The managers may decide to restrict the owner's perquisites in some unforeseen way.

To avoid complications, structure the equity plan so that the owner has the right to buy back the equity of managers at any time. It's important to have a clear and fair formula for determining the price at which the stock will be bought back. This will assure managers they will be compensated for the effort they put into the company, even if they leave. It will also help to avoid bitterness and possible litigation if they go elsewhere.

Finally, structure the plan so that the principal can buy back the stock held by managers if they leave voluntarily, or if they die, to keep the stock from falling into outside hands.

Source: Philip Kimmel, partner, Hertz Herson & Co., New York.

Part III

**THE GREAT BOOK
OF BUSINESS SECRETS**

Marketing
And Sales
Management

Chapter 24
Marketing Management Wisdom

Much Better Marketing

■What's the most serious marketing error you see companies committing?

The biggest mistake is basing marketing on what management wants to do rather than on what it can do. There's often a macho atmosphere in the boardroom, and everyone follows the manager who comes up with the biggest dream or biggest objective. It doesn't seem to matter if the dream is unattainable or the objective unreasonable. Ironically, rich and successful companies are the most likely to fall into this trap.

Xerox is a classic example. Since 1969, it has probably spent close to $2 billion trying to build a computer and office-systems business. Though the marketplace accepts the company as a great maker of copiers, it rejects Xerox in other businesses. The losses continue to mount. And since Xerox diverted its attention from copiers, competitors have been able to chip away at Xerox's share of that market.

Xerox, for all its expertise and money, fell into the trap of following a grandiose marketing dream instead of concentrating its resources on what it was eminently capable of doing.

■What examples can you cite of companies with the right approach?

Domino's Pizza and Federal Express. Domino's entrepreneur Tom Monahan first devised a way to improve home delivery of freshly made pizza. Then, while other pizza vendors advertised price and toppings, Domino's focused very narrowly on what it could do best—deliver the pizza…fast. It did what it was capable of, pushed its ability…and won.

Federal Express initially tried to be Emery at a discount, and it ran ads that essentially said, we can do it cheaper. That didn't work, mainly because a growing number of competitors could also offer discounts. Then Federal Express focused on what it could do better than the competition—guarantee next-day delivery. It did what it was good at, pushed it…and won.

Wrigley is another company that's consistently rejected the temptation to expand in other fields. Instead, it focuses on just what it knows it can make and market best—chewing gum—and its market share has increased.

These companies follow what we call bottom-up marketing. They didn't dream up a grandiose marketing strategy and then try to devise tactics to carry it out. Instead, they knew what they could do tactically…and let that determine their strategies.

■But how can a company expand and still maintain a narrow focus?

The only real way is the Procter & Gamble route, in which a company creates a new product with a separate identity and then focuses narrowly on that product's unique advantages.

Apple Computer followed that track. When Apple moved into the business computer market, it didn't try to convince buyers that Apple computers were suddenly office machines. Instead, it created MacIntosh as a separate line with unique business-computing features.

■Marketing people have a tendency to tamper with product image. How can a CEO keep them on track?

Part of the problem is that top executives don't always have much control over marketing. They hire middle managers to handle it while they sit back and dream up elaborate five-year growth plans. But to be effective, a top executive has got to worry about planning for today, not five years from now.

■How can CEOs stay in closer touch with marketing?

It's no secret. They simply have to spend more time at the front. They've got to get a feel for what's actually motivating their customers. When the head of Sears Roebuck, for example, visits a store, he lets the manager know several weeks in advance. That's not how to do it. CEOs should put themselves in a position to see things as they really are.

Getting back to Xerox...if the head of that company had gotten out to see customers, he would have known very well that the name Xerox meant copiers, and not computers. Then if the company still wanted to get into the computer market, it might have created a product with another name and marketed it on the basis of that product's unique advantages.

So, not only should a CEO maintain periodic contact with customers, he should encourage his senior managers to do the same. These senior people are typically isolated, and subordinates feed them information they believe their bosses want to hear.

■Are focus groups useful?

Only to a limited extent. The problem is that researchers too often try to sell their pet ideas in the conclusion of a focus group report. However, the raw data from focus groups can be useful.

So when you get a report back from a focus group, spend time with the raw data. That's where you can get into the mind of the customer.

■How helpful is direct-response advertising in keeping a company in touch with the marketplace?

Direct response is by nature helpful because the ads ask customers or prospects to send in coupons or to phone or write for more information. This feedback clearly tells the company which tactics are working. And from that information, a company can build on those attributes of a product that customers respond to most. Those are the attributes that will distinguish the company from its competition.

Source: Jack Trout, president, and Al Ries, chairman, Trout & Ries, Inc., marketing consultants, Greenwich, CT. They are coauthors of *Bottom-Up Marketing*, McGraw-Hill, 11 W. 19 St., New York 10011.

Marketing In Inflationary Times

Not too long ago, companies that were almost right could usually count on a second chance in the market if they had good trade relationships to carry them through a major mistake. Not so when inflation has raised the stakes. And greater sophistication on the part of both foreign and domestic competitors has reduced the odds for success. To keep up with the shifts, management must avoid inflation pitfalls and make whatever changes are necessary in its comfortable ways of marketing.

Biggest inflationary trap. Looking at the company's sunk cost (the cash already invested) in a product as the controlling factor in marketing it. Beware of the manufacturing mentality in marketing: I sell what I make. We have to find a way to sell more of these widgets. Instead, have the courage to decide that the profitable market for widgets has disappeared. Instead of reflecting on sunk costs, look for ways to use capacity more profitably. Consider getting rid of widget-making machinery in order to: Invest in new machinery that will improve productivity for other product lines or switch to products that can be sold at a higher margin because the company has a productivity edge on competitors or the product is more desirable to the consumer.

A crucial calculation. Determine costs and profitability on a line-by-line, item-by-item basis. With both inflation and interest rates at near-record levels, it is essential to know which businesses are making money and which are draining resources. Too many companies don't know. Service companies, too, must analyze which clients are profitable.

Get rid of deadwood. That used to mean people. Now it means rooting out anything that is a losing proposition for the company. A major impediment is thinking that what currently is in place is permanent. Almost every company has some product it would be better off walking away from—typically a high executive's pet project that everyone else is wary of touching. Don't worry whether or not some assets can be sold. Simply put a padlock on the door.

Targeting. Marketing research is yielding fewer and fewer distinct answers to marketing questions just when inflation-impacted marketers need specifics most. The old pattern consisted of a single brand-product in the lead, followed by a couple of pretty good brands and a bunch of cats and dogs. Now, the top two or three brands in any category are virtually at parity in quality, image and, often, in marketing approach. Too often, conventional surveys rate one product 4.57 (on a scale of one to ten) and another 4.65. Neither wins. And neither company can make an informed decision.

Find the precise set of characteristics that define a product's bliss point. Then decide how far the company can back down on features and costs before it loses too much consumer appeal. Computer models are being used by national companies to make these analyses. The idea is to search in an open-ended way for the optimum combination of product characteristics. Don't just focus on finding the best of a given bunch of products.

For example, it's wasteful to spend extra money to improve product quality if inflation-impacted consumers of that item are motivated more by nutritional features or price.

Test-market savings and a dramatic reduction in the time required to go from product concept to actual marketing are added benefits. During an inflationary period, this is almost as valuable as more precise positioning.

Source: John H. Lewis, president, Weston Group, Inc., Westport, CT.

Recession Wisdom For Marketers

Management must run an especially tight ship during a recession, but it's a big mistake to inflict false economies on the marketing effort. Instead:

■Hire top sales and merchandising people who may be available from other companies. Fine talent often enters the job market as other companies cut back. Use this opportunity.

■Strengthen sales promotion. Best bets: Price promotions and creative deals. Also look for relatively inexpensive ways to create new excitement (slight changes in product or package design).

■Get more leverage from the advertising budget. Don't drastically reduce it. Companies that keep an advertising presence emerge from recession faster and stronger. Use the fact that the company is maintaining its ad budget to get more and better service and merchandising help from the media.

■Don't be afraid to introduce a promising new product into a soft market. This could help the company establish a solid springboard from which to take off when the market rebounds.

Source: Malcolm Moses, Malcolm Moses & Associates, Merrick, NY.

Price-Setting Essentials

Companies that can't quickly revise cost estimates and hike selling prices are likely to see their profit margins abruptly erode in today's climate of high interest rates and soaring production costs.

Simplify the price-setting system and review it often. Before setting a price, determine these factors:

■The upper price limit for the product. To calculate the ceiling, use market research to get an accurate reading of what price level is possible. If the research is prohibitively expensive, guessing can be effective. But make estimates on the high side so prices can be lowered later.

■The floor price, which is the minimum that doesn't result in a loss at a specific level of production. Simplify the identification of fixed costs (supervisors' salaries, rent, etc.) that do not vary with production, and variable costs (raw materials, direct labor, etc.) that do. Relate the costs to volume.

■Identify nonprice-related aspects of the product. These help differentiate the product from its competitors so it needn't be sold on price alone. Emphasize other values, such as quality, performance, service, prestige of ownership, warranties, delivery time, and packaging.

Source: Seidman & Seidman/BDO, New York 10023.

How To Respond To A Competitor's Price Cut

When price competition flares, the worst management move is emotional retaliation. Instead, stay ready for sporadic price cuts by rival companies and exploit the opportunity to strengthen the company's market position.

The first step is to assess the price cutter's position.

■Is the competitor aggressive or desperate? A well-managed rival may be cutting prices to increase market share. That could pose a serious threat and require immediate action. But a drifter in the industry may be liquidating inventory to raise the needed cash. This spoils the market temporarily, which the company may have to live through.

■Does a price-cutting competitor have the capacity and other resources to usurp a significant share of the market? Assess its present facilities and supply sources.

■Does the price-cutter enjoy a cost advantage? Review the degree of integration and comparative costs of labor and transportation. Zero in on a competitor's greatest area of efficiency as a spur to reducing your own company's costs.

Build on knowledge of the market to develop the best counterprice strategy.

■How price-sensitive are your company's customers? Most sellers overestimate the effectiveness of a competitor's price decrease. Astute buyers value long-term relationships above transitory savings. They may even fear that the price-cutter's quality will be poor, the service sloppy or the supply uncertain. Reinforce these apprehensions, if they are warranted. And a temporary deal, cash rebate, or other incentive helps keep customers loyal without remorse.

■Are other competitors starting to discount also? Don't lead the way.

■Can the company's distributors absorb the price differential?

■Does the price cut attract additional buyers or generate additional volume? Be alert to profitable extra business that could be booked at a lower price.

The company's options:

■Do nothing for now. This is probably the best tactic if the price cut is merely a test of the market or a forced liquidation.

■Threats of retaliation or a lawsuit may scare off the aggressor. Try to avoid letting a competitor maneuver the company into a strategic change solely for defensive purposes.

■Nonprice moves. This could be the most effective strategy if customers prize reliable quality or delivery, extended credit terms or warranties, above all. Most forms of nonprice superiority are more secure from competitive threat than lower prices.

■Put a fighting brand into the lower-priced market to slug it out with the price-cutting aggressor. This keeps intact the company's present price structure and image. (The new entry may even boost the regular brand's volume.)

■Bracket price. Maintain (or even raise) the price of the brand under attack. But offer another brand below the aggressor's price.

It is essential to monitor customers' and competitors' reactions to the company's counterstrategy closely. Have a contingency plan ready.

Source: Dr. Harold W. Fox, professor, Ball State University, Muncie, IN.

Know Yourself—Know Your Markets

Identifying new markets and spotting emerging competitors are often easier if management continually redefines the company's line of business in current terms.

An overly broad definition is useless. Calling a pencil manufacturer a communications company will not help. But defining it as a low-cost writing-instrument maker might be successful.

Test the new definition against this checklist:

■Matches management's values.
■Appropriate for several segments of buyers.
■Distinctive.
■Consistent with the company's experience and image.
■Fits into other operations.
■Durable demand under changing conditions.
Source: Dr. Harold W. Fox, professor, Ball State University, Muncie, IN.

Getting More Out Of Marketing Consultants

Companies should retain marketing consultants to conduct annual audits of over-all marketing operations, not just to tackle special problems or projects.

Hire a consultant for two or three days to 1. Review overall marketing operations and 2. Write a letter citing the company's marketing strengths and weaknesses.

Ask for an estimate on all the work the consultant believes he could do to improve particular marketing functions.

Alternatively, the next time the company calls in its marketing consultant for a specific purpose, ask him to audit the overall marketing operations as a secondary assignment.
Source: Jack M. Doyle, Jack M. Doyle Advertising, Inc., Louisville, KY.

Ten Ways To Increase Marketing Productivity

In its focus on production efficiency, top management often overlooks potential improvements in the way the company reaches, penetrates and services its markets.

Aim for a lower cost of marketing as a percentage of revenues and a rate of sales growth that outpaces increases in sales and marketing manpower.

Steps to better marketing:

1. Target market segments and geographical regions more selectively.

2. Increase market leverage and flexibility by strengthening the market information base.

3. Reorganize sales territories to reduce travel time and yet maintain customer contact.

4. Encourage salespeople to specialize so as to serve key market segments or classes of trade better.

5. Minimize sales and promotional support for marginal areas. When direct selling is not justifiable, use distributors.

6. Focus more resources on national-account selling.

7. Do not reject out of hand potential selling methods or channels that have not been traditional in your market, such as offering salespeople double or even triple commissions for sales above quotas.

8. Avoid advertising in saturated markets. Concentrate dollars on local media and point-of-sale ads, perhaps shift from 60-second TV spots to 30-second.

9. Tighten control over advertising production costs.

10. Improve product manuals and set up 800 telephone lines so customers can resolve minor service problems themselves or with minimal help.

Source: Earl L. Bailey, director of marketing management research, The Conference Board, New York.

Biggest Marketing Mistakes Companies Make

Few, if any, companies can claim to be doing everything right in marketing. Even the most successful companies sometimes err. Most common marketing mistakes:

■In-fighting. Energies that should be spent serving the customer are too often spent fighting for turf with other departments.

■Neglecting customer responsibility. Functional departments such as engineering, finance and manufacturing are not held accountable for customer demands. These demands must be communicated by marketing to all departments—and all departments must be involved and committed to satisfying the customer.

■Failing to measure customer satisfaction. Profits, sales billed, orders received, backorders and market share are important measures of success, but what's often forgotten is the most important measure—customer satisfaction. Measures of customer satisfaction, defined in company-relevant terms, must be as important as more traditional measures.

■Failing to ensure top management commitment. Marketing is too important to be delegated just to the marketing department. The marketing department rightly encompasses sales, advertising and market research. But the whole company must be involved in customer satisfaction. Only the chief executive officer has the clout to get this message across.

■Failing to deliver. Once customer satisfaction is defined, the critical issue is insuring its delivery. The key is to make sure that everyone in the organization knows that "cheating on the customer" is a cardinal sin.

Source: H. Michael Hayes, Ph.D., Director of the Graduate School of Business, University of Colorado at Denver, 1475 Lawrence St., Denver, CO 80202. Dr. Hayes worked at General Electric for almost 30 years before joining the faculty at the University of Colorado, and has written extensively on the subject of management and market planning.

Decision-Making Help From The Competition

Competitive analysis can be used as an integral part of management decisions and a major factor in all strategic planning.

It's important to keep current on industry statistics. An analysis of the competition usually doesn't require elaborate intelligence-gathering systems. Often more useful is applying common sense to readily available information and asking intelligent questions.

■What do competitors' products show about their understanding of the marketplace?

■Has the competition left a gap between what they are offering and what customers and potential customers really want?

■Are competitors diverting cash or technical resources to new or different product areas?

Approach the marketplace conceptually with flexible thinking. This tactic might have alerted dairy companies to beware of market losses to soft drinks or warned bread marketers that yogurt was a threat to the traditional lunchtime sandwich. The moral is know where to look for competition.

Source: Connie A. Cox, Cox, Lloyd Associates, Ltd., New York.

Chapter 25
Product Development

New-Product Traps

Over 70% of new-product development work revolves around product improvements, line extensions, brand extensions, flankers (products in a similar, broad category), additional flavors, additional sizes, etc.

There's tremendous pressure to extend existing brands because companies have invested a great deal of money in them and they want to make the most of that investment.

Unfortunately, much new-product development money is wasted because companies fall into the dangerous traps involved with introducing new products to today's tricky markets…

Trap: Going too far afield from the company's traditional image. Cadillac found this out the hard way with its downsized Cimmaron. And Revlon recently announced its intention to market a deodorant under the name *No Sweat*. Though the company is banking on its powerful name recognition in the cosmetics market to introduce this product, it is definitely running the risk of tarnishing its image as a marketer of glamour products.

Trap: Misreading the buyer for a new product. Companies must start by asking…Is this a product that anyone needs? Is it fulfilling a need that's not being fulfilled now? Who's the likely buyer for this product? Some products have multiple buyers and the company must take into account the differing needs of each category of buyer.

Example: A company made a new line of small connectors to link up office computers with other equipment. Problem: The end users, the office managers to whom the company was marketing, were really not the key decision-makers for this product. Most companies depend on systems contractors to hook up an office equipment network. The contractor and his distributor are the real decision-makers for the product.

The company also must anticipate how buyer attitudes may need to change to accept a new technology.

Example: Some of the first automatic teller machines (ATMs) didn't do well because customers simply weren't ready to deal with them. Chemical Bank's *Pronto* home banking system also fell victim to being ahead of its time. People weren't ready to bank by home computer. Sears and IBM's new *Prodigy* service is the latest entry in this field. One tactic they're using to try to overcome the indifference of computer owners is to market it as a gift to give new home-computer owners.

Sometimes, too, there may be a need but it is impossible to fulfill that need for a reasonable price.

Example: A decade ago, when telephone answering machines first came out, they were so expensive that only self-employed people could rationalize buying them because they couldn't afford to miss calls. When prices came down below

$100, however, many more buyers could justify their need for an answering machine.

Trap: Underestimating the level of competition for a new product.

Example: A company manufacturing a product for one industry decides to use plant capacity to manufacture a modified version for another industry. Capital costs are high and there are only three competitors. Problem: Each competitor dominates one of the three possible positioning alternatives that are relevant to buyers' needs, and decision cycles are lengthy. Without a way to differentiate, business will be difficult to build and sustain.

Trap: Flawed new-product communication. Sometimes new products fail simply because they're not communicated properly. Customers may refuse to accept a brand extension that doesn't fit their image of the company or its products. This can be a special problem with service products because they're intangible. Without a physical product, the name of a new service, the identity of its parent and the way it is communicated are crucial in persuading customers to buy.

Solution: Understand very well what the brand name means. When insurance companies began to diversify into other financial services markets, for example, they reached for names that conveyed the strength of the parent insurance company but avoided confusion with insurance products. Example: New York Life conceived NYLife Investments and NYLife Realty to promote its investment and real estate products.

Because services are easily copied, service products need powerful and distinctive brand names to imprint them in people's minds. But that can sometimes backfire. Marine Midland Bank called its ATM machine MoneyMatic in the beginning. The name was so successful that it was on its way to eclipsing the name Marine Midland...but, eventually, the company changed the ATM's name to MarineMachine and the access card to the MarineCard. This had the added benefit of tying together all of the company's products as well as new products such as MarineEdge and MarineGain.

But it's not always advisable to put the corporate name on every product.

Example: When Holiday Corp. launched the innovative Embassy Suites concept, it gave it a different name to position it as separate from the Holiday Inn hospitality concept.

Trap: Internal inefficiency. Common: Development of the new product takes so long that the company loses its competitive "window." This means lost opportunity costs, as well—because the people who devoted 18 months to product development could have been developing something else.

Example: GM's Saturn project, meant to bring the hottest space-age car to market first, has taken so long to gear up that Japan's leading car makers have brought models such as the Infiniti, Lexus and 300ZX to consumers way ahead of GM.

Solution: Management must examine how long it's taking new products to get out the door and look for ways to expedite the process. New, computerized tools vastly speed up design and engineering work. Multifunctional teams are much quicker than moving a product idea from function to function.

Example: When IBM decided to develop a personal computer, it assigned a team and removed them from all other new-product development. Layers of bureaucracy were eliminated and team leaders had the ear of top decision-makers. New-product development teams always work best when there's clear direction from, and a good connection with, the top. It's harder and takes longer for new-product ideas to make it from the bottom up.

Trap: Introducing no new products because of fear of cannibalizing existing successful ones. Fortunately, however, more managers are realizing that if the company resists putting out new products for this reason, a competitor may do it for them and take that business away from their existing products.

Example: Diet Coke may have taken sales from Tab, but it has been a driver of growth for the entire Coke franchise.

Source: Mark J. Deck, director of KeyFactors Group, the new-product development practice of Temple, Barker & Sloane, Inc., management consultants, and Lippincott & Margulies, Inc., identity and image consultants, both subsidiaries of Marsh & McLennan, 33 Hayden Ave., Lexington, MA 02173.

Assessing New-Product Risks

Things to make sure about before more money is committed. Will the product:
■Truly fulfill a recognizable need?
■Deliver a demonstrable advantage over competitive products?
■Lend itself to future upgrading and improvement?
■Be cost and value competitive?
Other points:
■Is money available for the product's promotion?
■Is the promotion designed to achieve a valid market trial in the shortest possible time?
■Has research been set up to feed back sales data and compare results with those of the competition?
■Has the company mapped a test-market plan capable of projecting national acceptance?

Source: John S. Bowen, president, Benton & Bowles, New York.

Clues To New-Product Success Or Failure

New-product success is likely if:
■The product is unique or superior to what's available now.
■The company knows the market and how to sell to it.
■The marketing and management people understand the product and feel comfortable with it.
■The market is large and growing, and demand is high for the qualities the product offers.
■The product requires substantial investment. That way everyone won't be jumping in to undercut it.
Failure is likely if:
■The price is high, but the product offers no economic advantage.
■The product is new and unfamiliar to the company.
■The market is competitive and customers are satisfied.
■Several similar products are being introduced in the same market.

Choosing Product Names

The ideal name:

■Communicates the product's main benefit (*Slender* diet drink, *Close-Up* toothpaste).

■Suggests the product's category to help position it in the public mind (*Head & Shoulders* shampoo, *Intensive Care* skin lotion).

■Is almost generic (*People* magazine) but doesn't go over the line and become so general the company loses it to competitors. The classic example of going too far is Lite, which Miller tried and failed to use exclusively as a trademark for its low-calorie beer.

Looking for a common pattern of success in products from the past won't help. Product naming was much more casual then, since there were fewer products on the market and the volume of communication was lower.

Avoid names that are:

■Overly broad. *Time* is a less effective name for a new magazine than *Newsweek*. Similarly *Fortune* is too general for a business magazine. *Business Week* is better.

■Coupled with a meaningless number (*Breck One* and *Colgate 100*).

■Based on a regional term or a place name.

■Without a specific meaning (General, Standard, Continental). Many such names are widely used, leading to consumer confusion.

Unless the product is the first and only one of its kind on the market, resist the temptation to give it a totally made-up name.

Source: A. Ries and J. Trout, *Positioning: The Battle for Your Mind*, McGraw-Hill, New York.

Product Counterfeiting Self-Defense Strategies

Today, counterfeiting is not just a problem for well-known consumer goods such as Cartier watches or Calvin Klein jeans.

The global demand for well-known brands has made producing counterfeit copies very profitable, in less-developed nations where it is sometimes a major industry, and within the United States, as well.

Recently, however, counterfeiting has spread from consumer goods to all sorts of manufactured products, including aircraft and auto parts and prescription drugs.

Frightening: More than two dozen airplane crashes have been blamed on faulty counterfeit aircraft parts. Ford Motor Company has warned that most counterfeit auto parts don't meet federal standards for safety.

Most vulnerable: Any manufacturer with a high-priced product...products with high profit margins...products that contain a lot of technology, such as computers.

Key: The counterfeiter circumvents research and development costs and has virtually no marketing costs. The counterfeiter merely finds a way to make a product that looks authentic. Our studies have demonstrated that it's often very hard for customers to distinguish a counterfeit product from the real thing by looking at it, especially with complex industrial products.

Trap: Sometimes a counterfeit looks better than the genuine article. Good test: The quality and performance of a product. But even that isn't infallible.

A celebrated 1983 case involved counterfeit Apple IIe computers produced in Taiwan, Hong Kong, Singapore and Switzerland. They contained pirated operating systems and were sold at greatly reduced prices. Apple finally got a judgment based on patent infringement.

Counterfeiting Hurts

Legitimate manufacturers are harmed by counterfeiting in more ways than just loss of revenue. (Annual revenue losses in the U.S. are estimated at $6 billion–$8 billion.) They suffer enormously from loss of buyer goodwill and brand image. When consumers unwittingly buy counterfeits and then are disappointed by the product's performance, they tend to blame the innocent manufacturer. Even rumors of counterfeiting can undermine consumer confidence. Sometimes whole industries or national economies can be affected.

Example: Kenya and Zaire farmers used counterfeit fertilizers one year and both countries lost most of their crops.

Fighting Back

The U.S. finally enacted a Trademark Counterfeiting Act in 1984 that makes counterfeiting a criminal offense and carries stiff jail sentences and fines, and makes convicted offenders pay treble damages and attorney's fees.

Problems: Counterfeiting is often perceived as a victimless crime. It doesn't receive priority attention from law enforcement officials and prosecutors who are more concerned with other criminal areas.

There's also controversy within the industry because the Act authorizes seizing goods and business records without notice. Some retailers fear that the law might be used to seize merchandise they obtained in the gray market—genuine products that are bought from foreign distributors instead of the regular U.S. distributors designated by the manufacturer. Often these "exported" products are priced lower than products marketed in the U.S. They're not intended to find their way to the U.S. market, but they're not counterfeit.

The U.S. government's efforts to promote an anti-counterfeiting code among members of the General Agreement on Tariffs and Trade (GATT), while partially successful, has not won support from some of the worst offending developing nations. But the U.S. Tariff and Trade Act of 1985, which allows for the suspension of tariff exemptions for countries that condone counterfeiting, has forced Taiwan and other East Asian nations to take remedial measures.

Bottom line: Companies that have a problem must find their own ways of combatting counterfeiting. This might include getting their own attorneys appointed as special prosecutors (as has been allowed by New York City's Second Circuit Court). Trade associations can lobby for laws that protect their particular industry.

Example: The Semiconductor Chip Protection Act of 1984 provides civil remedies against the copying of the unique patterns of connections etched on electronic chips.

Best Defenses

■Code the product. There are now many forms of advanced technology that let companies secretly identify their products as genuine by means of magnetic bar codes, special inks, holograms or various types of digitized fingerprints.

Example: Levi Strauss has significantly reduced its blue jean counterfeiting problem by weaving a unique pattern into its labels. Caution: Counterfeiters can learn to duplicate codes and protective measures, so the company must be prepared to change codes frequently.

■Change the product. Sometimes it's possible to make engineering or some other changes that render the product more identifiable and less vulnerable to counterfeiting.

■Track dealers closely. This is by far the most effective—but most expensive—way to fight counterfeiting. Bogus goods are often sold through legitimate outlets. Carefully monitor the company's distribution network to make sure merchants aren't dealing with questionable sources. This may require hiring investigators. For the most part, however, careful tracking and strict reporting and identification systems will discourage distributors and dealers from counterfeit activity.

Helpful: Maintain frequent and close contact with distributors and dealers. Distributors may handle counterfeit merchandise because it's more profitable for them. Try to counter that temptation by offering rewards to anyone in the distribution channel who discovers and reports counterfeiting activity.

■Develop a reputation in your industry for standing ready to legally protect your company's patents and trademarks. Go after offenders aggressively.

Source: Dr. Ronald F. Bush, chairman, marketing department, College of Business, University of West Florida, 11000 University Pkwy., Pensacola, FL 32514.

Choosing the Right Distributor

The length of time a product has been on the market could be a critical factor in choosing the right distributor. For example, middlemen who do the best job during the early market-development stages could be all wrong when it comes to handling more mature product lines, and vise versa. This is particularly important in industrial distribution.

Give top priority to the technical specialist at the beginning stages. That's when the marketplace is adapting the product line to new applications. The technical specialist's emphasis on (a) large end-users, where most new products gain initial acceptance, and (b) engineering levels where the purchase decision is ultimately made.

Consider adding general-line distributors, as market growth flattens out and differences among competing products diminish. By reaching many more small end-users, these all-purpose middlemen help increase market saturation.

Inventory specialists may be best for the company during the later stages of product maturation. These distributors, with their emphasis on large-contract "buys," are most efficient when competitive pressures reach their peak and cost becomes the user's prime buying yardstick.

Source: Frank Lynn, president, Frank Lynn & Associates, Chicago.

Reappraising The Package

■What emotional appeal does the package project through color, type, size, shape, and graphics?

■Does it highlight the product's best strengths against competitive products?

■Does it attract attention?

■Is the endorsement linkage between the brand name and corporate name strong enough?

■Are new packaging materials available that may improve appearance, reduce costs, or both?

When To Drop A Product

Take a critical look at products that produce the smallest sales. Consider whether some of them should be discontinued. Advantages:

■Profits will represent a higher percentage of sales and a higher return on capital.

■There will be lower inventories, thus less cash will be tied up in inventory and less borrowed.

■Management's time and attention can be focused on more profitable items.

■Management is forced to consider why a product is failing.

■Listen to arguments for giving a slow-moving item one more try, perhaps trying to boost its image by repackaging or reformulating it, or giving the item a new ad campaign. Look for ways to turn losers into winners.

Chapter 26
Marketing Research

When Is Research Necessary?

A common pitfall is launching a market research project when one isn't really necessary.

Stick to the proper use of market research, which is to get information when there isn't enough available.

Situations that justify research:

■To help choose between different strategies.

■To supply more data when management is internally divided on a policy, plan, or goal.

■To find out precisely why the market share is falling or distribution networks are weakening.

■To define the reasons why a particular product or service is doing very well, and to apply the responsible factors to other areas.

■A new product is being considered.

■A new market is being evaluated.

Source: *Sales Manager's Bulletin*, Waterford, CT.

Market-Research Strategies

Should mail questionnaires or interviews (individual, group, or telephone) be used?

Use mail when:

■The target group is small, well defined, and has a common identity.

■The research questions can be expressed clearly and simply and are important to everyone in the target group.

■A mailing list is readily available.

Personal interviews are best when:

■The researcher wants detailed, specific information and doesn't know who has it.

■The company isn't sure what it's seeking. A personal interview permits follow-up questions.

Group discussions are best when:

■Vague psychological areas are researched. What's a product's image?

■Fresh ideas are being sought. In a group, people encourage, react to, and build on each other's ideas.

■The focus is on exploring complex or hidden motivations.

Telephoning is best for:

■Measuring of ad impact.
■Quick, informal studies of short, specific answers.
■One-shot checks of product recognition and brand preference.
■Specialized studies involving a small number of trustworthy respondents.
Source: G.E. Breen, *Do-It-Yourself Marketing Research,* McGraw-Hill, New York.

How Market Research Can Mislead You

The average market-research questionnaire is never justified beyond the usual explanation: It's always been done this way.

What to watch out for: The almost universal temptation among researchers to add extraneous questions. These merely complicate tabulation and delay giving managers the few basic answers they need before going into test markets.

Typical example: A new product description, followed by a choice of five boxes:
■Definitely would buy.
■Probably would buy.
■Might or might not buy.
■Probably would not buy.
■Definitely would not buy.

What's wrong with this approach: The results are too vague. One division or company (not noted for new-product development) might be discouraged by only 24% "definitely would buy" responses and might drop its plans. Another, more aggressive company might add together the 24% "definites" and the 31% "probables" and forge ahead, overconfidently thinking it had a 55% mandate from consumers. Still another manager might conclude that the 24% "definites" were solid, but that perhaps only half of the "probables" should be counted.

What the manager really needs to know: Whether consumers would definitely (not probably) buy or try the product (not repurchase or switch brands). Or, would they not? Other categories just confuse the respondent and becloud the results.

Another common mistake: Questions that lead consumers to assume they are being asked to switch brands. Actual purpose: To find out whether or not they would try the new product. Avoid questions such as: How would you rate this product for economy? How do you think this product would compare with your present brand? These questions are patently absurd since the true answer is: I don't know. I haven't tried it yet. If the respondent guesses, how valid is that judgment?

Worst abuse: Questionnaires burdened with downright mischievous open-end comments, which must be transcribed verbatim and so take months to collate and analyze. By that time, no one cares to read the results.

The ideal new-product questionnaire should:
■Be no more than one page long.
■Expose respondents to the product concept quickly, before they become bored answering questions.
■Then ask in simple terms: Would you buy this product or not?

Beyond the answer to that question, the only other helpful information is the factors that were important to the consumer in making the decision.

Source: Gerald Schoenfeld, principal, Gerald Schoenfeld, Inc., New York.

A market survey in which no more than 25% of the results are surprising is probably on target. When 75% of the results surprise company managers, start worrying that the assumptions being tested are really off base.

Overpromoting the product can invalidate a market test. If a comparable level of promotion cannot be sustained nationally tone it down.

Source: Louis Harris, public opinion researcher, New York City.

To Boost Market Research Response

Keep the survey short...Use multiple choice answers...Enclose a gift—a dollar bill, a discount slip for the next purchase...With your survey include a self-addressed, stamped envelope.

Source: *Service Advantage: How to Identify and Fulfill Customer Needs* by Karl Albrecht, Dow Jones-Irwin, 1818 Ridge Rd., Homewood, IL 60430.

Chapter 27
Export Marketing

How To Find Export Markets

Unlike large corporations, many small companies don't have the resources to pursue overseas sales. There are several low-cost steps that companies that are not exporting can take on their own or with the help of export-assistance organizations to explore international possibilities.

How to tell if a product can attract a foreign market:

■Find out whether competitors are exporting. If they are, chances are good that there's more room in the overseas market.

■Consult the company's trade association. Most have economists who are familiar with foreign markets. A few have export specialists.

■Tap the Commerce Department's information system. It lists products being exported and countries that are buying them.

When a company believes it has a potential export market:

■Determine the price range of the product overseas.

■At several possible price levels, get estimates of production, marketing, and shipping costs. Remember that higher export overhead often makes the initial return on investment lower for a company's overseas sales.

■Begin making contacts with prospective buyers in target countries.

Professional assistance is available from:

■State and local government agencies. Many have offices that help companies develop export operations. The Regional Export Assistance Program, a division of the World Trade Center, offers low-cost assistance to companies in New York and New Jersey.

■Marketing consultants. Most large U.S. firms also work in the international field. Many of their knowledgeable staff members are available after hours. Retired export managers in the U.S. and overseas make good consultants.

■The U.S. Department of Commerce's Worldwide Information and Trade System. It can put U.S. companies in touch with specific foreign companies that are likely prospects.

When a company isn't big enough for its own export division, consider hiring an outside export manager who knows the major foreign markets and relevant shipping and tariff regulations. The National Association of Export Management Companies, 99 Church St., New York, NY 10007, puts American manufacturers in touch with export management companies. There is no charge.

Source: Gregory Landenburg, international marketing consultant, New York.

Before You Venture Into A Foreign Country

The proper way to handle business dealings abroad differs, often sharply, from country to country. But there are basic steps every company must take well before it actually ventures into any foreign market:

■Study the country and its business customs.

■Know the market potential. (One U.S. company actually started a frozen food venture in a major country in the Far East before it realized that most homes in the market area did not have freezers.)

■Accurately assess the competition. Newcomers from the United States often don't realize the strength of rivals already on the scene.

■Most companies don't establish an international business until their sales reach the $30-$50 million level. Exceptions are that some high-technology businesses may have a strong international market from the outset. And some service businesses never go international.

The best source of information is the Commerce Department. Also helpful are the Export-Import Bank, Small Business Administration, and the Overseas Private Investment Corporation.

Get To Know The Export Market

Before wasting time and money trying to crack international trade markets, there are simple questions to ask. Specifically:

■Which countries restrict your company's products because they are produced locally?

■Could customs duties price goods out of the market?

■Is franchising or licensing an effective alternative?

■What U.S. financing is available to potential foreign customers?

■What is the likely profit margin and profit potential?

Several government and trade organizations will assist anyone trying to export products. For those addresses and further details, send for the free publication, *How to Export—A Step-by-Step Guide*, Washington Researchers, 918 16th St. NW, Washington, DC 20006.

How To Get Organized For Selling Abroad

Essentials if the company is preparing to take its first plunge into international waters:

■Foreign-language ability. Set up an international section in the customer-service department. At least one staff member must have a full (reading, writing, and speaking) capability in each new market's native tongue.

■Foreign-currency savvy. Prepare to accept foreign currency in payment of invoices. If marketing plans include East European countries, where all local currencies are nonconvertible, develop a rapport with a key currency broker in Vienna.

■Foreign-sales personnel. Post native company-trained employees in each territory. Top managers must be at home there. Other staffers should at least be ex-residents. Knowing nuances of local culture, idiom, and politics can be as vital as language expertise. Count on the competition (foreign and domestic) to know this. Foreign nationals hired after the sales program is underway (without company training) could be worse than none.

■Metric systemization. Whether or not the company has converted to metrics for U.S. marketing, it's a must in markets that use nothing else. Metrication of product specifications, invoice data, trans-shipment distances, and all forms of communication involving numbers is required.

Source: *Textile World*, New York.

Cracking The Japanese Market: How Day-Timers Did It

Day-Timers, a maker of diaries, calendars and other time-management aids, used a key principle of marketing—look for the niche—to carve out a Japanese market.

It began when Day-Timers' president, Robert C. Downey, discovered Japanese businessmen were receptive to American ideas on productivity. Example: They were enthusiastic about a grid that Downey devised for tracking the time spent on various executive tasks.

Finding The Niche

The company found its niche among Japanese middle managers. Key: The Japanese are workaholics. Many work 70 hours a week. But most of them are under intense stress, because it means neglecting families and other personal interests. They were, therefore, excited about a product to help them get their work done faster.

One preliminary problem confronted Day-Timers, a direct mail company. There are apparently no mailing lists in Japan. However, Japanese department stores have enormous lists. And Day-Timers learned that, in Japan, everything is negotiable.

The basic product—a diary planner—was unchanged from the U.S. version. The only thing printed in Japanese were the instructions, and the company made sure they were very detailed and precise for Japanese customers.

The Final Lesson

But such success takes time. Two years elapsed between the time the idea was born and the time the company actually began marketing in Japan. You can succeed in Japan if you have a product or service to fill a gap in the Japanese market. Patience, understanding and a willingness to listen to how business is done there are all vital to success.

Source: Adapted from *Nation's Business,* February, 1989 (©1989, U.S. Chamber of Commerce) 1615 H St. NW, Washington, DC 20062.

Eastern Europe—Traps & Opportunities

While many opportunities in Eastern Europe already exist for Western businesses, great caution is required. Biggest traps:

■Currencies are not readily convertible into dollars—and most countries have limits on repatriation of profits. Most currencies will face devaluation as economies become more open.

■Labor costs which appear low can actually be quite high—once relatively low productivity and benefits and entitlements are added on. And, labor regulations make it difficult to cut the work force.

■Limited purchasing power. While the profit potential from 140 million people who have had little or no access to Western products appears enormous, the market will be limited for at least a decade until current low personal incomes are improved by economic growth.

■Lack of a transportation infrastructure poses problems for shippers.

■Objectives are sometimes incompatible. Eastern European firms want to export, while many Western companies are attracted to the vast untapped markets inside Eastern Europe.

Other Problems

■Ground rules for business deals are murky and subject to sudden revision.

■Valuing assets is difficult because of the long absence of market forces.

■Trained management talent is in very short supply.

■The Mideast problem adds a wrinkle as Eastern Europe grapples with soaring energy costs.

Outlook: It will take at least five to 10 years of economic dislocation before most Eastern European nations begin to benefit from restructuring.

How to proceed: Eastern European hotels are overflowing with Americans who mean well, but are working with uninformed assumptions about the opportunities and risks.

Better: Do some intense homework first. Visit commercial consulates in the U.S., country specialists at the Commerce Department, experienced executives, professionals and consultants who have established offices in Eastern Europe.

Aim: To develop a list of contacts at the national level and within the local governments who can help you locate potential partners. Plan your agenda and visits with government officials and prospective business partners. Confirm and reconfirm interview dates before leaving the U.S.

Useful Steps

■Designate a company specialist to keep abreast of developments.

■Take part in a specialist tour or trade mission.

■Attend seminars where qualified speakers can add to your knowledge of particular countries.

■Commission market research surveys and market-entry studies. These can save the company fruitless trips, time and money.

■If a country looks promising for exporting, attend a major trade exhibition. This is the most effective way to promote products in Eastern Europe.

Strategic Considerations

Reexamine the company's long-term goals and see how they would be furthered by having an Eastern European connection.

Would an Eastern European joint venture, for example, serve as a back-door entrance to the unified Western European market after 1992? (The European Community will be granting preferential trading relationships to most of Eastern Europe.)

One other consideration: The rapid revival of cultural and national expression since the destruction of the Berlin Wall revealed the fallacy of Eastern Europe as a "bloc." While they share a legacy of communism, each country has its own distinct history, culture, language, economy and priorities.

Hungary

With a history of entrepreneurship, Hungary is the most advanced in the dynamics of a free market of all the East European countries. Its $2/hour average labor rate may rise, but won't rival Western rates in the near future. Result: It has already attracted about 1,500 Western joint ventures. The reopened Budapest Stock Exchange is the only exchange in Eastern Europe. Budapest is like a gold rush town.

Caution: With only 10 million people and the highest per capita debt of any of these countries, Hungary has better prospects as a manufacturing location than as a large-scale market.

U.S. investment in Hungary totals $350 million. Almost half of this is General Electric's investment in Tungsram, the Hungarian lighting products company. McDonald's and Citicorp are already well-established. Another $500 million of U.S. investment is on the way. In addition, heavy hitters like General Motors and Ford are coming. Hungary welcomes Americans because it does not want to be dominated by the Germans. Total U.S. investment could soon hit $1 billion.

Many Hungarian companies are going private via government sell-offs to foreigners. Examples: Chinoin, the pharmaceuticals company and Novofrude, a major computer software firm. Hungary now has a state agency to act as the intermediary between Hungarian companies, the various ministries that have been in charge of them, and prospective private investors.

Likely scenario: Foreigners will be allowed to invest around 60% in state-owned companies, the government will keep 20% and another 20% will be sold on a bargain basis to employees. Key: This would give employees an immediate ownership stake in enterprises that must undergo restructuring and layoffs.

Basic services in Eastern Europe are still underdeveloped. It can take hours to make a telephone call. U.S. telecommunications companies are very aggressive, and it is possible that the eventual solution will be cellular systems that leapfrog wire technology.

Czechoslovakia

With a solid infrastructure and outstanding labor and managerial traditions, Czechoslovakia could be the sleeper of Eastern Europe. It's already second only to the former East Germany in gross domestic product. Its education level rivals the U.K. and it was among the top 10 industrialized countries in the world before World War II. But it must overcome extensive pollution and hazardous waste problems, and, more important, a degree of inertia that is apparent in the wake of sweeping changes.

The country is slowly opening to foreign investment. A national investment bank will prepare projects for foreign investment, but the necessary legislation is not yet fully in place. Biggest opportunities: Investment in basic manufacturing facilities, motor vehicles, upgrading machinery, construction, textiles, food processing equipment, agricultural products and some consumer goods.

German Unification

The former East Germany is in the fortunate position of already having a hard currency—the super-strong deutsche mark. It will also develop more rapidly than other Eastern economies because unification with West Germany will yield hefty economic assistance. But the eastern sector of Germany faces many problems. Out of 8,000 existing business entities, 30%–40% will go out of business, causing higher unemployment. Another 30% are viable—but the rest are on the edge.

After state enterprises started paying employees in West German marks July 1, 1990, they were faced with laying more people off or placing them on part-time status. And officials estimate that a quarter of a million people too many are employed in agriculture. Unemployment could climb into the millions before the transition to a market economy is complete. There are also problems of who owns East German land and buildings. Possible claims on property by West Germans are currently holding up many construction projects. Now that unification has taken place, however, legal reforms to resolve this will be forthcoming.

Opportunities for Western companies: Too many U.S. companies view former East Germany as a hands-off situation. But, if you are underrepresented in Western Germany, the eastern region could be an entry point for the "new" Germany. Those with operations in or exports to West Germany will have an easier time taking advantage of the East's rapid development. Western input is also badly needed in machinery, agricultural equipment and electronic components manufacturing.

Poland

Under the Solidarity-led government, Poland has already undertaken the most painful reform measures of any Eastern European country. But the political situation isn't yet fully settled, and the country faces a monstrous $40 billion debt. Poland's prospects remain more a question of hope than reality.

Like the other Eastern European countries, Poland has infrastructure and pollution problems and primitive banking and telecommunications systems. But its 38 million population is well-educated and the government desperately needs Western capital to develop export-oriented industries.

Best opportunities for Western companies: Agricultural and food processing machinery, chemicals, paper, construction materials, office equipment, telecommunications, tourism, medical and environmental technologies.

Source: James E. Searing, director, international business services, Ernst & Young, 787 Seventh Ave., New York 10019. Ernst & Young's *Viewpoint* magazine has published a special issue on the free market revolution in Eastern Europe, available at the address above.

How To Move Into Europe

At the end of 1992, the 12 nations of the European Community* will unify trade laws and eliminate remaining trade barriers, creating a $4 trillion market of more than 320 million people. This means that marketing strategies for non-European businesses selling to that enormous market must be dramatically changed. U.S. companies that want a piece of the action should start taking immediate steps.

*Belgium, Denmark, France, Greece, Ireland, Italy, Luxembourg, the Netherlands, Portugal, Spain, the United Kingdom and Germany.

Step #1: Market Research

Many U.S. companies will fall into a costly trap. They'll think that since Europe and the United States have many similarities, they can just take their products across the Atlantic and be welcomed with open arms. But the European marketplace is very different from its American counterpart...and it will change even more by 1992.

Shrewd move: Hire a European market research firm to probe for readily exploitable opportunities there. American market researchers—no matter how competent they are—won't be as effective. Reason: Basic market research may give a good idea of how well a product will do today in any one of the 12 countries. But after 1992, that product may suddenly be on the shelf with competing products from elsewhere in the EC...or, luckily, it may itself find a market niche elsewhere...or the product could see new distribution channels opened or closed. Moreover, EC commissioners in Brussels are still writing the new trade regulations. Only an experienced European marketing research firm will be able to factor these major elements into its research.

Step #2: Finding Distribution

If the research concludes that your company has a product or service with potential in Europe, the next step is to find a distributor. For historical reasons, distributors often play a larger role in marketing a product in European marketing than they do here.

In the U.S., for example, we often have several competing distributors, or companies can distribute directly to a retailer. That's not always the case in Europe. Smart moves:

■Contact the industry's European trade associations in areas where market research is favorable. Find out how the distribution systems work and how they're likely to change after 1992.

■Then talk with several distributors. Screen for those with experience in selling similar foreign products. Ask for a complete rundown on what's needed to introduce your product—the paperwork connected with export to Europe, tariffs, obligation for warranties, and, of course, what percentage the distributor will get.

■Check out prospective distributors more thoroughly than you would in the U.S. Especially important: Ask major European retailers about them. Look for aggressive distributors who have a good reputation with retailers and who stick with a product in difficult times.

Step #3: Test Marketing

Like anywhere else, testing is essential. But anticipate big problems here.

Retailers control the European marketplace, and they won't jump into action to put a new product on the shelf. Even distribution will probably be slower. In the U.S., a company that wants to test a product can have it on shelves in several cities within a few months and get meaningful results a couple of months later. In Europe, test marketing typically takes two or three times longer.

Today, virtually all advertising is national, not regional, because most media are national. Result: Even if you test a product in, say, three German cities, you may have to buy national advertising. Apart from the unnecessary expense, what happens to customers in other cities who see the ads but can't buy the product? Later, they may ignore the ads when the product does go on sale in their area.

Fortunately, regional marketing through targeted promotions is becoming increasingly available in Europe, but it's nowhere near the extensive level of the United States.

Best strategy: Test market in one of the smaller European countries, such as Belgium or Holland. Results might not be quite as reliable as they'd be with a bigger sampling, but costs won't be prohibitive. And generally, such tests will reveal simple cultural differences that can save a company substantial time and money when it does go multi-national with its product. Examples:

■Tang entered the British market a few years ago only to discover that the British don't drink orange juice for breakfast, let alone an orange-juice substitute.

■Campbell and Lipton have had difficulty overcoming a cultural bias against dehydrated soups.

■Acceptance and purchase of life insurance is dramatically different in some parts of Europe.

Recommended: To bolster European market testing, use focus groups. Participants can be useful not only in pinpointing cultural biases but in thinking of new uses for old products.

Step #4: Setting Up Shop

Experience shows that American companies are generally more successful in the European market when they have permanent representatives there. It's tempting to let U.S.-based executives handle a European operation—especially when it's still small—but that idea simply doesn't work.

In fact, a Europe-based staff is especially necessary in the early stages, when the company is building valuable relationships with distributors, retailers, bankers and potential partners. And since most problems occur in the early stages, it's essential to have a top executive on the spot to handle them.

Brussels, Frankfurt, London and Paris are usually the best cities for European headquarters since they're the major media and business centers. That can be especially important since European retailing is consolidating. Many major retail customers are likely to have major offices in these cities by the time the 1992 unification occurs.

Step #5: Hedging Your Bets

Trade barriers generally declined throughout the world over the last two decades or so. But the trend could change. In the coming decade, the EC could erect new barriers against the U.S. and Asian exporters.

U.S. companies with a long-term interest in the European market should consider manufacturing or assembling in Europe, either on their own or as a joint venture with a European company. Manufacturing costs are especially low in Spain and Portugal, and the influx of manufacturers is likely to produce a boom economy in those countries.

Source: Dr. Don E. Schultz, professor of advertising and direct marketing, Northwestern University, 1813 Hinman Ave., Evanston, IL 60208.

Chapter 28
Marketing And The Law

Six Ways To Minimize
Product Liability Risks

■Strongly warn users against any possible product abuses that could result in injury.

■Periodically review all product claims for misleading statements.

■Establish a consumer complaint procedure and explain it carefully to all employees who handle customer telephone queries and letters.

■Handle all complaints systematically. Errors made by switchboard operators and other clerical staff in handling complaints can increase a company's vulnerability in a product liability suit.

■Set up worst-case contingency plans for receiving product liability complaints.

■Distributors should negotiate hold-harmless agreements to put liability for distributed products on the manufacturer.

Source: Richard S. Betterly, D.A. Betterley Risk Consultants, Inc., Worcester, MA.

Criminal Antitrust Violations

Corporate antitrust violations are criminal offenses. The executives can be sent to jail. Criminal antitrust actions brought against individuals have increased 300% since 1977. The average fine in 1980 was $27,000. The average jail term was three months.

Offenses most likely to result in criminal action are price-fixing, allocation of territories or customers, boycotts, tying agreements, and willful violations of the law.

The best legal strategy for a defendant is to quickly convince the prosecutor and court that the offense is regretted and will not be repeated. Then try to plea bargain. The prosecuting attorney will not initiate discussions about plea-bargaining. They are more likely to accept a deal offered by the defendant before they have spent a great deal of time developing the case.

Source: Robert P. Beshar, attorney, New York.

Preventing Illegal Pricing Practices

Courts now punish top corporate officers for negligence when subordinates collude with competitors on prices. An established preventive system may impress a judge with top management's effort to abide by the law:

■Have lawyers tell salespeople what the laws allow and what they prohibit. Make the sessions constructive and realistic. Stress what can be done under actual field conditions.

■Help price-setters observe the law. Explain and enforce specific codes of conduct. Reduce pressures to maintain a particular price.

■Avoid opportunities for collusion. Centralize pricing. Control contacts with competitors.

Source: Harold W. Fox, professor, Ball State University, Muncie, IN.

Proving Intent In Price-Fixing Cases

Court rulings and judicial rebuffs make it tougher to harass and convict business executives. The government now has to prove not only that criminal activities did take place, but that defendants also intended to curb competition.

Exchange of information is not proof of price fixing and can even serve legitimate business purposes, at least as far as federal antitrust law is concerned. But be aware that some states have tougher laws.

Pitfalls In Fighting Foreign Competition

The government has streamlined the procedure for fighting foreign companies that dump goods on the American market. But U.S. companies should be careful in using it. If a trade association gets into the act, a complaint against dumping can look like an effort to curb foreign competition, and that is illegal. The Justice Department may become suspicious if:

■The trade association denies membership to the subsidiaries of foreign producers.

■Dumping charges are brought merely to harass the foreign companies.

■Signals go out to overseas producers that U.S. companies will not complain as long as foreign prices remain above a specified level.

■Illegally restraining competition can result in making the company vulnerable to a treble damage penalty. Convicted companies are also exposed to liabilities for loss of sales to U.S. distributors and from customers who paid higher prices.

Source: Carl A. Cira, Jr., U.S. Justice Department, the World Trade Institute.

Suing Market Research Firms

Market research firms have been sued for malpractice when new products failed after the researchers predicted success. To guard against lawsuits, some firms now include in their contracts a statement that their research results are indicators of market trends but not a guarantee of success, and that they are to be used only as a tool, to supplement a company's knowledge of the marketplace and of its own products and services.

Source: *Marketing News,* 250 S. Wacker Dr., Chicago 60606.

Losing Your Trademark

A trademark can be lost if the company using it doesn't follow federal labeling requirements. The Trademark Trial & Appeal Board said that because the owner of the mark "Peridyne" had sold the substance for two years without complying with the rule that package labels must include ingredients and the manufacturer's address, the trademark had been abandoned.

Source: *TTAB No. 15,243.*

Chapter 29
Direct Mail Marketing

The Public's Reaction To Direct Mail

How the public really feels about direct mail:

■Most people enjoy receiving a variety of mail.

■They separate their mail into six categories: personal, incoming money, bills, magazines, catalogs, direct-mail advertisements.

■Many people enjoy getting "junk" mail and use the term generically.

■Consumers don't mind being on mailing lists. They're quite willing to throw away mailings they don't want.

■The most popular kinds of direct mail: catalogs, free samples, coupons. Least popular: requests for donations, duplicate mailings, advertisements that have nothing to do with the recipient's interests.

■Catalogs are seldom thrown out without being looked at.

■Bill inserts are read with interest.

■Contests, while popular, arouse hostility in some consumers, particularly men.

■The person handling the mail in the home usually also pays the bills. In most American homes, this is a woman.

Source: Goldring & Co., Chicago.

Direct Mail Guidelines

Direct marketing presents opportunities for big and small marketers. There's no guaranteed system for success, but here are guidelines recommended by Bob Stone of Rapp, Collins, Stone & Adler Advertising, Chicago:

■Best mail order products: Items not readily available in retail stores. Items not available by mail at a price as low as yours.

■Recommended markup: On a single item, sell at three to four times cost. Items sold together in catalog can be marketed profitably by selling at twice what you pay for them (preferably 2$^{1}/_{2}$ times).

■How to get started: Test items individually first. Then build catalog around those that sell best.

■Mailing lists. Stick to lists of people who have bought by mail. Best prospects: Names that appear on two or more lists (a good list broker can be very helpful).

■Best pages in a catalog: Backcover; inside front cover; pages 3, 4, 5; inside back cover; center spread; page facing order form.

■To get bigger orders: Accept credit cards. (Average charge order from a catalog is 20% larger than order requiring check.)

■When to use TV for mail order: Best as support medium for saturation mailings or newspaper inserts. Small TV budget can increase responses from prime medium by 25%. Best items to sell directly via TV: Merchandise that lends itself to visual demonstration.

More Effective Selling Letters

Use direct-mail experience to improve business letters. Specific suggestions:
■Use an opening that promises the reader a benefit (a free booklet, time or money saving, etc.).
■Ask a question that gets the reader to agree with the points in your letter.
■Get news into the message.
■Keep the opening paragraph short. Alternate long and short paragraphs.
■Address the reader as an individual.
■Get to the point quickly.
■Don't annoy the reader—and lose him—by telling him obvious things about his own business.
■To carry a reader through the entire letter, use conjunctions liberally. They work particularly well at the opening of sentences and paragraphs.
■Keep the tone personal, low-pressured, friendly, sincere, informal.
■After writing the first paragraph, ask yourself: Is that what I'd say after the handshake if I were calling in person?
Source: John D. Yeck and John T. Maguire, *Planning and Creating Better Direct Mail*, McGraw-Hill Book Co., New York.

Don't Use Directories For Direct-Mail Lists

Don't copy names from a trade or professional association directory for business and professional mail promotion, because every directory is substantially out-of-date as soon as it is published. (Rates of address change in some directories vary from a few percent to over 50% in a single year.)

Best strategy is to rent the list directly from the trade association or professional society. The rental cost is usually about $40 per thousand.
Source: *Book Marketing Handbook*, R.R. Bowker Co., New York.

What Makes A Mail-Order Catalog Successful?

■Merchandise that's useful, interesting, attractive and with easily perceived value.

■Prices that are as low as possible. Exceptions: Higher prices can be charged when the merchandise can't be found elsewhere or convenience outweighs the cost.

■Products with a common theme. Merchandisers should appeal to a particular interest group or a specific life-style. Example: L.L. Bean's outstanding catalog of outdoor-oriented goods.

■Merchandise that's artfully displayed. Color isn't necessary but factual descriptions are.

■Money-back guarantees.

■Testimonials from satisfied customers.

■An order blank that's easy to fill out according to simple instructions in easy-to-read type.

■A free service for phone orders. Payoff: The order-taker can suggest other items while the customer is on the line.

Source: Julian Simon, author of *How to Start and Operate a Mail Order Business*, in *Direct Marketing*.

■Catalog life is extended by using a toll-free number. Reason: Prospective buyers will phone to find out if merchandise is still available.

Source: *Direct Marketing*.

■Projecting direct-mail response: Half the total response to first-class national mailings comes in five days once it starts. With third-class mailings, half comes within the first 13 days of returns. Slower: In the summer and at Christmastime. Faster: With regular-size envelopes (No. 10) rather than the larger ones.

■Best months for business-mail-order companies: Nonseasonal mailers get the best responses in January, February, September and October. (They are about equal.) Weak months: June and November. Worst of all: Pre-Christmas.

Source: *The Business Mailer Quarterly*.

Before You Rent A Mailing List

Two kinds of lists can be used for direct marketing:

■Compiled lists: A list of names developed from published sources, such as directories, membership lists, professional associations, etc. Strength: May be best way to identify specific type of customer for the product. Weakness: No evidence the listed name ever bought anything by mail, a big factor in getting a profitable response.

■Response lists: Names of individuals, companies, organizations that have bought a product (book, equipment, magazine) or a service (attended a seminar on a particular subject) related to the one your company sells. Strengths: Prospects have defined themselves as interested in the area and as being able and willing to buy by mail. Weakness: May not be able to identify qualified list for your company's product.

Both kinds of lists are available from list brokers. For information on brokers, write to Direct Mail/Marketing Association, 6 E. 43 St., New York 10017.

Costs: Compiled lists run $25 to $30 per thousand names. Qualified lists average about $40 per thousand, but range from $25 to $100. The broker's fee comes out of this charge (usually it amounts to approximately 20% of the list rental cost).

Source: Walter Prescott, president, Prescott Lists, 17 E. 26 St., New York 10016.

Chapter 30
Telephone Sales

Planning Your Message

Plan and tightly organize the sales message. The wording and progression of the message are even more important in telephone marketing than in print, radio, or television selling. When a canned phone pitch is boring or insincere, the problem is that it has been poorly planned and delivered, not that it follows a set format.

■Begin by grabbing the listener's attention and getting past the natural tendency to say no right away. Use the listener's name several times within the first few seconds. Ask an easy question, to which the listener must answer yes. Example: Can you hear me okay?

■State the reason for the call within 15 seconds, the time when the prospect's attention begins to wander and the person wants to hang up. Be brief and phrase the reason so it offers a benefit to the listener.

■Ease into the fact-finding phase, the heart of the call, with closed-ended, easy-to-answer questions that help the salesperson control the conversation. Then, shift to open-ended questions to find out the prospect's attitudes.

■Recommend and explain whatever course of action seems best to follow up the call. Example: Let me suggest that I call you monthly to keep you up to date on what's coming on the market.

■Close with a firm question designed to win the prospect's agreement to the recommendation.

Source: Bill Good, Telephone Marketing Associates, Salt Lake City, *Real Estate Today.*

Mail And Phone Efficiency

■Fold outgoing mail to fit into standard business-size envelopes (No. 10) instead of putting material flat into larger envelopes. Reason: Saving on postage and envelopes. More important: They also reach their destinations faster, because they can be handled by the Postal Service's automated sorting machines. If a large envelope is essential for a first-class mailing, stock a supply of authorized first-class envelopes with green diamond borders.

■Green diamonds on the borders of oversized envelopes help the post office's employees identify and expedite first-class mailing. The distinctive marking makes such mail stand out among the piles of plain large envelopes, which usually get processed at the much slower book or bulk rates. These special envelopes are available at stationery stores. They can, of course, be imprinted with the company's standard 1050 and address information.

■Window-envelope mail can be delayed in the mail if not properly designed. Best: Start the window one inch from the left side of the envelope. Leave 1/4 inch of white space around the address inside the window. Postal Service automatic-processing equipment rejects design variations. Make sure the address is typed in dark black letters and centered in window. Faded carbon addresses cannot be read by optical scanners.

Source: *DM News.*

■Expand the phone system without adding new equipment by giving some employees a call-waiting feature. This allows them to receive a second call on a line they are already using. By assigning an employee one line to use for both incoming and outgoing calls, it is possible to eliminate one other line from that phone, freeing it for someone else.

■Reduce phone abuse by having new employees sign a form authorizing a paycheck deduction for unauthorized calls. What to charge them for: Personal calls on company time (except for urgent situations). Calls made in a manner that is substantially more costly than company policy allows.

■Phone can be altered so employees can receive calls on any incoming lines but can call out on only one line. By having telephone lines billed separately, it is possible to know which person is making what calls.

Source: *The Encyclopedia of Telephone Cost Reduction Techniques* by Herbert Alan Jordan, Add-Effect Associates, Wayne, PA.

Telephone Sales

Selling by telephone, as old as the technique is, is still in its infancy. But a pattern of success has already emerged. The elements:

■The product should ideally be reasonably priced and familiar. New products do not sell well by phone.

■Success of the phone campaign is often determined by how well the product is matched to the age and sex of the person called.

■Callers should use short scripts.

■The pitch should be made to the person on the list, not to anyone who answers.

■Some days and times are better than others. Friday night and Sunday morning are generally poor.

■Add-on items lend themselves to phone sales.

■Offers should have a money-back guarantee.

Source: Joseph J. Libman, president, Ring America, Chicago.

Best Hours To Reach Prospects By Phone

■Chemists and engineers: 4–5 p.m.

■Contractors and builders: Before 9 a.m., at noon, or around 5 p.m.

■Dentists: 8:30–9:30 a.m.

■Druggists and grocers: 1–3 p.m.
■Executives: After 10:30 a.m.
■Housewives: 10–11:30 a.m.
■Lawyers: 11 a.m.–2 p.m. and 4–5 p.m. Avoid court hours.
■Physicians: 9–11 a.m. and 1–3 p.m. Those in suburbs can be called between 7 and 8 p.m.
■Professors and schoolteachers: After 4 p.m. or between 6 and 7 p.m.
■Salaried people: At home, 8–9 p.m.
■Stockbrokers: Before 10 a.m. or after 4 p.m. Eastern time. Avoids stock exchange hours.
■Insurance brokers and agents: 9–10 a.m., around noon, and at 4:30 p.m.

Source: *How to Increase Your Sales by Telephone* by Earl Prevette, C. & R. Anthony, Inc., 300 Park Ave. S., New York 10010.

How To Win At Telephone "Tag"

Telephone tag, the seemingly endless cycle of calls and returned calls that are missed, is one of the more time-consuming frustrations of executive life. Beat the frustration by organizing your telephone tactics.

If the person you want to talk with isn't in, and you do want him to call you back:

■Leave a detailed message of the subject of the call.
■Note a time span when you'll definitely be available.
■Make a phone appointment—a specific time when the party can reach you.
■ *Tell the secretary that no reply will be assumed consent or agreement.*

If you don't want the other party to call back:

■Ask for a specific time when he/she will be available, so you can try again.
■Find out if the person can be paged.
■Request that the secretary relay the information to your secretary, keeping the bosses out of the phone process.

Source: *Execu-Time*, Box 631, Lake Forest, IL 60045.

Phone Problem Solver

Important name and phone number to keep up-to-date: The vice president in charge of your area at the telephone company. If there are any serious problems, go to the vice president, who knows everybody and the structure of the operation. (The president, who's uninvolved in operations, does not.) If there's a problem, call immediately, and you'll get amazing results. The contact is especially important when you're changing from one system to another, moving, etc. If you can't reach the vice president, take the problem up with the vice president's secretary, who can be just as effective.

Chapter 31
Advertising Strategies

Market-Testing A New Ad Campaign

Market-testing is the only sensible way to determine whether additional advertising, a switch in media, or new copy will boost company sales. What to do:

■Develop a new theoretical advertising plan. Company managers decide how much they are willing to risk on growth. For example, a company with $20 million in sales and a $4-million gross profit may be willing to spend $2 million on advertising. Industry average advertising-to-sales (A/S) ratios are usually dependable standards to make sure the budget is in line. To introduce a new product, increase market share, or combat competition, the firm may consider exceeding the industry A/S ratio.

■Work out a test-market translation plan. Normally, this is a 10% microcosm of the national plan. Budget $200,000 (instead of $2 million). Target six cities that cumulatively represent 10% of the country, as a whole, and offer fairly typical demographic characteristics. Age, income, geographic location and city size should be well mixed. (Cities widely used for such tests are Syracuse, Denver, Phoenix, and Madison, WI.)

■Test and monitor results. Measure product sales six months before and six months after the test is run (impossible for new products) in order to provide a more accurate projection of results if the national plan is put into effect.

Results may seem less promising than they are if the company does not have many distribution outlets in the test city. To strengthen distribution use the TV ad schedule for the upcoming test to convince store buyers to stock up for the campaign.

Source: Jim La Marca, president, La Marca Group, New York.

Executive Involvement In Advertising Decisions

Few bosses spend time on advertising in proportion to the size of the advertising budget. Yet the best way to ensure that the company is getting the best advertising for its dollars is to get involved. This can be accomplished by personal contact with the creative people at the ad agency doing the work. They need the benefit of the chief's familiarity and experience with the products. But remember, there can also be too much participation in advertising by the chief executive officer.

Remedying Ad Failures

Just because the pre-market tests document high memorability of ads and the company uses media that reach the largest target audiences doesn't mean ads are producing maximum sales, because frequency and exposure intervals of ads may affect consumer response more than creative impact or media selection.

Careful tracking of response to various frequency and exposure patterns are needed for cost-effective advertising: On a market-by-market basis, use different approaches with the same media budget and audience rating level. Extend or shorten periods in which the ads run. Intensify or dilute concentration of ads during specific periods. Compare sales patterns in each market. Keep on fine-tuning to maximize results.

Source: Gene Dewitt, media services director, McCann-Erickson, New York, *Advertising Age*, Chicago.

Setting An Ad Budget: How Much Is Enough?

Although there are no definitive rules, there are useful criteria that can help financial and marketing executives determine how much to spend on advertising. It's important to listen to an ad agency's advice, but formulate overall strategy at the company.

The basic problem: In general, the more money spent on effective promotion, the greater the sales. But there is a point of diminishing returns, at which extra ad dollars will not produce additional profitable sales. And there is no way to measure the precise effects of advertising spending.

The size of the ad budget is affected by a variety of factors: the size of the geographic market, distribution of buyers, type of product advertised, and competitive spending.

Most companies use one of the following approaches:

■Percentage of sales. The budget is based on last year's sales or anticipated sales for the coming year. It is a popular and easy method but not always the best. Trap: It lacks the flexibility needed to take advantage of unusual marketing opportunities that may arise.

■Fixed amount for each unit produced. It has the same defects as percentage of sales, except more money becomes available as more units are produced.

■Competitive spending. A useful guide when the average is based on a number of competitors, but competition may be wasting money. A copycat company may commit the same mistake.

The best method is based on identifying both advertising objectives and tasks.

First determine the communications objectives an advertising campaign is designed to achieve.

They should:

■Be specific and quantitative. For example, an 8% increase in sales, 12% increase in market share, 40% brand awareness.

■Include a position in the advertising media best suited to convey the brand message.

Once management agrees on the goals, estimate the cost of these tasks. The total appropriation can be adjusted to fit into the company's financial resources by modifying objectives.

The objective and task approach is the most logical method to determine an ad budget. The difficulty lies in estimating the level of effort needed to achieve objectives. This can be overcome by experience and by measuring productivity. Systematic testing of results at varying budget levels would be helpful.

Percentage-of-sales is still the simplest and most widespread method used by companies to arrive at an ad budget. (Frequently, it is expressed as advertising-to-sales ratio—A/S.) Advertising as a percentage of sales varies greatly by industry and product:

■Industrial products, airlines, autos, oil, utilities and retail chains have low ad budgets relative to sales (usually under 2% of sales).

■Convenience and package goods: Soft drinks, tobacco, soaps, drugs, cosmetics and toiletries generally have high ad budgets as a percentage of sales (can go as high as 25%).

Source: James La Marca, president, La Marca Group, media consultants, New York.

Common Mistakes That Waste Advertising Dollars

■The ad budget is allocated to national media when the company's sales are geographically more limited.

■One broad marketing plan is used for all markets when individual ones should be developed based on brand-development potential on a market-by-market basis.

■Seasonal purchase patterns are ignored.

■It's not known which media best influence target customers. Rectify this by including media usage questions in all consumer research.

■The company's media buyer overpays for broadcast time when it is highly negotiable.

Source: James La Marca, president, La Marca Group, media consultants, New York.

When To Use Comparative Ads

Stacking a product directly against the competition's brand in a comparative ad can confuse and mislead consumers. Still, such ads can be effective if used carefully.

As a rule, products with practical rather than psychological benefits are most suited for comparative ads. The ad should depict the benefits in normal daily use.

Use comparative ads when:

■A new or unknown product needs public awareness. Demonstrate advantages over the market leader; psychologists have found that a low-status object gains in importance when compared to a high-status one.

■The goal is to plant doubts about a rival product. If the ad is convincing, loyal users of the competing product are likely to try the challenger at least once.

■A product has good distribution but low market share. Strong comparative ads can make the item better known but usually at the expense of other brands, not the market leader.

Avoid comparative ads when:

■The product is vulnerable to counterattack by the market leader.

■Its only advantage is price. Rivals can neutralize the entire ad campaign simply by lowering their prices.

■The product's benefit is one of marginal consumer interest.

Don't plan a comparative campaign on the assumption that it will attract attention merely by tackling the leader. The novelty of comparative ads has worn off. What they say is the key.

Source: *Advertising Age*, Chicago.

Chapter 32
Working With Ad Agencies

Rating Ad Agencies

Key factors:
- Past record.
- Related experience.
- Ability of personnel on the account.
- Agency fee.
- Time needed to launch campaign.
- References from other clients.
- Importance agency attaches to satisfying clients.
- Awards and other professional recognition won by agency.

Assign points to each criterion on the basis of how important the company believes it is for a project. A company may feel that a good track record is worth 10 points and creative ability is worth 15.

Source: Bob Chang, Harshe–Rotman & Druck, *Sales & Marketing Management*, New York.

Choosing A New Ad Agency

- Ask the agency what it feels makes great advertising. It should be similar to the customer's view.
- Review projects done specifically by members of the team who will handle the new account.
- Determine how past creative work met a customer's objectives. Did it stand out from the clutter?
- Weigh the advantages of an out-of-town agency with a strong creative service against the negatives of working only via telephone, plane, and mail.
- Evaluate the charges beyond the 15% agency commission on ad space or the 17.65% fee on services.
- Run a background check to be sure the agency pays suppliers promptly, since top talent may be unwilling to work for a slow-paying outfit.
- Identify the long-term clients and review for steady growth. A heavy client turnover could be a sign of agency problems.

Source: Rich Flaskegaard, Minnesota advertising executive, *Advertising Age*, New York.

Why Clients Switch Ad Agencies

Major contributing factors:
■Dissatisfaction with billing procedures. A major complaint is inaccuracy. Financial misunderstandings usually occur when the agency operates on the fee system. When a client starts to complain about billings, it is a signal of unhappiness with the agency's overall performance.
■Frequent turnover of agency personnel leading to continual changes of key employees.
■Lack of creativity. Another major complaint is lack of innovation by the agency.
■Poor agency management. The advertising agency is perceived by its clients as lacking in depth and in the managerial resources it needs for growth.
Source: Robert Boyd, Northern Arizona University, Flagstaff, AZ, *Ad Week*, New York.

What Ad Agencies Need From Clients

■Early consultation, before plans and ad budgets have been firmed.
■Prompt, accurate responses to the agency's questions.
■Treatment with respect, even when differences occur.
■Reasonable deadlines from clients and the willingness of clients to meet their own deadlines.
Source: Don Hauptman, creative consultant, *Direct Marketing*, Garden City, NY.

Getting More Out Of Agencies

Companies can use their advertising agencies as marketing consultants to conduct annual audits of overall marketing operations, not just to handle advertising production and placement.

Specifically, have the advertising agency, working as marketing consultant, spend two or three days to: 1. Review overall marketing operations. 2. Write a letter citing the company's marketing strengths and weaknesses.

Ask for an estimate on all the work the agency believes they could do to improve particular marketing functions.

If the company's advertising agency doesn't offer this service, the next time the company calls in a marketing consultant for a specific purpose, ask him to audit the overall marketing operations as a secondary assignment.
Source: Jack M. Doyle, Jack M. Doyle Advertising, Inc., Louisville, KY.

Chapter 33
Advertising Copy

Principles Of Effective Copy

■Get attention by stating a believable promise in a few words. Or illustrate the product and its advantages in a photograph.

■Hold the reader's attention with titles, subheads, illustrations and a good first paragraph.

■Create desire by piling up product benefits.

■Make copy believable. Include specific figures, testimonials and guarantees.

■Prove it's a bargain by giving specifics on price reductions and building up the value of the product.

■Create a reason to buy now. Use a special offer for promptness.

■Close ads with a paragraph that makes it easy for customers to act. But shop-worn phrases like "Write today" or "Order now" are too weak. What stirs prospects to action? Coupons (especially those offering a premium); 800 numbers; explicit buying instructions, including the actual words to use in the response; details about an easy-payment plan.

Not every ad can contain all elements, but aiming for them is the first step toward copy that works.

Source: John Caples, vice-president, BBD&O, New York.

Basic Advertising Appeals

Universal human desires motivate people to read, to believe, and to buy. Build advertising appeals on these basic wants: to gain, to save, to do, and to be.

People want to gain health, popularity, praise from others, pride of accomplishment, self-confidence, time, improved appearance, comfort, social and business advancement, security in old age, leisure, increased enjoyment, and personal prestige.

People want to save discomfort, money, worry, embarrassment, work, and doubt.

People want to do things that express their personalities, satisfy their curiosity, and attract others' affections. They want to be able to resist domination by others, emulate the admirable, acquire or collect things, and to improve themselves in a general way.

People want to be creative, efficient, recognized authorities, good parents, up-to-date, first in things, gregarious, sociable, hospitable, proud of their possessions, and influential over others.

Making Advertising More Meaningful

Successful advertising should hinge on the unique selling proposition (USP), i.e., the particular merit that distinguishes a product and makes it meaningful to consumers, for example, the "Think Small" theme of Volkswagen, one of the most successful unique selling proposition campaigns in advertising history.

Current advertising tends to focus on mood and feeling, rather than on the quality of a product. Also, the emotions that are projected tend to be similar. For example, the scenes of happy old people, teenagers, babies, and dogs, generally associated with Pepsi-Cola ads, are now imitated by many other companies, with the result that consumers don't distinguish among products being advertised. Some advertisers end up supporting the opposition.

Why the USP is important today. As the economy gets tougher, advertisers will have to focus increasingly on the consumer's need for the product.

Main focus of the USP. It demonstrates what the product can deliver that no other product can. A common mistake that companies make is to limit the emphasis of their advertisements to the product, without a broader regard for larger consumer interests.

Strategy. Say the company makes furniture. Instead of representing itself as being in the furniture business, it should project the image of being in the home-environment business.

The difference. In the new definition (along with an offer to give customers decorating advice), the company is selling a reassurance that the consumer's choice of purchases will be expertly guided. In addition, the manufacturer is promoting the belief that its customers' homes will be more beautiful and fashionable as a result of buying the company's furniture.

Source: Jan Hedquist, president, Rosser Reeyes, Inc., New York.

Keys To A Successful Small-Space Ad

Get a powerful headline that makes a promise…be specific (don't say "more," say "20% more")…address the reader as "you"…use testimonials and endorsements …offer a guarantee…use a coupon…repeat the offer in the coupon or the last line of the ad…use a photo or drawing of your product. Often helpful: Designing the ad on a slight slant within its border to break through the linear look and clutter of other ads on the page. This will make the ad stand out.

Source: Richard Siedlecki, Richard Siedlecki Direct Marketing, Ventura, CA.

Unforgettable Tag Lines

Advertising tag lines, those repeated slogans used to identify a product or a company, work wonders only when their catchy recall establishes the product and leads prospects to it repeatedly.

Three forgettable flops:

■Ford wants to be your car company.

■NBC: Proud as a peacock.

■Because the wine remembers. (Can you remember which wine?)

Ones that work:

■Don't the squeeze the Charmin. (There are more consumers who perceive Charmin to be softest than there are those who don't.)

■Merrill Lynch is bullish on America. (The biggest bull market in U.S. history brought Merrill Lynch Pierce Fenner & Smith the sharpest growth any stockbroker ever experienced.)

■Have a Coke and a smile. (Inviting and memorable.)

How to create a winning tag line of your own? Don't force it. And do not dream it up first, then build a campaign to fit it. A good tag line is likelier to turn up by chance in a campaign that is already under way. It's often hidden somewhere in good copy or in a headline and needs only to be recycled.

But face the prospect that a really good tag line may not be forthcoming. A tag line is good only if: 1. It can significantly strengthen the marketing strategy and 2. It can stand alone to suggest the campaign to your market in a kind of shorthand message.

Timing is essential. Unforgettable tag lines, good or bad, don't achieve that status overnight. And never without careful multimedia planning plus hefty spending. The keys are repetition, longevity, and wide exposure. It's a tough task without big spending, but not impossible. Low-budget campaigns that are stretched out can bring it off. A combination of packaging and point of sale (where appropriate) is helpful.

Source: James I. Greene, president, Creative Associates, Inc., Dallas, *Adweek*, New York.

Effective Trade Advertising

■Get the real prospects to indicate their interest in your company's product or service far in advance. The best way to do this is to offer free literature. It takes very little ad space to make the offer. And every company has something already written to offer in the ad.

■Make it easy to respond. Offer a toll-free or collect telephone number. It makes the prospect feel that the advertiser wants to do business.

■Show names of salespeople. Customers prefer calling a person. And salespeople appreciate the ego massage.

■List the company's telephone number and address. No matter how big or well known the advertiser is, chances are the customer does not know the company's phone number and address. Make it easy for the real prospect to make contact.

■Know the ad's target. It costs the same to reach both the big and little firms. Ads that work pick up where the sales force can't go, because of some geographical, financial, or another reason.

■Use the word "free." It is magical. Don't take it for granted that everyone knows ad literature is free—say so.

■Don't bury the company and the offer. Make sure the offer, address and phone number are in large enough type to be read easily.

Source: Freeman R. Godsen, Jr., Smith & Hemmings, Los Angeles, *Adweek*, New York.

How To Test Advertising Effectiveness

■Does the ad get through the "clutter" of other ads? Does it rivet the viewer's (or reader's) attention within the all-important first three seconds? A common error is the failure to recognize that the ad's true competition is other ads, not other products.

■Does it zero in on just one or two ideas to leave with the viewer? Frequently, the ad lists so many reasons for buying the product that the viewer becomes confused and doesn't remember any of them.

■Is it relevant to the way the viewer sees himself and his own needs and desires? Be careful though, running an ad written for one need where customers have entirely different needs.

■Does it leave the product's name clearly in the viewer's memory? Or is the ad so "cute" that people remember the cuteness but forget the name of the advertiser?

Source: Nicholas VanSant, VanSant Dugsdale Advertising, Baltimore, *Marketing News.*

Print Advertising Checklist

■Most important point—does the headline clearly promise a well-defined benefit? Readers respond to simple, direct information. They tune out headlines that are cute, boastful, or exaggerated. Good headline: Eight attractive ways to solve your storage problems. Bad headline: It has everything.

■Is the ad cluttered or hard to read? Don't use light type on a dark background and don't superimpose words on pictures. Lines of type should be short enough to read easily. Avoid using fancy type, copy or art that's tipped at an angle, color for color's sake.

■Without being clever or mysterious, does the body of the ad tell the reader how, what, where, when and why?

■Do the illustrations back up the sales point?

Many ad professionals strive for creativity above all else. But flashy ads usually don't work.

Source: Robert B. Parker, *Mature Advertising*, Addison–Wesley Publishing Co., Reading, MA.

Chapter 34
Wise Buys In Advertising Media

Why Local Media Are A Good Buy

Advice for advertisers whose budgets are keeping pace with the inflation in media costs or whose product sales are falling short of targets: Fall back from national or regional advertising support to a local-marketing approach.

Concentrate advertising dollars in areas where business is strongest.

Spot TV is relatively soft right now. The biggest bargain is the late fringe viewers, between 11:30 p.m. and 2:00 a.m.

Radio is also hot. Strengths:

■Power to deliver good levels of a target audience.

■Reach and frequency are excellent for a reasonable out-of-pocket cost.

■It sells.

However, the radio audience is so segmented that no one station delivers a meaningful number of potential customers. Therefore, the advertiser must buy at least four stations in major markets to get meaningful impact. In certain markets, 10 or 11 stations are sometimes needed to do the job.

As an example, to reach 60% of the women between 25 and 54 years of age in the New York metropolitan market five times within a four-week period, time must be bought on five to seven stations.

The cheapest way to buy TV and radio times is to use buying services that own banks of time on desired stations, which they can sell at attractive rates.

But this trade time can usually be preempted if the station finds a cash buyer for the same time.

Solutions:

■Write tight specifications, with penalty clauses, into the company's deal with the buying service.

■Monitor the service closely to assure that the purchased ad time is being delivered.

■Tie a trade deal with a cash purchase to give the company some insurance against being preempted. The station will generally treat an advertiser who pays some cash better.

An economical way to buy print is through 3M's Magazine Network, Inc. (MNI). It has been around for a decade, but is now catching fire. MNI offers advertisers selected editions of many magazines (including *Time, Newsweek* and *U.S. News & World Report*) on a market-by-market basis. The cost is a fraction of what it costs to buy the entire circulation.

MNI delivers a wide range of special-target audiences such as high-income individuals, working women, urbanites, executives.

Source: Bruce Hoenig, senior vice-president and director of media, Avrett, Free & Fisher Inc., New York.

Shrewder Newspaper Advertising

■Ask for a discount if the ad will run more than once. Papers usually give a reduction of 5%–15%, depending on how often the ad appears.

■Don't automatically buy a full-page ad when seeking maximum impact. If well designed, even a quarter-page ad can dominate a page.

■Always include the company logo. Leaving it out squanders much of the benefit that comes from advertising frequently.

■Think position. For an extra fee, many papers guarantee space on a page with proven high readership. Or negotiate the premium position without a premium charge.

■Ask the newspaper sales representative for readership survey information to help decide which section of the paper is best for the ad.

Source: S. L. Dean, *How to Advertise: A Handbook for Small Business*, Enterprise Publishing Inc., Wilmington, DE.

Advertising Space At Bargain Rate

Advertisers can save up to 75% on remnant space. That's unsold space the magazine must fill as an issue's deadline approaches. To reserve the best, tell the space sales rep to put the company account on the remnant buyer list. The usual saving is 40% of the rate card. Be prepared, though. Remnant space must be filled quickly. Have ads ready for the moment when space is available. There are even some brokers in remnant space. Remember though, that remnant space is not available to current advertisers and there's no ad agency commission.

TV Time At Bargain Rate

The cheapest way to buy TV and radio times is to use buying services that own banks of time on desired stations, which they can sell at attractive rates.

But this trade time can usually be preempted if the station finds a cash buyer for the same time.

Solutions:

■Write tight specifications, with penalty clauses, into the company's deal with the buying service.

■Monitor the services to assure that the purchased ad time is being delivered.

■Tie a trade deal with a cash purchase to give the company some insurance against being preempted. The stations will generally treat an advertiser who pays some cash better.

How To Get Your Product On National TV For Next To Nothing

Giving away your product as a TV game or talk show prize gives it exposure to a national audience at a cost that's a small fraction of the cost of buying a comparable amount of TV advertising time. Any nationally sold consumer product or service is a candidate for this exciting form of promotion.

How it works: Through an advertising agency that handles these promotions, your company offers its product for use as a prize to the producers of a show you think will give it the best audience (your ad agency will be able to tell you which shows have the kind of audience you're trying to target). The agency writes promotional copy to be used on the air and creates any visual material, including videos, you want to accompany the product on the show. There are two categories of prizes…

■Major prizes. They include merchandise valued at $500 or more. Manufacturers pay nominal placement fees—about $200 per broadcast—for acceptance of these products by the producers.

■Minor prizes. Merchandise worth $25 or more. Placement fees for these prizes are much higher…often in excess of $4,000 per broadcast.

The placement fees also vary from show to show. Products offered as prizes on *Wheel of Fortune*, for example, carry the highest placement fees. The fee for a minor prize on a single broadcast of *Wheel of Fortune* is over $4,500 (about $200 for a major prize). On *The Price is Right*, the placement fee for a minor prize is only about $1,000, and about $200 for a major prize.

The Payoff

For this fee, plus modest ad agency charges for writing the promotion copy and marketing services, your product gets national TV exposure of eight to 20 seconds (the average for most prize mentions is 10 seconds). With *Wheel of Fortune*, this exposure covers more than 30 million American homes.

Typical campaign: A $1,000 video camera given away to *Wheel of Fortune* contestants on, say, 40–50 broadcasts and to contestants on 40–50 broadcasts of *The Price is Right* in the same period would cost a total of about $25,000 in placement fees, costs for media agencies, creative work, etc. Payoff: The product can be seen about one billion times by consumers.

■Comparable cost for 80–100 prime time 10-second network TV spots: Over $550,000.

Added bonus: Some TV shows now allow manufacturers to air toll-free phone numbers when their products are being mentioned. Measuring consumer telephone response can provide valuable information about the effectiveness of your campaign.

Source: Allen E. Barkus, president, Ted Barkus Advertising Co., Inc., 1512 Spruce St., Philadelphia 19102.

Smart Ways To Buy Radio Ad Time

■Don't buy from combined figures on audience ratings. Get the station's breakdown of those figures by age group. Most stations lump the 18–49 age group together for sales purposes. But if your company is selling home improvement products, the rock station, with all of its 18–49-group listeners under 23 years of age, isn't the place to spend your advertising dollars.

Beware of ratings that are distorted by temporary promotions which are timed to increase audience during ratings periods. Tip-off: Too-dramatic gains.

■Choose the type of station most appropriate to your purpose. The rock station is a good place to recruit young people. Top middle-of-the-road stations are good for product selling. FM stations used as background music in offices and plants reach that captive industrial audience.

■In choosing the time at which your spots are to be aired, don't overlook lower-cost weekend radio. The weekend audience is less predictable, but it's there.

If your dollars are going to buy more expensive "drive time," specify when the ad will run.

Why? Actual commuter rush hour is generally 7 to 9 a.m., but radio stations often charge prime drive-time rates for ads run from 6 to 10 a.m.

■Save high costs of buying during special broadcast by buying ad "adjacency" which runs immediately before or after the show.

Source: Walter G. Young, vice-president of John E. Hayes Co., in *Industrial Marketing*.

Chapter 35
Sales Promotion

Promotion Pays Off

Cents-off coupons, cash refunds, sweepstakes, and other promotions have been growing almost twice as fast as national advertising during inflationary times.

The reason is that promotion is very price-oriented. And inflation drives consumers toward every possible way to save money at the supermarket. Some 70% of households send in for cash refunds, as compared with 40% a few years ago. Fully 80% regularly redeem coupons. And this is not a low-income phenomenon. Families with over $25,000 in income and relatively high education levels are the smartest shoppers. They also are more apt to see the newspapers and magazines in which coupons appear.

To promote effectively:

■Recognize that consumers are eager to try brands that offer coupons, but they are simultaneously moving to nonbrand generic products (now 14% of supermarket sales) if the product is used in quantity and if there is little real difference among products.

■Use cash refunds to load up customers with several packages of a product instead of the single package they usually buy.

Source: Louis J. Haugh, managing partner, Westport Marketing Group, Inc., Westport, CT.

Sales Promotion Ideas

■Sampling. Free samples distributed by mail or door-to-door.

■Coupons. In the product package, by mail, or in newspapers and magazines.

■Trade coupons. Offered by retailers rather than the manufacturer.

■Trade allowances. Special payments to retailers for advertising and displaying the product.

■Bonus packs. Such as buy two, get another free.

■Price-offs or cents-offs. Should allow at least 15% off the regular price to be effective, more for weaker brands.

■In-, on-, and near-packs. Such as packaging the product in a reusable drinking glass, or several brands of cereal packaged together.

■In-the-mail premiums when one or two labels are sent in. Can be free or with an additional charge, usually less than $5.

■Contests (including sweepstakes).

■Mail-in refunds. A customer who sends in a label gets either a cash refund or a coupon for another purchase.

Source: William A. Robinson, William A. Robinson, Inc., Northbrook, IL.

Premium Considerations

■The most effective promotions are those that tie the premium to the sponsoring product. For example, tea bag manufacturer using an automatic-dispenser vacuum bottle; breakfast food and a digital alarm clock.

■Customizing (the consumer's name on a shirt; favorite football team on an athletic jersey) increases the premium's appeal. But that's only if it doesn't stretch delivery time out too far.

■Price—for self-liquidators, do not charge more than 50% of retail value.

■Offering a number of premiums in the same ad can backfire. Ad ends up looking like a mail order catalog. The better way is to focus on the most appealing one.

■Consider shipping costs. Consumers don't like paying postage and handling charges in addition to the basic price. Low-value items that are heavy or fragile to ship are a bad idea.

■Trends: 1. Higher prices. (Recent analysis: Price to customer was over $5 in 37% of the cases.) 2. Longer delivery times. (Average now is 39 days.)

Source: *Incentive Marketing*, New York.

Basics Of Promotion Advertising

Promotion advertising differs significantly from consumer franchise-building advertising. The latter is long-term in nature and aimed at giving customers reasons to buy. Promotion advertising is short-term. It pushes for the order by providing incentives (coupons, rebates, premiums and contests).

Print is the usual medium for promotion advertising. Some big-budget companies use broadcast advertising to get consumers to look for the promotion at stores or in newspapers.

As a general rule, resist the inclination to include extraneous points in the promotion ad. Focus on a simple call to action. Including other ad copy is dangerous.

Typical calls to action:

■Redeem this coupon and save money.

■Buy this product and get a $2 refund.

■Win $100,000 in the product sweepstakes.

■Buy this product and get this other item for only $4.95.

Remember that a sweepstakes cannot legally require a purchase. It is generally used to focus attention on the brand and reinforce key copy points. A sweepstake's ability to move products at retail is limited, but it can lead customers to make a purchase.

Most promotion events are price- or value-added-oriented. As such, promotion copy must appeal to the wallet rather than emotions. But this doesn't mean the ad can't look like the franchise-building ad. Graphics should retain the brand's inherent appeal to its target group. Most promotion ads have higher readership scores than straight brand-sell ads. A promotion ad generally attracts a wider audience to the product.

It's essential to keep the offer simple. Example: Save 25¢ now with this coupon. To be avoided: Save $1.50 when you purchase six of the products/sizes listed and send in proofs of purchase with two cash-register tapes from a supermarket. (To say the least, consumers would be confused.)

The art, copy, and terms in promotion ads should get the same clarity and attention to detail that other advertising does.

Source: Louis J. Haugh, managing partner, Westport Marketing Group, Inc., Westport, CT.

Trade Show Space Considerations

■Storage: Some back-to-back booths have storage space created by columns; others don't. If you need storage, make sure it's nearby, if not in the booth itself.

■Booths near a freight entrance may have to be set up late and dismantled early.

■Water and gas: If you need these utilities, make sure they're available. If they are available and you don't need them, make sure your space won't be reassigned at the last minute to a company that does.

■Obstructions: Check plans for columns, changes in ceiling height (usually indicated by dotted lines), changes in floor level shown by ramps or stairs, utility control boxes that must not be covered by an exhibit.

■Layout: On most diagrams, heavy lines indicate back walls of exhibits, light lines are space limits.

■Traffic pattern is important in picking a trade show booth location.

When people have a choice, they tend to turn right as they enter an exhibit hall.

Pick a spot that maximizes the booth's visibility to a visitor walking in this counterclockwise pattern.

■Best corner: One that permits the visitor to see your booth before he turns.

■Setting up a trade show booth: Do not crowd it with equipment. Space is needed for demonstrations, ashtrays, wastebaskets, and for your salesmen to mingle with prospects. Prospects are reluctant to stop if they feel they will crowded.

Avoiding Trade-Show Rip-Offs

Defensive strategies: 1. Arrange for unloading and assembling of equipment beforehand. Schedule work precisely, hour by hour. (Enables those in charge to detect goldbricking, etc., and possibly head off extra charges.) 2. Make early contact with the show manager and local service unions. They have the power, not the exhibit hall staff. 3. Attend exhibitor meetings and discuss mutual problems. Solidarity gets better results than individual complaints. 4. Construct displays with safety devices such as unbreakable plastic cases for valuable items. Weld working parts of vital equipment. 5. Sell marketable items at the end of the show to reduce thefts.

Source: Ron Hardaway, AT&T, New York, and director of the National Trade Show Exhibitors Assoc., Rolling Meadows, IL.

Chapter 36
Managing Your Salespeople

Setting Sales Budgets

The basic method is for top management and operating sales managers to submit their own proposed budgets. Where there are great variances, differences are analyzed and a compromise is worked out. Areas of common agreement are automatically accepted.

But using the costs of the existing sales force as a starting point in budgeting doesn't take into account changing company objectives or marketing considerations.

Not allowing for enough time lag between sales efforts and the initial order is a common error. Expenditures of time and money don't always show up in actual orders within the same budget year.

An "investment" approach to sales budgeting rather than "expenditure" approach is a good solution. This way management can use return-on-investment in appraising sales efforts. The cost of training and the nonproductive period of new salespeople can be more accurately measured over the longer term. The cost of selling new products and entering new markets is extended over a longer payback period.

Source: *Checking Up on Your Sales Force*, The Sales Executives Club of New York.

Sales Quotas That Work

Past sales figures continue to be the best guide to quotas. Six factors that are also important:

1. Economic trends (national and regional).

2. Number of competitors selling in each territory and their performance.

3. Size of the actual and potential market. Whether or not the count is increasing or decreasing.

4. Anticipated levels of sales promotion and advertising.

5. Plant capacity and probability of production slowdowns.

6. Amount of time it takes to reach customers, close the sale, make the delivery, and collect.

Source: *The Effective Manager*, Boston.

Improving Sales Performance

Salespeople can often turn in a good performance simply by focusing on their strengths or coasting on the regular orders of a limited number of good customers.

The problem is that management is satisfied and neglects to search for areas of potential improvement.

Even top performers may be ignoring potential customers in their territories. Or they may be downplaying less popular items in the company's product line. Suggestions:

■Consider assigning additional salespeople to search for new customers, even in a star performer's territory. They may be able to develop new accounts without taking a penny from the regular salesperson's commission.

■Make joint sales calls routinely with the salespeople to be sure they aren't ignoring products or sales techniques. Be wary about barging in on customer negotiations. It could undercut the salesperson's authority.

Source: William Exton, Jr., William Exton Jr. & Associates, New York.

Mistakes In Managing The Sales Force

One of the more serious signals of marketing problems is frequent changes in sales strategies…one month it's a contest for sales reps to win a trip to Aruba…the next month, quotas change…then, it's a special bonus of some sort.

Problem: These are usually desperation tactics—symptomatic of a lack of solid marketing strategy. Management is simply relying on salespeople to go out there and somehow find customers wherever they can. This approach may generate some short-term successes, but will eventually bring management back for more fixes, once that push is over.

Trap: Falling into a pattern of reactive responses to competitive pressures—lurching from crisis to crisis by relocating sales reps, adjusting product lines, etc.

Reality: There's no substitute for a carefully planned, long-term marketing program that the company sticks with—and one it can adapt to the changing times sensitively and intelligently. That's the key to a successful sales force.

Source: John R. Graham, Graham Communications, 40 Oval Rd., Quincy, MA 02170.

Chapter 37
Sales Methods

The Intelligent Way To Prospect For Clients

Too many salespeople approach a territory with the notion of selling to every possible account. But the servicing of smaller accounts and all-inclusive prospecting is too expensive today. Instead, identify and go after a segment of the market. That's more productive than all the various individual accounts that might buy a product.

A segment is a group of users and prospective users that differ in size but are in the same general business. It's better to concentrate on selling to the segment that offers the highest sales potential than to try selling to all businesses in a territory that might buy.

Identifying the best segment to prospect, and getting to know its particular needs and product uses, sharpen the sales effort significantly.

Questions to ask when prospecting segments:
- What new segments or categories of business can use the product?
- What is the company's present share of the market in each segment?
- Which segments represent the greatest potential?
- What businesses within the segment haven't been sold yet?

Always do as much research beforehand as possible to avoid the soaring costs of making personal calls to find prospects. It's often possible to identify the accounts and determine their needs and ability to pay before contacting them.

Get supportive market data. The kind depends on what sort of product is being sold. For consumer goods, get population and income data. For industrial goods, sales and employment data. The best data sources are the U.S. Department of Labor, Bureau of Economic Analysis Data (available from the U.S. Department of Commerce).

Once customer contact is made, be sure to determine who has the authority to buy. In today's complex organizations, more people are getting involved in buying decisions.

Source: Dr. Robert Vizza, dean, Manhattan College's School of Business, Riverdale, NY.

Computers Increasingly Valuable Sales Tool

More and more companies are arming their salespeople with laptop computers and sales automation (also called contact management software). Among the Fortune 500 companies, there are few sales reps who aren't currently automated or in the process of becoming automated. Main reasons for switching to computers…

■Increase sales. More, better, up-to-date information "on-line" in the salesperson's hands means closing more sales faster.

Examples: Knowing what's in stock without having to place a separate call to the factory. Knowing the time of the month the contact makes his decisions to re-order.

■Increase efficiency. A sales rep with a laptop computer can automatically pump out a personalized form letter instead of having to write the letter from scratch. He can do a spreadsheet on potential dollar savings for a prospect. He can get his mail more efficiently—electronically, rather than on paper.

■Cut costs. If salespeople can enter orders directly via their own computers, rather than read the numbers to an order clerk at headquarters, the company no longer needs the clerk. Further, the order will be more accurate when the salesperson enters it than when the clerk enters it.

What Good Software Can Do

Think of sales automation software from a salesperson's viewpoint. Some things the software can accomplish:

■Management of contacts. The program stores contacts' names, addresses and telephone numbers. The best programs store alternate contacts at different addresses. They can also automatically dial the contact's phone number and can store notes, such as what the sales rep promised the contact the last time they spoke. In addition, they will store form letters and personalized letters.

■Communications with contacts. All communications back and forth with various contacts can be stored, including letters, confirmations, proposals and contracts. All this can be called up on the computer screen.

Impact: A salesperson can walk into a contact's office, sit around a table with the contact, review the file, write up a contract and sign it there and then.

■Order entry. The salesperson can place an order, via his computer, from the contact's office and can track down the status of an order on the computer. When will it be delivered? Is it in stock? What's the Federal Express shipping number? These questions can easily be answered by computer.

■Communications with the company. Memoranda from the sales manager to the sales reps in the field informing them of specials can be handled by computer. Technical information, such as specifications, compatibility, warnings, etc., can also be made instantly available by computer.

■Sales history. A complete history of the company's dealings with a particular customer, and an analysis of that history, can be stored in the computer. This gives the salesman a clear picture of the customer's buying patterns.

There's no off-the-shelf program that will perfectly match the company's needs. Some, however, will come closer than others.

If you have the money, buy a customized program.

Alternative: Buy several of the more popular programs. Play with them and figure which one most closely matches the company's needs.

Do's And Don'ts Of Automating

■Don't force hardware on the salespeople. Involve them in the process of finding the right machine. Present the sellers with at least six company laptops. Let them take samples on the road to play with. Let them decide which one they want.

All laptops are compatible with IBM desktops. So there's no question of which will run what programs. They all will run all programs.

What is really needed is a 286 or 386 machine. These are faster than the first MS-DOS laptops.

■Don't force programs on salespeople. Involve them in the process of finding a package. Let them see what you've found. Show them suggested screen layouts. Solicit their input. The more they can contribute, the more they'll feel it's theirs. Since many sellers are prima donnas, the company will not want to alienate them by shoving technology down their throats.

■Don't write your own programs. People who write these programs are experts in the field. They know what they're doing. Better: Pay a dealer (also called a VAR, or Value-Added Retailer) to modify an existing program for you.

■Set down specific rules about entering data. At some stage, the company will want to use the sellers' prospect databases, for instance, to send company newsletter offers, etc. To be of use to the company, the information must be entered into the computer in a standardized way.

Major Problems

The rewards of automation are potentially immense, but the company must not underestimate the time and effort. Two main problems:

■Data conversion and integration. All companies have information in one form. Getting from that "form" to the laptop and back is a "big" issue. It needs to be thought out well in advance. Otherwise, it can be an expensive and time-consuming proposition.

■Learning and discipline. Salespeople must learn to use the computers both to retrieve and to send information to the company. And they must maintain the system. Although none of this is easy, if they see it benefits them, their customers and their sales, they won't mind cooperating.

Source: Harry Newton, publisher, *Inbound/Outbound* magazine, New York 10010.

What To Know About Your Accounts

What to know about an account before the next call on it:

■Its business, products, market, and primary customers.

■How big it is. Its ranking within the industry.

■Who does the actual buying? Who makes the decisions to buy? Who influences these decisions?

■How often the company buys. Quantities ordered.

■Total sales for last year.

■Its primary competition. Approximately how much business your company is doing with them.

■The financial standing of the account.

■What plans it has that could affect the use of the products being sold.

■What problems immediately concern it.

■What value customer places on the products now being bought.

What to know about the person being called on:

■Job responsibilities and purchasing authority.

■The business problems the buyer needs solutions for.

■Where the buyer fits into the organizational structure.

■Some of the buyer's personal interests and his business background.

Source: Robert F. Vizza and Thomas E. Chambers, *Time and Territorial Management for the Salesman*, Sales Executives Club of New York.

Reasons For Lost Sales

To turn a weakening sales situation around, know what's causing the trouble. The first step is to isolate the problem. Key questions:

1. Are sales of all products down? Just a few?

2. In which areas are sales down? Use specific breakdowns such as urban, suburban, rural, residential, college, inner city, recreational.

3. Are sales down for all types of accounts? Is the decline limited to chains? Independents? Some other classification?

4. Where did the business go? Was it lost to a competitive product? Another size of the same product? One of the company's own products? A cheaper product?

5. When did the decline start?

6. How serious is the drop? Is the change due to seasonal factors? Did a similar decrease occur at the same time last year?

Source: *Managing a Sales Team*, Lebhar–Friedman Books, New York.

Chapter 38
The Sales Call

Planning More Effective Sales Calls

■Decide on the objective of the call. ("Make a sale" is not good enough unless all the preliminary groundwork has been done. Asking for the order at the wrong time is as bad as not asking at all.)

■Review everything known about the customer (purchases from competitors, results of previous calls).

■Identify the product benefits that are not available in competitors' products and are special to the prospect.

■Focus on the selling points that will best illustrate product benefits. Write them, in advance, in a logical order.

■Prepare a file of spec sheets, photos, testimonials, test data, etc., that fully supports the sales story.

■Anticipate general areas of resistance. Plan how to counter each one.

■List all the specific sales objections the customer could raise. Arrange them in order of importance.

■Prepare at least two answers for each anticipated objection.

■Write out the pre-closing summary. Decide on the closing strategy to use.

Source: *Sales Manager's Bulletin*, Waterford, CT.

Asking For The Order

One of the reasons for the failure to ask for the order is that some salespeople actually don't know what words to use at this most crucial point in the sale. Their fear of a turndown is so pronounced that obvious courses of action open to them become clouded.

The salespeople who has experienced something akin to panic when faced with the necessity to ask for the order might, with profit, consider some of the general courses of action that follow:

1. Show, by words and actions, that you expect an order.

2. Use questions; get the customers to commit himself point by point.

3. Suggest a course of action that will, ultimately, have but one possible destination—an order.

4. Seek areas of agreement and use these to launch your close.

5. Ask for a larger order than you expect to receive so the customer can "compromise" and reduce the order to the size you actually hoped to get.

6. Simply ask for the order!

Examining the possibilities of these general courses of action, we should consider first the course of action which is most obvious; i.e., the last mentioned—ask for the order. Essentially, when you ask for the order you are using a test question to determine how effective your presentation has been. You are about to find out whether you have gained and held the customer's attention; whether you have gained his confidence; whether you have established a need and caused him to see it as a high priority need. If the customer rejects your bid for an order at this point, it means that you must identify the area in which you have not yet been successful.

Take note what we did not say, "You must identify the area in which you have failed." You have not failed until your customer has made the purchase from some other supplier.

If the customer does not agree to buy when you ask for the order, you should listen intently to the words he uses. These can provide you with clues that will suggest the course of action you should now follow. For example, he might say, "I'm not ready to buy just now." This is far from saying, "No, I am not going to buy from you." He is implying that he will probably buy—later. Just how much later depends upon you. By judicious questioning you may be able to identify the reasons for his delay. We usually delay or procrastinate when we have unpleasant decisions to make, or when we are in the middle of a tug-of-war between two opposing decisions. We can be made to act in one of two or three ways:

1. If we are shown that the cost of delay is higher than the cost of taking action.

2. If we can be shown that we have more to gain by taking one action rather than the other.

3. If we are shown that taking one action will be far more costly than taking the other. Therefore, when the customer indicates that she "is not quite ready to decide," she has given you a valuable tip, and it now becomes your task to decide which of the three foregoing actions will be most valuable to pursue.

If you are, frankly, "scared stiff" when the time comes to ask for the order, keep in mind that the task will not become any easier if you delay. Once you have made your presentation, you face the one best time to ask for the order. To delay may be fatal to the sale.

Only a few weeks ago, a chap approached us to obtain a contribution to an institution. As we listened to his presentation, we found our interest in the project increasing. We had, mentally, decided to give a rather large contribution. Unfortunately for the institution, the chap never got around to asking point-blank for the order. His delay gave us time to think the matter over, and as we considered other similar demands on our resources, we decided to reduce the contribution by better than 70%. This 70% was lost because the "salesman" did not ask for the order when our buying mood was at its peak. All that was needed was a "little push" on his part and the sale would have been his.

So, in considering ways of asking for the order, don't overlook the most obvious, the most direct route. "May I have your order now?" The chap who failed to ask us for our order was afraid to ask for the size contribution that we—and he—had in mind. This could not help but have an effect upon us. It leads us to think, "That is a rather large donation—in fact, too large...I'll reduce it." Don't be afraid to ask for a large order—the customer always has the option to reduce it; and this, in fact, causes him to feel that he is dominating the selling situation, that he is not being "high pressured," that he is making the decision, not you.

You can also use the seemingly "indirect" approach in which you imply that you are going to get an order: "May I phone your order in now so that we can insure immediate delivery?"..."What model (color, size, etc.) do you want us to deliver?"…"Where do you want us to deliver it?" (or "install it," etc.)…"How soon would you like us to provide you with drawings?"

In each of these examples, you have given the customer a choice. Certainly, he can always react with "Wait a minute—I haven't given you an order yet." "Don't rush me." If your indirect bid for an order elicits this type of response, you can always answer with, "Gosh, I'm sorry. I had no intention of pressuring you. I just thought that the advantages of (this product or service) were so desirable that you'd want to move quickly…but if there is something I haven't covered, or if there are questions I have not answered, I'll be glad to do so, because I'd like to see this in your plant" (or "in your home" or "on your shelves," as applicable to your product or market).

So…what has been lost by asking for the order? Not a thing. You have backed off graciously; you've put him at ease, reaffirmed your desire to serve him further and given him a chance to ask questions. You've also made him feel that he is dominating the selling situation. You have followed the principle that you should act as though you expect the order.

A radio announcer concluded his commercial with, "Buy several of these suits for the summer." This approach is based on the tendency a potential purchaser has to think, "I may buy one, but I'm not about to buy several." The announcer's goal may well have been to sell us just one. His words are supported by the same solid psychological grounds that prompt us to "overstate the customer's objections." He will almost inevitably say, "I didn't say that. What I said was…" And he will go on to understate his previous objection—giving you something with which you can successfully cope.

There is but one obvious danger in asking for too large an order (in the hope that he will reduce it to the size of order you really had in mind). If you do not handle this with care, he may get the idea that you are not aware of his real needs. Your recommendation must be reasonable.

■Use questions; get the customer to commit himself point-by-point. "I see that you feel this is a good price, Mr. Burke?" Burke replies, "Yes." "And you feel that it meets your production requirements?" Burke answers, "I'm sure it will." "Well, Mr. Burke, production means money to you and delay means expense, so will you let me send in your order now so you can start benefiting from the installation as soon as possible?"

The foregoing is a simple example to indicate the nature of this technique. It can be used far more subtly in the sale of sophisticated equipment, and the questioning can be more extensive than that indicated in the example. You can ask questions on a number of points that have been covered in your presentation. They should be aspects on which you know your customer will be sold and, therefore, you can anticipate, with certainty, that his answers will be uniformly "Yes." With every "Yes" reply, he is making it more difficult to respond with a "No" when you finally, point-blank, ask him for the order.

■Suggest a course of action that will, ultimately, have but one possible destination—an order. "Mr. Kramer, I'd suggest that you consider buying this basic unit now and then add other units as your production needs increase. If you agree, I'd suggest that we get this first unit ordered today."

"Mr. Draper, I'd suggest that you order (quantity) feet of this cable now, as a starter." In this approach, the customer has the freedom of choice. He can reject the quantity you recommend but may still give you an order.

■Seek areas of agreement and use these to launch your close. "I certainly agree with your views, Mr. Rogers, on heat dissipation problems, and our men in the lab feel the same way. You're going to be delighted to find that this unit won't raise the temperature a degree in your (plant, store, home, etc.). I'd like to suggest that we get an order in now. You're going to get a lot of satisfaction out of seeing your ideas on heat dissipation proven through performance."

Once again, you have given the customer the feeling that he has dominated the selling situation. At the same time, you are not manipulating him. As has been said so many times in this book, you are merely moving the customer to a decision…a decision which you sincerely feel is going to be in his best interests. He will decide favorably if you have earned his confidence and supplied him with sufficient proof, assurance and attention. You are not working against his interests. Keep in mind that as a rational being he will not make judgments that are opposed to his vital interests.

Twelve Keys To Positive Selling

1. Don't make promises that can't be kept. The customer never forgets. Follow through on all commitments.

2. Don't knock competitors. It's counterproductive. Most buyers become intrigued with a product under assault.

3. Don't question a customer's final decision to buy competitive merchandise. Instead, increase your own selling efforts.

4. Don't get too close to buyers. Habitual socializing can be risky. When a buyer begins to expect such treatment, withdrawing it becomes painful.

5. Don't complain to buyers about job or domestic problems. Complainers quickly change from friends to nuisances.

6. Don't overwhelm buyers with technical information. They are more interested in what a product or service can do for them, not so much how.

7. Don't try to impress customers with professional qualifications, education, social status. Some buyers resent those who appear to be snobs. Learn about each buyer's personal history and adapt the conversation accordingly.

8. Don't ignore personal sensibilities. Never smoke unless a buyer lights a cigarette first. Do the same with drinks at lunch. If a noontime nip with a key customer is necessary, be careful about seeing other key customers after that.

9. Don't overdress. Extreme fashions call attention to the wearer. Conservative clothes are always safe.

10. Don't be a gossip. They are universally distrusted.

11. Don't used canned presentations. A prepared pitch is best, but try to preserve spontaneity.

12. Don't misrepresent the product. Know the warranty terms and how much backup to expect from the supplier.

Source: P. J. Koerper, *How to Talk Your Way to Success in Selling*, Prentice-Hall, Englewood Cliffs, NJ.

Identifying Buyer Attitudes

It helps to match the sales pitch to the customer's attitude and personality. Basic customer attitudes to identify:

■Mainly concerned with the product itself. Usually wants substantial proof of its usefulness, quality and value. Bone up to provide all this information.

■Prefers buying from a salesperson he likes. Win his confidence.

■Indifferent to both product and salesperson. Earning the customer's trust might result in a sale.

■Tentative. Buys only generally accepted or status items. Focus on the product's reputation.

■Concerned with making a sound purchase from a trusted salesperson. Logical presentation. Answer questions with facts.

Source: *The Grid for Sales Excellence*, McGraw-Hill, New York.

Negotiating With Buyers

A negotiating session is an exercise in persuasion. Sellers who do their home-work enhance chances of success. Before making proposals to potential customers, consider:

■Personality. Introverts generally require details. Extroverts may be bored with them.

■Behavior. The buyer's actions in previous negotiations.

■Age. If the buyer's is very different from the seller's, some values are also likely to differ. For example, people who experienced the depression of the 1930s tend to drive for security all their lives.

■Need. The extent to which the buyer needs the item being sold.

Source: John J. McCarthy, *Electrical Wholesaling*, New York.

Winning Over A Customer

How to win the customer's faith, and how not to lose it:

■Avoid exaggerated claims for the product or unrealistic promises.

■Anticipate objections. Prove that the product can solve them before the customer brings them up. At the least, the purchaser is impressed by the salesperson's understanding of the situation.

■After the sale. Show a continuing interest in the customer.

■Attack head-on any post-sale problems. If the boss complains that the salesperson worries more about the customer than the company, show how it works both ways. Confidence earned helps the salesperson in the future, and thus enriches the company.

Responses To Four Common Sales Stalls

■I haven't had time to think about it. Response: I know how busy you are, but just a few minutes can clear the whole thing up. For example…

■I've got to talk it over with my partner. Response: Fine, a wise decision. Now let's get the whole thing boiled down so your partner can clearly understand it.

■The price is too high. Response: I know some companies that sell for less, and I'll explain why they do.

■Business is bad right now; I'll have to wait. Response: I'm sorry to hear that, but we can work out satisfactory terms. Tell them how to make business better.

Source: *How to Sell in the 1980s*, Prentice-Hall, Englewood Cliffs, NJ.

What Closing A Sales Call Really Means

A common misconception is that closing a sales call means simply getting the order. In reality, closing is accomplishing the objective of the sales call. That may or may not be to get the order on that call. Other closing objectives include:

■Getting approval to survey the company's needs.

■Presenting a written proposal.

■Demonstrating the project.

■Answering objections.

■Finding out the firm's buying and decision-making structure.

To be sure all the objectives of the call are met:

■At the end of the call, agree on the aims of the next one with the buyer. Some salespeople rely on their flexibility and experience instead of planning the next call.

■At the beginning of the next call, restate the agreed-upon objective. This tactic heads off any problem if either the buyer or the salesperson is unable to deal with the matter that day.

Before setting the objectives, analyze the decision process the buyer has to go through. What does the buyer need to know and do? Who else has to agree to the purchase? This will establish call objectives most likely to advance the buyer's decision-making process.

When it comes to time spent on calls, more is not better, particularly on a call where a decision to buy has been made. This often produces conflict and anxiety. The longer the salespeople stay, the more likely buyers will change their minds. Anything the salespeople say may provide an excuse to back out.

When the moment for the sales close comes, maintain silence. It makes buyers focus on the fact that it is their move now and time for a decision.

Source: Dr. Robert F. Vizza, dean, School of Business, Manhattan College, Riverdale, NY.

Part IV

Administration And Office Management

Chapter 39
The Efficient Office

Designing The Office

With office rents skyrocketing, many companies are asking designers for ways to put more employees comfortably into less space.

Good design reduces employee turnover and boosts productivity. For example, studies show that carpets, in preference to vinyl tile, reduce absenteeism and the correct light level makes the employee work more efficiently.

Another advantage of a good design is that office ambience enhances the company's image among employees and customers. A futuristic design may stimulate a creative mood among employees of a high-technology firm. Elegant offices enhance the image of a cosmetics company.

Office warmth can be created by color, texture, and enough furnishings to make the office space look like it's being fully utilized. Sometimes a large picture or bookcase can substitute for some furnishings.

Use a sensible approach. Many companies try to standardize offices and furnishings according to rank. Instead, tailor the design to the individual executive's tastes, but standardize elements such as decks and carpeting. Give the executive some choice in upholstery, wall color, artwork, and accessories.

Money-saving luxuries:

■Reduce overhead lighting. Thousands of dollars could be saved by switching to low-bright ceiling lighting, and most offices are overlighted anyhow.

■In open-space designs (i.e., areas of large, unobstructed spaces, with no built-in offices), let some of the window light filter into the inner areas. Daylight is humanizing. It makes employees feel like performing better.

Open-space design:

■Pro: Allows for greater density.

■Con: Makes privacy more difficult.

Originally, the open-space concept used plants to separate work areas. But sound carried too far and offices looked like tangled jungles. Thus, movable partitions were installed to break up open spaces. One aid: Build rooms where sensitive meetings can be held in privacy.

Source: Jack Lowery, Jack Lowery Associates, New York.

Eight Ways To Cut Space Costs

1. Consider local space sharing with the possibility of sharing the services of a receptionist, secretaries, cleaning personnel, utilities, base telephone charges, etc.

2. Prelease space from the developer of a building under construction when the developer is pinched for cash. Companies have a better chance of negotiating downward at that time.

3. Rent the rear of the premises on bargain terms. This can more than off-set the remodeling expense. Leave an access mall to the low-cost quarters, then let the owner rent the front space to small shops at a premium.

4. Rent executive offices in a prestigious building, but maintain the bulk of operations in a low-rent district.

5. Consult a designer before renting space, to avoid costly mistakes. Companies seldom consider proper storage space, and they often ignore the space needs of noisy or dust-sensitive equipment (such as computers).

6. Lease more space than you currently need if you expect to grow; sublease what you do not presently need.

7. Audit the office or plant space you plan to lease. A survey found that in 95 percent of the cases covered, the firms had less space than they had signed up for. (Errors averaged 4.5 percent but went as high as 12.5 percent).

8. Periodically check your list of office, plant, and warehouse space. Rearrangements may produce space suitable for 1. Better use, 2. Cost savings, 3. Subleasing.

Cheapest Ways To Break A Lease

It may be necessary to get out of a lease when space projections turn out to be more optimistic than actual needs. Some ways to get out at least cost:

The sublet:

This is the "cleanest" method—that is, to rent the space to another tenant. To do this requires some smart negotiating when the primary lease is drawn up.

Every lease should contain carefully formulated sublet provisions. Rarely will the landlord resist that. But he will insist on the right to screen the prospective tenant. Be sure the provision to screen contains a section that says any rejection must be based on "reasonable" grounds. The word "reasonable" is purposely vague.

If the landlord gets sticky about what is reasonable, the leverage is on the side of the tenant. He can claim the landlord is acting in an arbitrary way and, as a result, refuse to pay rent for "just" cause. He can then move—inviting the landlord to sue if he wishes. Usually, the landlord accepts the sublet tenant at that point and the primary tenant wins by default.

If the landlord wishes to push the suit, the tenant's greatest potential loss is the payment of rental dollars during the disputed period. Courts generally do not saddle the tenant with the landlord's legal expenses for the suit.

The lease should also state that the landlord must decide on the suitability of the tenant without unreasonable delay. Rarely is this provision in a sublet section. It is a good idea to include it.

The cancellation clause:

Many landlords will accept a tenant cancellation clause at specific periods in the lease. Say you take a ten-year lease. You could negotiate to have the right to cancel any time after the third year by paying some prearranged penalty, which usually gets smaller each year. That clause should be used in conjunction with the sublet clause, since if you are able to sublet the space you should not have to pay the cancellation penalty.

Walking away:

If the space is rented for a business operation that is physically separate from the main office (in another city or another part of town), set up a subsidiary to rent the space. Retail chains do this all the time.

In general, if the space is rented by a new company (even though it is owned by a well-known parent), the landlord will request that a security deposit accompany the lease. The size of the security will depend in part on the amount of site preparation needed for the new tenant.

Should the tenant have to withdraw early, all he has to do is move and leave the security deposit behind. The ethics of such a move are in the gray area, and few major corporations would want to use this device, but it is something that one should be aware of.

Leveraged ploy:

If a landlord becomes unreasonable, a smart tenant brings in any subtenant, even a less than desirable one. If the landlord rejects the subtenant, the primary tenant cries "foul," and uses that as justification for claiming the lease has been breached. He refuses to pay rent and notifies the landlord of plans to move out.

Once the landlord realizes this ploy is being used, he may back down and try to bring in a more acceptable tenant or let the primary tenant bring in someone else. Timing and bluff are critical elements of this ploy.

Be sure the original lease states the type of business to be conducted in the space in the most general way. If the statement is too specific, the landlord may use that as a way of rejecting a subtenant.

How To Size Up An Office Building

Signs of a good building:

■A minimum of five separate thermostat controls per floor (one for each side, one for the interior). Reason: Temperatures vary by 20 degrees from side to side.

■Bathrooms, halls, and public areas that have been cleaned before the building opens each day.

■A telephone in the elevator connected to an answering service, in case of breakdowns.

■Provisions for heat or air conditioning to be available after business hours on days when overtime is necessary. Also: Lights that can be kept on after the evening cleaning crew has left the offices.

■Maintenance personnel on duty during working hours.

Source: Paul A. Berman, Paul A. Berman Realties, Inc., Hackensack, NJ, writing in *The Office,* 1200 Summer St., Stamford, CT 06904.

Construction Contract Traps

Construction contracts generally provide for a performance bond or other financial guarantee by the contractor that the construction will be done as specified and on time. But clients can unwittingly invalidate this guarantee by materially changing the contract. Contracts frequently contain a clause which stipulates: All changes must be approved beforehand by the surety (the bonding company or other third party making the guarantee).

Even without the clause, if the contractor's performance bond does not specifically include the terms and conditions of the contract, the surety may only cover costs for work left undone, and not for the bills unpaid by the contractor for completed work.

Source: Marc J. Lane, attorney, Chicago.

Service Contract Protection

Contracts for service are not covered by the Uniform Commercial Code unless the contract says so. To bring a service contract under the code, add language such as:

"The parties to this contract recognize that the Uniform Commercial Code does not normally apply to the performance of services as distinguished from transactions in goods. However, the parties agree that the Uniform Commercial Code shall apply to this contract, and any dispute arising under this contract shall be resolved under the provisions of the code."

Destroying Old Files

Destroying old files can protect businesses in potential litigation, reduce the cost of document storage by hundreds of thousands of dollars and keep confidential information private. How to do it: Schedule the destruction of broad classes of files once they reach a certain age. Destroy all related papers on schedule. If the destruction isn't performed routinely, courts may rule it was done to conceal information in a pending suit. Give executives and others who handle confidential information shredders for their offices, and require them to destroy drafts of documents and informal communications once they're no longer needed. Retain only documents required by regulatory agencies or essential to the functioning of the company.

Planning Tips For Office Routine

Make your office run smoother with these techniques:

■Arrange routing lists alphabetically. This avoids hierarchical irritations that arise when one person's name is placed below someone else's.

■If there is a way to avoid written memoranda, use it. Eyeball-to-eyeball response is important in gauging how information is received and how it will be acted upon.

■Brevity is the essence of good communications.

■Boil down ideas and reports to less than one minute, if possible.

■Try not to hire assistants, even when the work load gets heavy. Assistants add a layer of bureaucracy, which reduces contact between managers and subordinates. They rarely expedite matters since they cannot make decisions in the boss's absence.

■Consider secretarial pools rather than personal secretaries. That way, letters can be dictated either to a machine or a person.

Source: Robert Townsend, author of *Robert Townsend Speaks Out*, Advanced Management Reports, Inc., New York.

Energy-Saving Tips

There are three categories of office energy-saving measures…

■Those related to the operation and maintenance of equipment.

■The building "envelope."

■The building's heating, cooling, lighting and ventilation systems.

The measures become progressively capital intensive/costly, as you move from the first to the third of these categories. Steps companies can take now:

Operation And Maintenance

■Install automated thermostats that have set-back capability. During unoccupied winter hours, the thermostat automatically reduces the temperature setting. In summertime, it shuts off air conditioning when the building is not occupied. Cost: Only $100–$150 per thermostat. But this will result in substantial energy savings.

■Keep the systems well-maintained. Cleaning and tuning boilers or furnaces can improve energy efficiency by 2%–10%, depending on how ill-maintained the system was to begin with. This simple measure is often overlooked. Cooling systems should also be tuned and cleaned.

Building Envelope

■Apply weather-stripping to doors and caulking to windows to reduce air leakage.

■Reduce ventilation air. Most air conditioning units bring in a great deal of outdoor air. By closing the dampers on these units, the amount of outdoor air being taken in can be reduced. This should not impair air quality, as long as minimum outdoor air, per building codes, is maintained.

■Install insulation. Roof insulation should be at least R-21. Wall insulation should be R-11 or greater.

Systems

■Install energy-efficient light bulbs. Most manufacturers make both regular and energy-efficient light bulbs and fluorescent tubes. The energy-efficient kinds cost more, but they more than pay their way in savings.

■Task lighting. Put extra light where it's needed, such as on drafting tables, and reduce the general light levels in the office.

■Convert to a more efficient air system. Conventional heating systems in older buildings may be either dual-duct or reheat systems. But they waste a lot of energy. A dual-duct system takes hot and cold air and mixes them to control the temperature in different offices. A reheat system first cools air and then heats it back up to the right temperature for each of the rooms. Better: A variable air volume system. This modulates the flow of air and does not waste energy in mixing hot and cold air or cooling and reheating.

■Take advantage of the incentives utility companies offer companies that introduce energy-conservation measures. Many utilities, particularly those in the Northeast and on the West Coast, offer substantial rebates for high-efficiency equipment. Some will give companies energy-saving materials, such as reflective solar film for windows, if the companies pay for installation.

Source: Rusi Patel, senior consultant, Arthur D. Little, Inc., 20 Acorn Park, Cambridge, MA 02140.

Chapter 40
Telecommunications

Getting The Right Phone
Equipment For Your Company

Most companies don't do their homework before buying telecommunications systems.

They rely too much on vendors to make the selection for them and to install the system. Result: The company ends up paying far more than it needs to—or getting less performance for the dollar than they could have gotten. Vendors, after all, don't tell everything.

Traps before the company starts to shop for a new system...

■Not knowing what the company is currently spending on its telecommunications systems. Avoid spending far too much for new equipment by using current expenditures as a benchmark for measuring the value of new purchases.

■Having no idea what a new system should do. Knowing what to expect of a new system will minimize the risk of buying one that is either not powerful enough or too powerful. Either way, this can be a costly mistake. Consult an independent expert for advice on the company's equipment needs.

■Not knowing the kind of wiring that will have to be installed. Knowing the type of wiring needed makes it easier to deal with vendors. Trap: A vendor may have its own wiring scheme proprietary to its particular system. This kind of wiring may not allow for future expansion, forcing the company to spend money upgrading the wiring at a later date.

Traps in the shopping process...

■Not getting competitive bids. Too many companies simply accept what their current vendor has to offer. They fail to do the homework that enables them to make specific requests for prices on the equipment they know they need.

■Only looking at the cost of the system itself. The amount of the purchase price is the minimum amount that will be spent on a new telecommunications system. Other costs that must be taken into account: Enhancements, growth, peripheral equipment and maintenance. More will be spent in these areas than on the original acquisition of a system.

When talking with vendors, ask about the availability and cost of peripherals, such as voice mail, data capability, and automatic call distributor systems, that may be needed in the future.

■Not understanding the price steps for growth of the system. For example, you buy a new cabinet (the system's central control unit) from company X and they tell you that you can expand the system to 500 lines. They tell you that the next 25 phones are relatively inexpensive. What they don't tell you is that you will need a whole new cabinet for the 26th phone at the cost of $12,000. The trap is not understanding the pricing changes as the system grows.

■Not considering pricing both during and after installation. The post-installation price of a phone can be as much as double the cost during installation. To cope with this price increase, buy extra phones during installation and stockpile them for future use.

■Failing to consider extra installation expenses. The four important categories of additional expenses that should be considered in purchasing a new system are...

■Asbestos removal or containment. This can quadruple the cost of installing a new system.

■Power needs. Special power lines and a back-up battery source may have to be brought in for the new system. This is not an expense vendors will tell you about.

■Heating, ventilation and air conditioning. For instance, a new system may need special air conditioning to run smoothly.

■Hook-up costs. The new system will have to be connected to the local telephone company's lines. New trunk lines may be needed, at additional cost.

Traps after the company has purchased a new system...

■Not calculating the cost of MACs (moves, adds and changes). Most companies overlook the cost of adding new phones, moving phones around and changing numbers and features. They often will simply ask a vendor to make these changes when necessary. Trap: Most vendors charge extra for each MAC. When you add a phone, they charge you. When you change a feature, they charge you.

■Not calculating the cost of training people on the new system. The estimated expense of man-hours lost in training must be included in the total cost.

Source: Neil S. Sachnoff, principal, TeleCom Clinic, a telecommunications and project management firm, 469 Tenafly Rd., Englewood, NJ 07631. Mr. Sachnoff is the author of *Secrets of Installing a Telephone System*, TeleCom Library Inc., 12 W. 21 St., New York 10010.

New Phone System: Lease Or Buy?

Should the company buy the new telephone system it so desperately needs, or should it rent the system? Here are some important factors to consider:

■Obsolescence. If it buys the equipment, the company gets to keep it—it has something to show for its money. But what will this equipment really be worth a few years down the road? Is it possible—or likely—that the system will be obsolete and its resale value negligible?

Leasing the phone system gives the company a hedge against obsolescence. It knows it won't be spending money on equipment it will quickly outgrow. The owner of the equipment takes the loss if it's obsolete when the lease is up.

■Tax breaks. If the company buys the equipment, it can write off the cost in depreciation deductions spread over the useful life of the equipment—generally seven years. Annual costs for insurance, maintenance, repairs, etc., are deductible as business expenses. When the company leases, the lease payments are fully deductible business expenses.

■Cash flow. No large cash outlays are required to lease a system. In addition, lease payments can be structured to fit a firm's budget. It's easier to do long-range budgeting for the company if it's making lease payments, as opposed to huge periodic outlays to buy new phone systems.

■Insurance. When the company buys the equipment, it must pay for insurance or bear the risk of loss. If it leases the equipment, on the other hand, the insurance cost is usually borne by the lessor.

■Legal issues. What if the company doesn't make it? Will it be stuck with expensive telephone equipment it can't unload? If the company bought the system, the equipment is an asset it can sell along with other business assets.

But selling may not be possible if the company leases the system. Lease agreements often restrict the company's right to dispose of the lease in the event the company goes bankrupt. The agreement may require the company to continue to make payments even when it's not using the phones.

Source: Laura Shanley, partner, and Lawrence W. Goldstein, senior tax manager, Ernst & Young, CPAs, 277 Park Ave., New York 10172.

Phone Deterrence

To keep employees from making too many personal long-distance calls, you don't need to install a costly computerized program to print out the details of outgoing phone calls from every extension. Simply tell employees that the company is monitoring outgoing calls. That's often enough to make most people reluctant to abuse the system.

Source: *Telephone Angles*, 4550 Montgomery Ave., Bethesda, MD 20814.

Tip-Off That Phone Bill Is Incorrect

Calls listed without a time or with the digits missing (5 p.m., instead of 5:00 p.m.) more often than not have been misbilled.

Source: Alan H. Jordan, telemarketing consultant, Wayne, PA, writing in *The Office*, 1200 Summer St., Stamford, CT 06904.

Monitoring Telephone Conversations

Telephone conversations on cordless phones can be monitored by Internal Revenue Service investigators seeking evidence of criminal fraud, according to a new advisory to agents. The official policy is that investigators do not need a warrant before such eavesdropping. Court permission is still required for tapping wired phone conversations.

Source: Revision to Sec. 9389.61(9), IR manual.

Fax Traps...Fax Fixes

While fax machines save great amounts of time and money, buying and using fax machines has become tricky.

Traps in today's fax technology:

■Legal problems. A fax copy isn't the legal equivalent of the original. If there are legal issues involved in sending or receiving a fax, consult the company's attorney.

■Offending fax recipients. Some companies still object to receiving unsolicited faxes, though they're becoming rarer. A few go so far as to get the sender's fax number and then burn out its machine by sending back a nonstop flow of overnight copy. Few companies, however, object to serious unsolicited faxes. If someone is difficult to reach by phone or letter, faxing can be an effective way of making contact on a legitimate business matter.

■Rushed fax-purchasing decisions. There are hundreds of fax models, with as many different combinations of features on the market today. Finding the right one for your company requires patience and thoroughness.

Cost Range And Features

Prices for fax machines range from under $500 to over $15,000—depending on the number and combination of features. A very functional middle-range machine for most companies should cost no more than $3,000. In this range, when the company shops for fax machines, keep these features in mind...

■Document feeder. This is a must for companies planning to use the fax for lengthy transmissions. Trap: Machines with feeders that handle more than 15 pages occasionally malfunction. Safeguard: Test the machine by seeing whether the feeder can actually handle its maximum limit.

■Paper cutter. Don't buy a fax without a paper cutter. If it doesn't have one, someone will end up manually cutting off each page of a transmission.

■Automatic dialer. This feature lets the user enter phone numbers so they can then simply punch a single button to dial any of several dozen frequent receivers.

■Memory. If you run out of paper while receiving a fax, memory lets the machine store it so you can print it out after you put in more paper. Memory also lets you send the same fax to several recipients without having to put it back in the machine each time you transmit.

■Image. Low-cost fax machines usually have thermal printers. Drawback: The image fades over time. If the longevity and quality of fax copies are important, buy a plain-paper fax that prints out documents much as the better photocopiers do.

Security

Fax machines, because they transmit replicas of diagrams, memos and other documents, make it much easier for sensitive data to leak out of the company. Safeguards:

■Group 4 fax machines. That's industry jargon for faxes that send digital, rather than analog, signals. This makes it harder for eavesdroppers to tap the fax lines. (These are the most expensive machines and they require a digital data line between transmission points.)

■Data encryption. This feature encodes the data and lets a fax machine transmit only to other predetermined machines with similar encoding devices. It makes tapping virtually impossible.

■Personal codes. Like secure computer terminals, some faxes are now available with a feature that allows them to be used only by people with the access code. Receivers must also key in an access code. Caution: Like office printers, plain paper fax machines have image cartridges which, when held up to a light source, can be read. If you're transmitting sensitive documents, destroy the image cartridges when empty or limit access to the machines.

Cost Controls

Companies have two options to deter employees from using the fax anytime they want...

■Activity reports. This feature prints out a report on each transmission—how long it took, where it was sent, and whether it was received.

■Personal accounting codes. Like some photocopiers, fax machines are also available with devices that require users to enter a code. The code can be used by accounting personnel to tell which department to bill for fax time.

Source: Lee Spenadel, manager, Ernst & Young's Network Services Practice, 787 Seventh Ave., New York 10019.

Chapter 41
Computer Savvy

Traps And Opportunities
In Computer Networking

Computer nightmare: The company finds out it can boost productivity by linking groups of workers to the same computer system. It spends thousands of dollars per employee on computers, wiring, software and a consultant. But productivity declines because the workers spend so much time unsuccessfully trying to figure out how the system works.

And this turns out to be a temporary problem—but part of a bigger one—because the system is obsolete in 18 months and the principal vendors have gone out of business.

How To Do It Right

Managers who got their start before computerization don't always understand the benefits of computer networking. Essentially, local area networks (LANs) can increase productivity when workers need to…

■Swap information as each of them works on a part of a joint project.

Examples: Engineers designing a turbine component…accountants preparing a fiscal report…editors working on a magazine layout.

■Obtain and store information at a central source, or database.

Examples: Insurance adjustors who need data on previous claims and also must file their own records in the same database…payroll departments who must constantly add information to their records.

The productivity payoff results when workers have instant access to data which they can swap as needed. Until recently, networking was possible only with sophisticated mainframe computers costing over $200,000. Today, companies can achieve the same productivity gains by linking common desktop computers, often at a cost of less than $5,000 per worker.

Ironically, the ease of networking is also a source of some of its problems. Reason: Most companies have PCs from several manufacturers, each with its own operating system…and workers typically use dozens of software packages. For smooth networking, hardware and software must all be compatible. And they must also be compatible with the software that controls the networking process itself.

Example: A company that wants to link an existing VAX computer with IBM PCs must invest in gateways. The technology isn't complex, but it is another part of a system that can go wrong if not designed and installed properly.

With so many stumbling blocks on the route to successful networking, companies should proceed carefully…

Step #1/Planning: Give end users a meaningful voice in planning networks. They're the best people in the company to decide what's needed.

Recommended: Name a LAN planning group composed of users, one or more of their department supervisors, and managers of the company's computer department.

Some companies hesitate to give users a big voice in LAN decisions, fearing they'll ask for unnecessarily expensive systems. In reality, they seldom do. And if they do, the computer department managers can put a brake on expenses.

More often, it's the users who veto an expensive system that the computer department recommends.

Example: Computer types often want IBM systems. End users usually opt for less expensive, but more efficient, LANs from Novell or Sun Microsystems.

Step #2/Expert advice: To set up a network, companies usually need to hire a consultant. Reasons: Since technology is changing fast, a consultant will know some of the latest alternatives. Also, an objective view is often needed to prevent specific departments or managers from putting their bias into the system.

Caution: Some less-than-ethical consultants promote specific hardware and software. Safeguard: When you hire a consultant, write a clause into the contract that states he doesn't represent specific manufacturers.

Good consultants are expensive, usually at least $500 a day and often as much as $2,000 a day.

Don't ask for quotes from vendors until the consultant and the LAN planning group agree on exactly what they want. If vendors are called in earlier, they'll try to sell the company features it probably doesn't need.

Step #3/The purchase: Before buying an expensive mainframe or mini-computer system, find out if company needs can be met with a network of PCs using the powerful 80386 chip. In many cases, they can.

Buy hardware and software only from vendors who have at least a three-year track record of good performance, and a strong service operation to support what they sell.

Don't buy a system that the company isn't willing to write off in three years, at the most. After that time, chances are good that the LAN will have to be substantially modified, if not replaced. Reasons: Network technology is changing fast. So are the networking needs of most companies.

The Future Looks Bright

For the last few years, LANs have been able to link workers on the same floor or in the same building. Now it's possible to link widely separated groups.

Example: Several pharmaceutical companies have begun to link research labs throughout the world.

This technology is moving within reach of virtually any company. Result: A business will not only gain the productivity boosts inherent in networking, but also many other cost savings.

Example: If a manufacturer wants designers in several plants to work on a new product, they no longer have to fly to a central location.

Source: Vincent Barrett, partner, Ernst & Young's Network Strategy Practice, 10201 Lee Highway, Fairfax, VA 22030.

Smart Computer Passwords

Hard-to-crack computer passwords that are easy to remember: Words from a foreign language...an uncommon family name...an obscure foreign town in its origi-

nal spelling…a misspelled English word (letters changed, added or repeated) two words with a non-letter symbol in-between, as in "do#this."
Source: *Computerworld*, 375 Cochituate Rd., Framingham, MA 01701.

Secrets Of Tight Computer Security

Sixteen of the nation's top computer experts were given the task of developing ways to make computers more secure against criminal intrusion and malfunction. Many of their recommendations could be useful to most businesses.

There are many very simple computer safeguards that even excellent companies overlook…

■Keep the company's computer programs simple. As programs grow and become more complex, chances increase that they'll become vulnerable to intruders.

That's an especially important lesson because many companies are tempted to write increasingly complex programs as their use of computers grows. That type of software, however, is likely to have flaws that can result not only in security breaches, but also in lost data or other faulty operation.

Example: Business programs often become less secure when programmers frequently modify existing software, adding on new pieces of programs as they go along. In doing so, programmers run the risk of putting new weak points into the finished product, as well as accumulating flaws in the original software.

Protection: Keep new software simple and written specifically for its intended application. If you do combine software, make sure programmers are aware of potential security problems—and solve them before putting the software in use.

■Avoid keeping the company's only copies of important data in the computer system. When a business does that, it risks losing the data due to computer malfunction, catastrophes such as fire or flood, invasion by a computer virus, theft of the computer or the chance that an operator will erase or alter the data either intentionally or by accident.

For most companies, those possibilities would be horrendous. But the risks can all be greatly reduced by separating computer data from the computer. In most situations, that requires nothing more than making back-up copies of data as they're generated…and storing them in safes or other locations that are locked and fireproof, often away from the company's premises.

■Use software that's proven to be free of problems whenever possible. There's always a trade-off for companies that want to buy the latest software on the market or that modify programs they've written in-house.

But in both cases, there's a greater chance of software error than there is in programs that have had time to be de-bugged through years of use.

■Programmers must write software in higher-level computer languages rather than the older, less sophisticated ones. Using higher-level languages, such as COBOL (Common Business Oriented Language), increases the reliability of the software and makes it less vulnerable to intruders. Software programs that are written in older, less-sophisticated languages are often technically cumbersome.

Working in these cumbersome languages can lead to flaws that hinder program-writing and invite security breaches. Newer computer languages, by contrast, enable programmers to automatically build greater efficiency and security into programs they write.

■Keep the company's computer staff up-to-date on developments in security. That's not always easy because American universities have largely ignored the subject. Until nearby institutions offer refresher courses, the company can retain computer consultants to bring the staff up-to-date on new ways to prevent security breaches.

■Don't rely on passwords without a safeguard against "dictionary attacks." Most business computers now require operators to enter a personal password before a program will respond. A "dictionary attack" is an attempt to find the password by trying every word in the dictionary.

Trap: It's easier than it might sound, thanks to smart thieves and the availability of dictionaries on disk. An intruder simply loads a dictionary in the computer, and programs it to try every entry as a password. The effort may take only a few minutes.

There are safeguard systems, however, that sound an alarm (or shut down the computer) when more than three password attempts, for instance, are made in a 30-minute period.

■Change the lock on "trap doors" in company software. Many computer systems have what experts call trap doors. These are ways for field representatives and maintenance personnel to get to the software's inner workings. Trap doors are usually guarded by passwords.

Example: Remember a couple of years ago when a "worm" shut down part of Internet, the international computer link for universities, government agencies and businesses? At the heart of the problem was a trap door in one of the Internet programs. Hundreds of computer experts knew about the trap door. One of them, a prankster, used the trap door to insert a new code, or worm, that caused days of confusion throughout the system.

Businesses face a special problem with trap doors. Reason: Software developers use the same trap door and password over and over again, even on new versions of the product.

Eventually, more and more people know how to get into the program. From that point, they can pirate data or plant flaws that cause the system to fail.

Safeguard: Change the password or location of the trap door in programs used for sensitive data. Often program documentation will explain how to do it, and most software developers will assist, if asked. Otherwise, the job can usually be done by consultants or knowledgeable in-house programmers.

Source: Dr. David D. Clark, senior research scientist, Laboratory for Computer Science, Massachusetts Institute of Technology, 545 Main St., Cambridge 02139. Clark is also chairman of the National Research Council's System Security Study Committee, which oversaw production of *Computers at Risk*, a study of U.S. computer security problems, National Academy Press, 2101 Constitution Ave. NW, Washington, DC 20418.

Computer Health Hazards

As office computers have become commonplace, so have problems for people who use them—eyestrain, headaches, back problems and injuries to hands and fingers. And though conclusive evidence isn't in yet, there is a possibility of injury from radiation emitted by computer monitors.

Unless companies take steps to avoid these risks, they jeopardize the gains computers are designed to achieve...not to mention risking an increase in medical claims and lawsuits.

How Injuries Occur

Companies have been slow in anticipating computer health problems because computers look similar to their benign forerunners—typewriters.

But computers are very different, and the difference is largely responsible for the injuries.

Examples: It's more difficult to read a computer screen than a typewritten page. Computers also let employees work at a steady, concentrated rate without the breaks that typewriting normally requires—changing paper and ribbons, using correction fluid, etc. Results: Eyestrain, headaches and muscle pain.

In addition, computer operators' hands remain in the same position for almost everything they do—scrolling to a new page, deleting a paragraph or even calling up a new file. If an operator has a modem and a speaker phone, he/she may even use the same hand position to make a call and take notes on the conversation. This can be injurious, as can repetitive motions.

Most Common Computer Hazards

■Eyestrain and headaches. These are typically caused by poor-quality monitors, glare from the screen and/or the failure of monitors to tilt to the optimum position for an operator to see both it and the keyboard. Solutions:

■High-quality monitors. The quality of letter image, known as definition, is far more important than whether the type appears in green or amber. The Human Factors Society, in conjunction with the American National Standards Institute, has developed standards for monitors. (A listing of those standards is available for $25 from the Human Factors Society at Box 1369, Santa Monica, CA 90406.)

■Adjustable monitor stands. These stands allow each operator to set the monitor at the best tilt and distance for his/her own specific use.

Worth considering: Adjustable workstation surfaces. These devices let operators raise, lower or tilt the entire work station surface to fit their individual physical needs. Price: About $1,200.

■Hand/wrist injuries. Brought on by repetitive motion or holding hands in awkward positions for extended periods, these injuries cause pain, numbness and loss of mobility.

Carpal tunnel syndrome, most likely caused by a combination of repetitive motion, excess force and awkward wrist posture, is currently the most publicized of these. It afflicts secretaries and others who spend long hours at a computer or typewriter keyboard. In this condition, compression of finger nerves leads to loss of feeling and possible paralysis.

The condition is frequently treated through surgery, but may recur if the employee returns to the same work conditions. Solutions:

■Frequent breaks for computer operators—ideally, five- to 10-minute breaks every two hours. Studies show that breaks work best when they're staggered, not when a whistle blows and the whole staff stops at the same time.

■Adequate training for operators, so they have the technical skills to do the job and they know how to prevent or minimize physical injury.

■The best keyboards, those which provide cushioning, auditory or tactile feedback and user-friendly key arrangements. Educated computer operators themselves are usually the best judges of keyboards. For a second opinion, consult the Human Factors Society. In a year or two, businesses may be able to buy a completely new type of keyboard that's designed to accommodate a person's normal hand position. (It's slightly raised in the center.)

■Adjustable work stations—consider the same ones recommended earlier for eyestrain problems.

■Make physical fitness a priority. Physically fit workers are less likely to suffer from computer-related ailments than those in poor health. A company wellness program is an effective way of maintaining employee health. Such a program can also catch injuries at an early stage, when the company can more easily correct the problem. Companies not large enough to fund a wellness program can now contract with private health services.

■Radiation injuries. This is still a very controversial area because evidence is far from complete. At this stage, dangers from lengthy exposure to extreme-long-frequency radiation emitted by computer monitors have not been conclusively ruled out. But the dangers haven't been convincingly demonstrated. Companies should keep abreast of research and get advice from legal counsel.

The Stress Factor

Even computer operators who work in the best-designed environments are prone to injury if they're also under stress. The most common causes are demanding supervisors and, ironically, computer programs that monitor operators.*

Signs of worker stress: High turnover, frequent absences, low job satisfaction.

If you suspect supervisors are at fault, consider giving them additional management training. If the monitoring system is causing stress, it usually pays to hire a consultant who can redesign it.

New monitoring systems now being developed promise to be almost user-friendly. The National Institute of Occupational Safety & Health, for instance, has experimented with monitoring systems that spot the types of errors that operators make when they're tired or under abnormal stress. When it spots these conditions, the computer advises the operator to take a rest.

*Most companies with large data processing operations have computer programs that automatically monitor the amount and quality of work performed by data processors. They do this by counting keystrokes in various periods of time. These programs are custom-designed by computer consultants and vary in price depending on the software and number of operators.

Source: Marvin Dainoff, director of the Center for Ergonomic Research and professor of psychology at Miami University, Oxford, OH 45056. A former researcher at the National Institute of Occupational Safety & Health, Dainoff is the author of *People and Productivity*, Carswell Co., 2330 Midland Ave., Agincourt, Ontario M1S 1P7.

Safer VDTs

■It's easy to redesign a workplace in which VDTs can be used safely. One organization, The Fund for the City of New York, changed its office layout so that employees sit an arm's length—28 to 30 inches—from their VDTs. They found that the electromagnetic radiation drops off sharply at that distance.

But radiation from VDTs doesn't just come from the screen—it comes out the back and sides as well. So the organization does not allow anyone to sit within 40 inches of another employee's VDT.

Even safer: Lap-top computers use safe liquid crystal displays (LCDs) that do not give off hazardous magnetic fields.

Source: Paul Brodeur, author of *Currents of Death: Power Lines, Computer Terminals and the Attempt to Cover Up Their Threat to Your Health,* Simon & Schuster, New York 10020.

If Your Computer Gets Wet

Water does not damage computer hardware provided the equipment is cleaned and dried within 12–24 hours after wetting. Most important: The wet components should be washed down with demineralized water to remove any contaminants and then dried with a fan or ordinary hair dryer.

Source: Ron Reeves, Factory Mutual Engineering and Research, Norwood, MA, quoted in *Computer Decisions.*

How To Protect Against Computer Viruses

While chances are slim that a company's computer system will be wrecked by the type of "virus" that attacked one of the country's scientific networks, there are many other ways for a virus to play havoc with business computers. And, as the number of computer experts increases, chances of a virus attack become greater. It's essential to take preventive steps to guard computers against such viruses.

Malicious Origins

For reasons perhaps best understood by psychiatrists, some computer programmers enjoy devising software that hurts the user. Some of these pranks, called time bombs and Trojan horses, are contained in harmless-looking software. But once these programs start operating, they can destroy files or other resident programs. Some of the programs will warn the user of what's going to happen or will flash "Gotcha" on the screen after the destruction occurs.

Viruses are a little different from these pranks. They introduce a flaw and take advantage of a computer's ability to replicate that flaw. Result: At first the harm is negligible, or even unnoticeable. But as the virus reproduces, the flaw becomes devastating. And there's no warning. If a company's PCs are linked in a network or to a larger computer, the virus can spread throughout the business.

How a company is likely to pick up a computer virus:

■From software written or modified by disgruntled employees. Companies are increasingly vulnerable because more employees are becoming sophisticated with computers...and businesses are designing more of their own programs.

■From commercial software. This has already occurred on at least four occasions, and in each case it was thought to be the work of disgruntled employees who worked for the software company.

■From software picked up from computer bulletin boards. These let computer users and hobbyists swap public domain programs and other information over telephone lines. Even though most companies don't use bulletin boards, individual employees can use company computers to access these bulletin boards.

■Through commercial databases. At least one major database has already had problems with a virus.

In the not-too-distant future, there may also be a threat from viruses that a competitor might plant in the company's computer system. (So far, this type of sabotage isn't known to have happened, but the threat is too, too real.)

Detecting The Virus

Problem: Viruses usually act slowly, so the first evidence of their presence goes unnoticed, even by experienced computer users. Subtle, first signs of the virus may include a change in…

■File dates, particularly those of the operating system (MS-DOS, UNIX, etc.).

■File sizes. Sophisticated virus writers, however, are able to prevent both file size and file date changes.

As the virus spreads, signs of its presence become a little more obvious.

Example: One virus eventually changed the names of diskette volumes.

Lines Of Defense

Overall approach: Since there are many ways for virus-contaminated software to enter a company's computers, the first line of defense is to screen all new programs. Recommended:

■Set up an office or department for testing all new software—whether it comes from outside the company or is written in-house. This screening can usually be incorporated into a department that companies should already be using to determine whether a proposed software change is actually needed.

Alternative: Hire a consultant to do the screening. For most businesses, however, it makes sense to hire a consultant just to set up the company's screening operation, not to run it. Exception: If a company uses off-the-shelf software and makes only minor modifications to it, it may be cost-effective to retain a consultant to screen the programs for viruses.

Several virus-detection programs are currently available to assist with the screening. The cost of both a testing computer and the screening software is usually under $10,000, a price within reach of even small businesses.

Caution: Screening programs aren't 100% effective…and they can't be, given the design of most business computers. But they will catch most software viruses and, as such, have already saved many businesses money and time.

■Make it company policy not to run software that isn't screened. Establish penalties for employees who violate the policy, and enforce the rules.

■Make it policy that data from a database can't be incorporated into an existing program. If a database has a virus, it can't hurt the company if the data is merely stored as information. But some programmers may see codes in the data that they think would be useful in company software. That could be dangerous because there's no guarantee that a line of database code isn't embedded with a virus.

■Run thorough background checks. Look into all employees who have access to company software.

■Separate the company's programmers. Keep them apart from employees who screen software and from those who use the programs. This not only reduces the chance of letting a virus in, but also helps protect the company against collusion among employees who would embezzle data or funds.

Source: John Panagacos, president, Boden Associates, a software development and consulting firm specializing in computer security, 11 Meadow Lane, East Williston, NY 11596.

Chapter 42
Protecting Your Company

Fire-Detection Devices

Key point in choosing fire detectors: A fire should be detected as early as possible, before heat builds up or flames break out. A developing fire produces invisible gases and smoke first. The detector should spot these.

A heat detector or flame detector may be worse than none since it provides a false sense of security. It allows the initial signs of a fire (invisible gas and smoke) to go undetected.

Invisible gas detectors:

■The high-voltage detector uses radioactive material to ionize the air.

■The low-voltage detector ionizes without radioactive materials, using a solid-state amplifier instead.

■The photoelectric cell units measure the level of light given off by a built-in source. If smoke blocks lessen the intensity, the alarm is triggered.

Remember though that all types of detectors have false-alarm problems, especially during a crowded meeting or cocktail party when many smokers are present.

Ban Smoking In The Office

Nonsmoking policies are easiest to implement in companies that have few smokers. A service company with a preponderance of younger employees, for instance, would probably have little trouble putting a ban on smoking since most of the employees already don't smoke.

A nonsmoking policy is harder to introduce in a company that has many older employees and/or blue-collar workers who are die-hard smokers.

The Best Nonsmoking Policies

■Give employees plenty of notice up front—two or three months' minimum—of the company's plan to ban or restrict employee smoking.

■Present clear explanations of the reasons for implementing the policy. Good reasons can generally be obtained from the company's health insurer.

■Involve top-level executives, preferably the CEO. Nonsmoking policies that come from the company's personnel department may be perceived as just another company policy not to be taken seriously.

■Offer stop-smoking programs for employees who need help. The company should include in its notice of the smoking ban a list of programs that employees can turn to. Some companies pay for the programs, some don't. Some pay only if the employee is still not smoking after six months. Some companies pay half up-front and half later if the employee successfully quits.

Most effective programs: Those that are given at the office. Smoke-Enders, for instance, will give classes at the company. The mere fact that the employer supports the program by holding it on the premises seems to enhance its acceptance and effectiveness.

■Make special arrangements for workers who continue to smoke. Many companies designate smoking areas—for instance, a section of the cafeteria. Some allow workers who have private offices to continue to smoke (but new employees filling these same offices would not be allowed to do so).

■Provide incentives for nonsmokers and disincentives for smokers. Examples:

■Keep health insurance free for nonsmokers, but smokers pay a portion of premiums. A $10-per-month charge for family coverage is often used.

■Offer nonsmokers reduced deductibles in the health-care plan.

■Charge smokers higher rates for life insurance than nonsmokers.

■Give nonsmokers credits toward flexible spending accounts.

Downside To Smoking Bans

Companies that have designated smoking areas may notice employees congregating there, taking longer breaks away from work.

What to do about this: Make it more uncomfortable for employees to smoke by moving the designated smoking area out-of-doors. Remind employees about the company policy to help smokers quit. Put candy bowls around the office.

There may be some initial grumbling by smokers about the company interfering with their lifestyle. The best way to counter this is to clearly state the reasons why the company adopted a nonsmoking policy. Good reason: There's strong evidence that smokers cost the company more than nonsmokers under a health-care plan.

Turnover is no longer a major problem since so many companies are introducing nonsmoking policies today that employees who want to leave will have trouble finding one that allows them to smoke freely.

Source: Ann W. Lemmon, consultant, Hewitt Associates, 100 Half Day Road, Lincolnshire, IL 60069.

Preventing Office Injuries

Statistically, one of every 27 office workers is injured on the job every year. And one of every 22 workers' compensation claims is for an office injury. Offices are booby-trapped with safety hazards, which many companies don't correct.

To make offices safer:

■Appoint a safety director to work with the insurance carrier to reduce hazards.

■Carry out regular safety inspections throughout the premises.

■Remove any penalties or stigmas associated with reporting hazards.

Common office hazards:

■Coffee spills and other items dropped on slippery, uncarpeted floors that might cause falls.

■Wastebaskets, desk or filing drawers, and any other objects left protruding into the aisles.

■Doors without glass panels to show what's on the other side (for example, a person standing there unseen, risking collision).

■Steel files that can fall forward because they are not bolted to the floor.

■Damaged or weakened file ladders and stools.

■Electrical extension cords stretched across aisles or between desks, frayed extensions, and broken plugs.

■Fans, coffeepots, and other appliances used by workers.

Source: *Modern Office Procedures*, Cleveland, OH.

Wise Safety Secrets

Du Pont Company has received the National Safety Council's Award of Honor for 41 of the past 46 years. Its record of lost workdays in 1987 was .04%...versus .62% for the chemical industry as a whole and 1.86% for all U.S. industry.

Investigation Is Key

While no company has yet been completely accident-free, it's a mistake to focus on preventing only the most serious accidents. Trap: Every safety incident—even a near miss—points up a weak link in the company's safety program that, unless remedied, will cause further problems—possibly worse ones—in the future. The company must therefore beef up safety measures in all of its operations. To do that, thorough investigations of all mishaps are essential. In fact, meticulous investigating is the essence of effective safety programs, because without accurate and detailed information about the causes of accidents, efforts to prevent them are a waste of time and money.

Objective of safety investigations: To identify and correct hazardous conditions, procedures or practices and then communicate the corrections to employees who may be at risk.

Guideline: Fully investigate any incident that involves a lost workday or could have caused a lost workday if the circumstances had been slightly different. Examples:

■Falling from a low scaffold causes an employee to twist his ankle. It could have been a broken leg...or worse.

■Tipping over backward in a chair. Not always serious, but any backward fall could cause head injury.

■Getting a shock from turning on a light switch. Shock from a switch having voltage potential of more than 75 volts DC or 40 volts AC is considered serious.

When an injury or near miss occurs, it's up to the line supervisor and his superior to decide how extensively to investigate. Usually second-line supervisors take the lead, gathering facts, reviewing safety procedures and rules and compiling the maintenance history of any equipment involved.

Our first step: Form a team of those involved in the incident...and the first-line supervisor...and higher levels of management (if indicated by the seriousness of the situation)...and the safety supervisor...and anyone else who can further the investigation.

If a contract with a particular union specifies having a representative at accident investigations, the company has no choice. Otherwise, the best policy is to include union participation on the team only when the union representative has information that will aid the investigation. Important: Management must retain responsibility for setting safety policy.

Speed Is Crucial

Launch the investigation promptly...within minutes if possible. It's important to investigate while everyone's memory is still fresh. Waiting allows witnesses to disappear or to influence each other. Given time, those involved may concoct stories to cover for mistakes they may have made.

Nothing related to the incident should be allowed to be lost, destroyed or discarded. It's best to interview the injured person at the site so he can explain exactly how it happened. If it's impossible to keep the site undisturbed until the investigation is completed, take pictures before things are moved around. Use a pocket tape recorder to make notes.

Set A Positive Tone

It's helpful, where possible, to explain up front that no disciplinary action is anticipated and that the company's objectives are to simply get the facts and determine causes so it can recommend ways to prevent recurrences. Recommended: Interview each witness separately and privately. Emphasize listening and learning, and be open-minded...willing to admit, if necessary, that training procedures, management or faulty machine maintenance might be part of the problem.

Example: A machinist who is not using a protective guard gets a metal fragment from a bench grinder in his eyelid. The plant doctor removes the fragment and there is no damage to the eye, but the shop supervisor convenes an investigation because of the potential for serious injury. The team talks with the injured worker and others in the shop, inspects the site and reviews grinder procedures. They find that the wheel guard was so scratched the machinist could not see to do his job. Therefore, he didn't use it. Recommendations of the investigating team: All grinders with scratched guards be taken out of service and replaced...regular grinder inspections be conducted...grinder rules be reviewed regularly with employees...and periodic checks be made to assure compliance with safety rules.

Many companies err by making only superficial investigations and focusing on the person involved in the accident rather than on the root problems that caused the dangerous behavior. What seems like carelessness, for example, may be the result of unrealistic demands for higher productivity.

Trap: When employees fear that the company only wants to find blame and punish, they may not report problems. This can result in serious accidents, as hazards go unchecked.

Another common mistake is the failure to follow through after an investigation. The company may, for example, come up with valuable recommendations but then not see to it that they're implemented. A manager should be put in charge of guaranteeing that recommendations are acted on.

Finally, communications often fail. In companies with multiple facilities, the lessons learned in one place may not be shared with other facilities. Solution: Networking between safety officials at different plants or supervisors on different shifts at the same plant. Site accident reports and recommendations (with all the specifics except names) should be made available to all supervisors and managers at all sites...not just to top management at headquarters.

Source: Harold C. Jacobs, CSP, and John T. Nieburg, CSP, senior safety consultants, Du Pont Company, Safety and Environmental Management Services, Box 80800, Wilmington, DE 19880.

Chapter 43
Security Measures

Where Employees Stash Stolen Goods

How thievish employees get loot off the company premises:

■Products are turned into "scrap" and then easily repaired after a worker is permitted to take the "spoiled" merchandise home with him.

■Company property is concealed in scrap barrels.

■Gas is siphoned from company trucks into private cars.

■Oversized lunch boxes hide company goods.

■Small items are concealed under clothing. Note: An arbitrator upheld a rule requiring men to tuck shirts inside their trousers before exiting via a guarded company gate.

■Valuable material—copper wire, for instance—is taken through the plant's gates on delivery trucks. The driver then hides the loot for a later pickup. Even dumpsters carried away by contracted sanitation companies have been used this way. Such scams always involve collusion.

■Merchandise is taken from a customer's order, thus they don't get all the goods for which they paid. The belief is that the customers won't check their shipment. In the aggregate, the small amounts stolen from a customer develop into large ones for the thief.

■Drivers leave products at a customer's house "by mistake" and retrieve them later. Note: This involves telephoning the receiver immediately from a pay telephone before he has a chance to check the delivery and call the company about the mistake.

■A hole is dug under a fence. Merchandise is then pushed outside and picked up after dark. Trap: No theft has occurred until someone takes possession of the material outside the premises. Successful prosecution may require surveillance until the offender picks up the merchandise.

■Shipping clerks send packages to confederates.

Source: Discharge arbitration hearings.

Body-Search Guidelines

Frisking employees suspected of theft is legal provided that employment applications say employees agree to be searched, everyone is told that the policy is to deter theft from the company as a whole (not because a single employee is under suspicion), and no groups are singled out for special attention.

Source: *Labor Update,* Pechner Dorfman Wolffe Rounick & Cabot, 1845 Walnut St., Philadelphia, PA 19103.

Searching Employee Desks

Employee desks can't be searched unless there's a pressing business need. A new circuit court ruling says that "...because (the employee) has a constitutional right to be free from unnecessary, overbroad or unregulated employer investigations...the search.. would be reasonable only if relevant to his job."

Source: *Showengerdt vs General Dynamics* Case No. 84-6231, 9th Cir. 1987. *Personnel Journal*, 245 Fisher Ave., Costa Mesa, CA 92626.

Security Secrets

■Inspecting lockers regularly to curtail theft is legal, provided workers are told in advance that it is company policy.

Source: *Safety and Security for Supervisors*, Business Research Publications, New York.

■Eavesdropping on an employee via a telephone extension is lawful in some situations. While federal law generally prohibits such invasions of privacy, courts have upheld the right of an employer to monitor conversations of employees suspected of giving confidential information to company competitors.

■Write customer identification information on the front of checks. Bank cancellation procedures often obliterate writing on the reverse side.

Source: Sklar Financial Control Corp., San Francisco.

■Petty cash rip-offs. Keep the petty cash box separate from other funds for accurate record keeping. Prenumber petty cash slips so that a missing slip can be detected. Also: Set a firm policy against cashing checks or making small loans to employees out of petty cash.

Source: *The Alert*, Kroll Associates, New York.

■Keep one bill with a known serial number in each cash register at all times. In case of burglary, the police can use that number to track down the thieves.

Source: *Mart,* Berkshire Common, Pittsfield, MA.

■Fake checks printed by counterfeiters differ from genuine checks in several ways. Make sure a check is perforated on one side, showing that it came from a checkbook. Reject checks that have shiny account numbers at the bottom. Reason: Fakes are not printed with magnetic ink, which is dull.

Source: *Florida Banker,* Orlando.

■Accept only checks with the correct local Federal Reserve number printed in small numbers in the upper right-hand corner. Example: The New York area number is 1-xx/210. (The xx digits vary by bank.) Counterfeiters rarely print the correct number.

■Odds on shoplifting. In a study of retail chains, 56% of employees and customers apprehended for stealing were prosecuted. Of these, 90% were ultimately convicted. False-arrest suits resulted from only 0.16% of the 280,000 apprehensions studied.

Source: National Mass Retailing Institute, New York.

■Warning calls from strangers can be dangerous. Case: An electronics dealer got a call at home from a self-described private security officer who said the company's side door was unlocked. When the manager rushed to the plant to lock the door, he was robbed at gunpoint. The best procedure: Call the police, and meet them at the scene.

■Internal theft prevention. Store all blank checks in a locked place. Have petty-cash slips sequentially numbered, just like checks.

Source: *Automotive News*, Detroit.

■People who never take vacations are not the only internal security risks. Watch those who come in early, work late, or come back early from lunch, especially if their jobs do not require it.

■Thieves rarely confess the full extent of their stealing. Rule of thumb: Double whatever the worker admits to.

Source: *Occupational Hazards*, Cleveland.

■Many older locks have their key code stamped on the outside. Anyone can look up the code in a locksmith's manual (readily obtainable for most makes) and obtain a new key. For security: grind off the code.

■Comparing signatures to detect bad checks. Slants, i's and e's are almost always the same in signatures by the same person. Instruct clerks to ask customers to write their name again and compare these three features if in doubt.

■Protecting your signature. Handwriting experts claim that careless signatures are as much to blame in successful forgeries as the skill of the forger. A good model signature is had to imitate and is worth cultivating. A safe signature is written quickly and continuously without lifting the pen to dot i's or cross t's until the end. The longer it is, the better, so use your whole name. Write your address and the date right below the signature to make imitation even more complicated.

Source: S. Gupta, Central Bureau of Investigation, New Delhi, India, in *Journal of the Forensic Science Society,* England.

■Sign your first name and middle initial on letters, but use your full name on checks. Instruct your bank to honor only the checks you sign in full.

Perils of Handling Suspected Shoplifters

Detention of a person suspected of shoplifting may expose the shop owner to a suit for false imprisonment under state law.

It may also give the suspect the right to sue the owner under the federal Civil Rights Act if he appears to be acting under state law.

This was found to be the situation in a recent case in which the owner was shown to have a prearranged plan with the local police department to come and assist him when he needed help, particularly when he was holding a suspected shoplifter.

The care with which suspected shoplifters must be handled is reflected in the view expressed by the trial court in this case, in which a woman had placed a jar of cold cream in her purse. The court said that while her deposit of the jar in her bag during shopping created some cause for suspicion, this fact didn't create reasonable grounds to detain the woman as a shoplifter before she had been given an opportunity to pay for the item.

Laws against shoplifting wouldn't be apt to have much deterrent effect if the view expressed by the court were to become widely publicized. A more practical approach would be to let the shoplifter pay for the goods. It's certainly better than suffering a $12,000 judgment, as resulted in this case. In addition, consider the time lost and the expense of being a defendant.

Source: *Smith and McClure v. Brookshire Bros., Inc.*, C.A. 5, 9/15/75.

How To Spot A Fake ID

Best identification: Photograph, physical description and signature. Employees who inspect identification cards should also use these safeguards:

■Repeat some information from the ID card back to the holder, but make a small mistake in repetition. Example: Is your address 733 Lake Dr.? (743 is the real number.) Impostors are often unfamiliar with details.

■Don't accept IDs that have the name of the state or issuing agency typed in instead of printed. A typographical error is almost always a sign of a fake.

■Check wear patterns on old cards. A genuine card will be worn mostly around the edges from handling. Some forgers artificially age cards, which gives a uniform look of wear all over the card.

■Look for raised edges around photographs, which is a sign that a substitution has been made.

■Feel for flaws in laminated cards, another sign of tampering.

■Compare the typewriter face on various parts of the card. Reject if there is a mismatch.

■Check the holder's signature against the one on the ID.

Beware: Birth certificates are poor IDs because they fail to describe the adult using them. Better: A driver's license, passport or credit card (that can be checked to see if stolen).

Source: *The National Notary Magazine*, Woodland Hills, CA.

Lie-Detector Tests

In 1988, the U.S. Congress passed legislation prohibiting companies from using lie detectors to screen for honesty in job applicants or employees.

While it is legal for companies to use lie detectors in trying to solve a workplace crime, the legal traps involved in doing so remain formidable.

Dr. John Furedy, one of North America's foremost experts on polygraphs, contributed research data that was instrumental in passage of this and other polygraph legislation. *Boardroom* interviewed him about the usefulness of lie detectors and about the precautions companies must take in using them.

■Don't we know enough about people and the technology now to make polygraphs work reliably?

No. Nothing has value in assessing the honesty of a person. Essentially, honesty is a very vague concept. People are honest to different degrees, depending on the circumstances. The notion of classifying individuals as honest or not honest—or as likely or not likely to be dishonest—makes no sense. Nothing can test for that.

It's a big mistake for managers to think they can really run a better company by hiring only honest people—and not hiring dishonest people—because honesty is so dependent on specific situations.

■American companies, which had been the world's biggest users of polygraph testing for such purposes, no longer can use them. What's an alternative?

The only truly effective way is to lead the company with honest values. Consistently increase the level of honesty within the firm through example...rather than relying on testing to eliminate the bad apples. An essential first step is to create loyalty for the company among the workforce. The best way to do this is to involve employees in sharing the profits generated by their work and improvements in the way they work. Beyond that, managers must set examples of honesty through behavior and what they demand of their subordinates.

■Can't polygraphs, though, still be used in an investigation of a specific crime—attempting to find out if an employee committed a specific theft, for instance?

Yes. The U.S. now makes a distinction between the use of polygraphs by companies for general detection of "honesty"—and their use in detecting deception about a specific act.

It might be possible to detect deception about a particular act by using a polygraph—whether or not an employee stole money, for instance.

Trap: The polygraph technique most widely used in the North America, the so-called Control Question Technique (CQT) does not do that. It comes nowhere near giving any reliable information about a specific issue.

It's called a test, which makes it sound like something standardized—an IQ test, for instance, or a test of knowledge. But it's no such thing.

■What is it?

It's a non-standardized interrogation. In less-friendly terms, I've described it as having a psychological rubber hose aspect. Results depend completely on how the operator works and the relationship between the operator and the person being examined. An operator who is friendly toward the person being interrogated can get a completely different set of results than a hostile interrogator might get. Any polygraph test worth its salt should be done in a blind way. The interrogator should have no knowledge at all about the person. But the CQT works exactly opposite.

It would certainly be a big mistake for a manager to ask an employee to take such a test, promise that the employee has nothing to fear if he is innocent, and then base his decision on the results of the test. Given all the scientific evidence now about the unreliability of the CQT, the chances of facing legal action if the person is fired as a result of such a test are considerable.

American managers are tempted by the apparent objectivity of the machine. They figure they can use the polygraph rather than make a difficult judgment themselves. It's easier to have a machine tell you, "the guy did it."

■What practice would you suggest companies use to root out dishonesty, instead of the CQT?

If the company has completely reliable evidence that an employee had stolen money—a videotape of the act from the company's security director, for example—that could be grounds for firing.

I believe it is also a mistake to fire a person on the single basis of dishonesty in a particular situation. As I've said, a person's honesty is dependent on circumstance. A decision to fire should be made on multiple factors—a number of things come together about a person's dishonest behavior, and you reach a threshold.

■You're specifically critical of the CQT. But is there perhaps another way to use polygraphy to detect deception?

Yes. It's called the Guilty Knowledge Test (GKT) and it was devised and validated years ago by one of the pioneer researchers on polygraphs, D.T. Lykken.

How Does It Work?

The details of the crime are held confidential from everyone possible. (In Japan, the police often use this technique because there is so much cooperation between the police and the newspapers.) The guilty person knows the details, of course. So, say you are investigating a murder in which the killer slit the victim's throat. You ask a series of questions such as—Did you kill Jake with a gun? Did you kill Jake with a hammer? Did you stab Jake in the heart? Did you slit Jake's throat with a knife?

For the person with guilty knowledge, the question about slitting the victim's throat will have greater significance than other questions. He'll give a larger response on the polygraph.

This technique has been tested for many years with good results. But I suspect that it is really most useful in very serious cases. In a typical business situation, getting a clear response is more complicated.

■What about all the advice we've read about detecting deception by people's body language, the way they shift their eyes, etc. Is there any scientific validation?

It has been demonstrated in laboratory tests that people can detect deception at a rate that's only slightly better than chance. But it's a very weak effect—instead of being right 50% of the time, an individual might be right 60% of the time. With such a slight advantage, the biases that any individual brings to an encounter with another person will figure very powerfully in coming to a decision about whether the other person is lying or not.

Furthermore, nothing at all emerges in the laboratory when you try to isolate exactly what the person is looking at in order to correctly decide that the other person is lying.

Managers should be very cautious and humble about making decisions based on what they think of as their own special ability to detect deception.

Source: Dr. John J. Furedy, professor of psychology, University of Toronto, Ontario, Canada M5S 1A1. He is co-author of *Theories and Applications in the Detection of Deception*, Springer-Verlag, 175 Fifth Ave., New York 10010.

Preventing Expense-Account Rip-Offs

Two new scams that employees are using:

■Car rentals. When returning a car rented on a personal credit card, the employee claims to have lost the contract. The rental agent makes out a new contract, leaving the employee with the original on which inflated time and/or mileage figures can be inserted for reimbursement purposes. To prevent this, have all rental charges billed directly to the company through a company credit card. Forbid employees to use personal credit cards for such business expenses.

■Airline fares. Employee trades in a full-fare ticket for a discounted seat and pockets the difference. Prevent this by tightening up the company's ticket-purchasing procedures to insure that it is getting the lowest fare to begin with. Make sure personnel who handle ticket purchases are familiar with the latest discount and promotional fares—they can save money on lower air fares.

Other rip-offs have been around for years and still work because most companies fail to check expenses under $25.

Old scams that are still widely used:

■Transportation between airport and town. Employee takes a bus and asks to be reimbursed for a taxi. The company should clearly state that the policy is to use the cheapest ride, except under special circumstances, such as rushing to a meeting. Require receipts, but recognize that these may be easily altered. Make it clear that such expenses, even if under $25, will be scrutinized. Then follow through with at least spot-checks.

■Double meal billing. Employee incorporates the cost of a hotel meal into the room charge on the expense account, then puts in for a fictitious restaurant meal. Deal with this by making sure there is a separate line on the expense-account form for room charges and another line for other meal expenses. Carefully double-check the completed form against the hotel bill.

The IRS requires the client to have an itemized bill from the hotel, but many companies never look beyond the employee's expense-account form.

Source: Harold Seligman, Management Alternatives, New York.

How To Protect Company Secrets

A common problem is that many employees aren't sure what's confidential and what isn't. Have someone in the know classify documents and stamp the degree of confidentiality on them.

Other ways to tighten procedures:

■Beware of those employees most likely to let secrets slip. Best candidates are those who socialize with competitors, compulsive talkers, and people who boast when drinking. Keep them off the list for classified documents.

■Don't discuss plans or developments with colleagues in nonsecure places. There's no way of knowing who's listening.

■Require all desks be cleared of confidential information at the end of each day.

■Account for every key to the office. Change locks when an employee who has had access to a key leaves the company.

■Don't throw sensitive material into office wastebaskets. Take it home and throw it out there. It's cheaper than buying a paper shredder.

Source: *The Effective Manager*, Boston.

Chapter 44
White-Collar Crime

Countering White-Collar Crime

The first line of defense against white-collar crime is never to trust any employee, especially not long-term workers who handle money or finances. If the company is up front about this, the boss and employee will work together better.

Basics of an antitheft system:

■Make sure receipts are quickly posted against specific invoices at all cash-collection points.

■Have two people deposit money in the bank at least twice a day.

■Cross-check deposit balances, slips, and receipts.

■Review the books on a regular basis, and make surprise checks.

■Require everyone to take vacations. For those in critical money spots, consider ordering surprise time off so procedures can be checked.

■Set up a paper trail whenever possible, with easily checkable invoices, check numbers, dates, etc., so that embezzlement charges can be made effectively.

Computer crime is on the rise. Prosecutors still do not have a handle on all the techniques. One common crime is clerks at computerized point-of-sale cash registers erasing cash receipts from the computer tape.

Computer safeguard efforts should start with programmers. If there is only one, hire an outside consultant to check that employee's work. Have printouts run with computer balances so a paper record is available. Reconcile balances often. Have supervisors check on computer operators. Check the supervisors, too.

Surprise audits by the firm's auditors are a good idea. It may also be smart to cross-check the auditors if they have been working on the books for a long time.

But if managers make charges they can't back up, they lay themselves open to a lawsuit. Therefore, call in police at the least suspicion, and let them quietly make a case. Then, don't be afraid to file criminal charges against the thief. Examples work wonders, especially in larger workplaces where everyone seems to want to get into the siphoning-off act.

Embezzlement sometimes starts with padded expense accounts. It is a good idea to be clear and tough about accounts. Require weekly reconciliation against advances, even if the employee is out of town.

Source: Lawrence V. Christ, assistant district attorney for consumer fraud, Johnson County Court House, Olathe, KS.

How To Guard Against Embezzlement

Be suspicious of embezzlement when bookkeeping employees:
■Are excessively sensitive to routine questions or protective of records.
■Continually work overtime.
■Refuse to take vacations or reject promotions.
■Allow ledgers to fall behind.
Suspicious cash-flow and production patterns:
■Collection of receivables declines without apparent reason.
■Debts are written off without good explanation.
■Raw-materials use increases but production does not.
Suspicious outside relations:
■Creditors ask to deal with a specific person.
■When absent, the employee receives many odd calls or visits from people who are reluctant to explain their business.
Source: *Alert*, New York.

White-Collar Crime Tip-Offs

U.S. companies are losing over $40 billion a year through kickbacks, embezzlement, and other so-called white-collar crimes. A substantial percentage of them can be traced to purchasing departments and could have been prevented if management had been more alert. Early-warning signals:
■A buyer dealing only with a few suppliers. Big orders go to only one or two of them while other potential suppliers complain.
■Refusal of a buyer to delegate his duties when he's absent.
■Sole evaluation of suppliers left up to a single buyer.
■Supply costs that have risen faster than the inflation rate for the industry.
■Purchasing records that are difficult to locate.
■Loading-dock scales that often malfunction.
■A purchasing officer's life-style that is conspicuously above that of similarly-paid employees.
Source: Jules B. Kroll, president, Kroll Associates, Inc., New York, *International Management*, New York.

Chapter 45
Insurance Savvy

Important To Check The Company's Insurance Coverage

Most businesses are seriously underinsured. Trap: They focus too much on the cost of insurance and too little on the cost of being inadequately insured in the event of a loss. Points to consider in evaluating insurance needs…

■Avoid a health insurance carrier that offers low rates for the first year—to attract business—then raises rates substantially in succeeding years.

■Avoid unreasonable exclusions and limitations in health coverage. Watch out for limitations on eligible hospital charges for room and board which are expressed as either a percentage of the bill or a fixed daily figure.

■Carry a minimum lifetime benefit of $1 million per person of health coverage with no restrictions.

■Carry liability insurance of not less than $1 million or an amount equal to the net worth of the company. Consider an umbrella policy to extend coverage.

■Is the business covered against theft losses by dishonest employees?

■Is it insured against untimely deaths of key employees?

■Is the company's disability insurance adequate? Would it allow employees to maintain their current standard of living in the event of a major accident or illness?

Source: Robert A. Bensman, Bensman Associates, Ltd., a benefit and financial consulting firm, 3100 Dundee Rd., Northbrook, IL 60062.

Group Insurance Overcharges

Some insurance companies may be overcharging their group insurance customers. Slight amounts can add up over the years. Because buying group insurance is so automatic, and complicated, the insurers usually can get away with it. But by knowing what the group contract is and how to negotiate with their carrier, most customers can cut costs by as much as 10% or more. Remember, the rate is not the annual cost of the insurance, it is only the advance premium. Most important: Get a breakdown of the premium charges. A common area where overcharge could occur is carrier retention. Only one out of a hundred insurance brokers really understands what goes into these surcharges, which are intended to cover a broad range of miscellaneous carrier costs. Insurers aren't eager to teach brokers either. Some of the costs included in retentions are:

■Carrier processing.

■Insurance company's profit.

- Contract and booklet printing.
- Carrier administrative service.
- Late payment.
- Pooling and conversion.
- State premium taxes.
- Commissions.
- Claim determination processing.

Many of these items should rightfully be picked up by the insurer.

Often as much as one-third of a year's premiums are held in reserve by the carrier to protect itself against the time when the customer terminates his or her policy.

Very often, the carrier pays little interest on this money. How to earn higher interest, or get the entire reserve refunded:

- Negotiate a lag time for premium payments equal to the amount held in reserve.
- Offer the carrier a letter of credit that guarantees payment for claims filed after the company switched insurers.

Signs that your company may be overcharged include:

- A retention percentage above 10% of annual premiums. Retention rates commonly vary between 8% and 12% of the annual premiums. In some cases, the higher retention is offset by a lower premium rate. Frequently, however, it is a gross overcharge.
- A reserve that exceeds 30% of annual premiums, or one on which little or no interest is being paid.
- A large number of small claims. It may indicate that a plan if misdesigned.
- A consistent retrospective charge levied by the carrier to compensate for an excess amount of claims. Negotiating the retrospective trigger level from 75% of premiums to 80% can save $5,000 on a $100,000 annual premium bill.
- A customer is dealing with a captive insurance agent of a specific company. No matter how smart the agent may be, the likelihood is that the agent is partial to his own carrier. Alternative: Have an independent broker examine the policy to see if there's a better deal elsewhere. The typical fee is $80 per hour. Depending on the size of the account, the total fee may be $1,500 to $3,000.

Source: Arthur Schechner, president, Schechner Corp., insurance brokers and group consultants, Millburn, NJ.

Another cost-saving idea is to self-insure claims and use a carrier only for catastrophic claims. Rationale: By self-insuring, the company can avoid paying the 10% or so retention fee that the carrier adds on to all claims. Since the retrospective trigger in the policy guarantees that the company will pay if there is an excessive number of claims, the company might as well pay the small claims right out of expenses and save the retention fee.

Reviewing Company's Insurers

Important: Take time to review the health of the company's insurers with your brokers. Many insurers have large holdings of junk bonds or real estate. Other danger signs: Low loss reserves, dividend cuts and poor financial performance as indicated in the annual study published by the National Association of Insurance Commissioners. Don't rely on A.M. Best, the insurance industry rating service, because some companies it rated A have gone bust. Better: Favor companies covered by State Guarantee Funds over those not covered, and independent brokers with access to a wide selection of insurers over salespeople who represent only one company.

Source: Mark Sameth of KSH Group.

Protecting Yourself Against Insurance Companies' Games

Nightmare: You suffer a calamity...a disabling accident...or a fire that destroys your home...or business...or a crippling disease.

It's a good thing you've faithfully paid your insurance premiums all these years. But...the nightmare has only just begun....

For no rational reason, your insurance company denies your claim. Suddenly, on top of your recent trauma, you are now faced with overwhelming debt...unrelieved stress...and a tough new enemy...your own insurance company. Here are answers on what to do from attorney William Shernoff, a consumer lawyer who specializes in helping victims who are abused by insurance companies...the "King of the Mountain" in getting claims paid.

Insurance Against Insurance Abuse

■Choose an agent with a high sales volume—in the event of a problem, he carries critical weight.

■Read your insurance policy carefully—pay special attention to the exclusion clauses. These are the phrases on the last pages of your policy that take away coverage listed in the first pages. Most claims denials are based on exclusions.

Most courts require that insurance-policy exclusions be clear and conspicuous. The burden is on the insurer to prove that the exclusion applies.

For group policyholders: Keep the booklet outlining your coverage—it frequently takes precedence over the fine print in the master policy.

■Review procedures for filing a claim before you need to. Many policies set time limits or require certain proofs of loss. But delay or mistakes in filing claims forms are not grounds for denial of an otherwise valid claim, unless the insurer can show that it has been damaged by your error.

■Keep scrupulous documentation of all materials relating to insurance claims: Medical bills, a current inventory of your possessions with photographs, photos and estimates of automobile damage—and any and all communication with your insurer, including phone calls.

What To Do If Your Claim Is Denied

If your insurance company denies your legitimate claim, you may have grounds for a "bad faith" lawsuit.

Examples of bad faith on the part of an insurer: Failure to pay a legitimate claim in a timely fashion...failure to meet the reasonable expectations of the policyholder...promotion and/or sales of useless benefits.

In addition, your insurer is responsible for the conduct of its agents—and the language of its policies. But before you sue, take these steps...

■If you have any dispute regarding the interpretation of policy language or if your legitimate claim is denied, insist on a written explanation.

■Don't assume the first denial is a final answer. Instead: Promptly write a letter of protest that is honest, straightforward and polite.

■Contact the agent who sold you the policy. It is the agent's duty to see that you have the correct coverage for your needs and to protect your interests. Often your agent will contact the company's claims department on your behalf. This may be all that is needed.

■If your claim is not satisfied, be persistent and keep going up the company's ladder. Start with the person who denied your claim. Save your telephone bills and follow up calls with a brief letter, restating the substance of the conversation. Persist if necessary by writing to the claims manager, supervisor or complaints department, requesting a reply. In most states, insurance companies are obligated to respond to your letters. Surprise: Insurance companies will often pay a dispute claim after hearing your side of the story.

■If you are still not satisfied, contact your State Department of Insurance. Unlike a court of law, the state cannot get you damages. But it frequently does get claims settled.

■Consider Small Claims Court if appropriate. Your damages include time lost from work, mileage, phone calls, postage, loss of use of the funds due you...and so forth.

■If all else fails, hire a good trial lawyer. In most cases, insurance claims will be handled on a contingency-fee basis. For a list: Association of Trial Lawyers of America, 1050 31 St. NW, Washington, DC 20007.

Source: William M. Shernoff.

Better Deals On Dental Plans

Many companies shy away from employee dental insurance because the plans are relatively more expensive than other medical insurance. This is because insurance carriers know that employees will use them heavily initially for overdue dental work.

Within two years, most employees will be caught up on dental repairs. At this point, the company should renegotiate the cost of the plan downward. Steps to take:

■Compile the records that show dental costs have peaked.

■Set up a companywide preventative tooth-care program to minimize future dental bills.

Source: Donald A. DiGiulian, DDS, publisher, *Dentographics,* Branford, CT.

Look To Other Insurers To Reduce Cost Of Disability Pay

Accident and sickness disability pay should be reduced by amounts employees are eligible to receive from other insurance. For example, many states now provide "no-fault" auto-accident insurance which pays hospital expenses of persons (pedestrians or motorists) injured by motor vehicles. The company's obligations should (where allowed) be reduced by what is paid by no-fault.

But workers sometimes neglect to apply for no-fault auto-insurance benefits because their employers have generous disability policies. Disability plans should be designed to offset insurance benefits receivable, whether actually received or not.

No-fault laws can reimburse employees for 80% of wage loss while disabled. Administrators of wage maintenance plans should take that into account.

Chapter 46
Purchasing Wisdom

Getting The Most Out Of Purchasing

Without regular attention from top management, a company's purchasing department is apt to fall into a rut. The buyers place their orders routinely. They call for upper-echelon help only when problems develop. To minimize that, check the operations' efficiency level by asking these basic questions:

■How often is a real effort made to find new vendors and fight price increases? Simply ordering from established suppliers is lazy, and often not cost-effective.

■Is management delivering the message that purchasing is an important corporate function? Is it provided with high-level guidance before problems crop up?

■Is there an amply budgeted training program? Buyers need to stay ahead of new developments to be effective. Seminars, conferences and special classes pay off.

■Is value analysis being put to use? This involves nothing more than determining which goods are needed and which materials or processes are best. And it will result in low-cost substitutions, more realistic specifications, avoidance of duplication.

■Does purchasing have easy access to engineering and other technical personnel? Without such in-house assistance, buyers can overwrite specifications or misjudge quality standards.

Source: Lawrence D. Miles, *Purchasing World,* Barrington, IL.

Better Purchasing Systems

Modern delivery systems are nothing new to Ernest L. Anderson, Jr., who for 30 years has been revamping company purchasing practices to cut down on wastes of time and money. He talked with *Boardroom* about the failings in typical purchasing systems and what top management should do about them.

■What's the biggest problem with most companies' purchasing practices?

Too much paperwork. If the system generates more than five pieces of paper for the total procurement transaction, something's wrong.

■Next biggest?

Too many sources. For most of their careers, purchasing managers have been told they must have at least three sources for every item they buy.

■Isn't the opposite—single sourcing—dangerous?

Remember the gasoline shortage a few years back? The people who got gas were the ones who had gone to the same gasoline station all the time. When the crunch came, they were the ones who were taken care of by the gas station managers.

Everyone knows from personal experience that's what happens—but we resist applying that knowledge to business.

■But how can a purchasing manager make sure he's getting the best price and service in such an arrangement?

That's the real management part of purchasing. To set the standards of performance for the supplier. The purchasing manager sets the specifications. The buyers can almost always dictate...and can demand delivery of 95% of the order in 24 hours, delivery of 98% defect-free merchandise, and whatever else is required.

■That's all? What about following up, expediting deliveries, etc?

There's no need for it in a well-managed purchasing system. You've negotiated the price and delivery specs with the supplier and signed a contract for 10,000 widgets a year at $1 each. If you're not getting your widget deliveries on time or they're frequently defective, the supplier is dumped for breach of contract. It's simple.

Once the purchasing manager has set the standards and negotiated the best cost—not price, cost—all the rest is ordering. And the purchasing manager should be out of the picture on ordering.

■What do you mean cost, not price?

Traditionally, purchasing people have only thought about price. Management has to insist that they think total cost—that means all the paperwork and inventory expense that add to the actual cost of purchased materials.

■Who does the ordering, then, if purchasing doesn't?

The user, of course.

■You don't mean the guy who needs the screwdriver?

Yes, I do. Management must understand that purchasing is a service function, not a control function. Purchasing assures the flow of material. But control over what's needed and when it's delivered should be in the hands of the users. The users should communicate with the supplier, order the amount required and set the time for delivery.

■But who controls how much they order?

The manager is in charge of the department budget. He okays the order. He can look in a catalog and see what the cost per unit is before he authorizes the order—something operating people don't always get to see.

■How does the user physically place the order?

Many businesses are using fax machines to order. Or, it can be done by computer. Businesses are using direct communication, user to supplier—well-designed systems that cut paperwork.

■How do you make sure that suppliers are delivering what they should—when they should?

Management by exception. The company's managers meet regularly and review supplier performance. If a supplier isn't regularly meeting his contractual obligation to deliver 95% of an order within 24 hours with 98% defect-free merchandise, the user tells the purchasing manager—the person responsible for the contract—that he has a nonperformance problem. Then it becomes the purchasing department's job to either get the supplier to perform—or find another supplier.

■So, if all goes well, there's no need to involve purchasing at all after the initial contract is negotiated. But don't many purchasing people dislike having others talking to their supplier friends?

Sure. That's the biggest resistance to these systems. But there's simply no need for purchasing to be involved with the mechanics of ordering. And they don't control anything beyond negotiating contracts and making sure suppliers deliver.

■Where, specifically, does the company gain efficiency and cost savings by using your system?

Top management must look at productivity in its purchasing operations just as it should examine productivity throughout the organization.

It's wasteful to make the clerical functions of purchasing into managerial responsibilities just to inflate the jobs. Equally senseless is pulling purchasing into the ordering process just because people in the purchasing department want to be the only ones who talk to suppliers. That's where paperwork piles up and poor delivery schedules, inventory pileups and cost overruns quickly creep into the system.

Source: Ernest L. Anderson, Jr., Anderson Associates, Inc., 5901 Chesapeake Park, Orlando, FL 32819.

Chapter 47
Cost-Cutting Methods

Cost-Reduction Reminders

■Materials. Look for materials that are cheaper to buy, easier to fabricate, offer a product improvement.

■Specifications. Consider eliminating manufacturing operations, cutting scrap, reducing rework, widening tolerances.

■Purchasing. Investigate quantity buys, market fluctuations, open contracts, any financing concessions from suppliers.

■Packaging. Costs may be reduced through redesign, new materials, different sizes, different quantities.

Source: *Purchasing Factomatic,* Prentice-Hall, Englewood Cliffs, NJ.

Four Ways To Fight A Price Hike

■Send the supplier a substantial purchase order, but specify the old price, as if the announced hike had been overlooked. The implied threat—accept these terms or risk losing the whole order, perhaps even the whole account.

■Ask for a reduction in price, without any reference to the proposed increase. This may lead to an eventual compromise at or near the old level.

■Acknowledge the hike, but claim an inability to pay more than the former price for this current order. The vendor will probably agree to continue with the old price, at least for a time.

■Turn the raise down, out-of-hand. Say that the company will go elsewhere unless the increase is rescinded. This is risky, even if the vendor feels forced to go along, because of the resentment stirred by the take-it-or-leave-it ultimatum. Then what? Someday, when the vendor holds the bargaining leverage, expect a move to get even.

Source: Dr. Chester L. Karrass, *Purchasing,* Boston.

Price-Protection Clauses

Three possibilities:

■Peg future increase to the seller's costs, seller to pass through higher costs on a dollar-for-dollar basis without tacking on a profit margin.

■Use a most-favored-customer clause. Specify that the seller can't charge any more than the most favored customer. Even if there's no easy way of actually checking, the seller can't be sure that they buyer won't accidentally find out. This possibility helps.

Don't Overpay Freight Bills

To avoid paying too much for your freight bills, follow these basic rules.

Pay only on the original freight bill.

Check the shipment weight appearing on the freight bill with that on the bill of lading. Figures are often transposed.

If possible, verify the accuracy of rates. Although this may require expertise you lack, you can set up in-house controls by asking vendors or carriers for quotations, setting up files of freight bills by vendor, and checking current against past bills.

Check to see if the bill is actually yours. Carriers often mix them up.

Not all freight is sent collect. If the letters "PPD" appear on the bill (usually near the total charge), it has been prepaid. Note: double-check the freight bill against the shipper's bill of lading. The carrier may have neglected to carry over the prepaid notice when he prepared his bill.

Only pay single shipment surcharges if the words "single shipment" or an abbreviation like "SS" or "SSCH" appears on the bill of lading. If it does not, you are not required to pay.

Obviously, check the arithmetic on the bill. Are extensions and totals correct?

Consignment Buying: How It Cuts Costs

A company that has some clout with its suppliers should consider buying on consignment. Basic tradeoff: The buyer agrees to purchase a certain volume of goods over a specified time. In return, the vendor stocks the order, at its expense, on the buyer's property.

This way the price is locked in, typically for one year. Inventory and carrying costs (including insurance) are paid by the seller. The buyer has immediate access to the goods.

When consignment works best:

■The buyer is able to estimate closely the amount needed over the entire period covered.

■The product has a long shelf life and will not become obsolete or need redesign.

■The order is large enough to be worthwhile to the seller.

Suppliers often don't understand the consignment method and rarely suggest it. But buyers should point out that consignment is a trade-off.

Advantages for the seller:

■Because there's an assured sale of a sizable order, the supplier may seek quantity discounts from its suppliers and may save by having one long production run.

■The seller locks up the business. Competitors can't get any of it for a year.
■Profit on the sale does not have to be taken into income and declared for taxes until the goods are actually accepted by the buying company.

Chapter 48
Purchasing And Suppliers

Using Suppliers' Knowledge

One advantage to a business slowdown: Faced with declining sales, suppliers will be more eager than ever to provide ideas and expertise. Be sure to encourage this knowledge sharing. One way is to post a sign prominently in the reception area soliciting their ideas. Be specific. Tell vendors to:

■Ask the company's buyers about the why and how of specifications. As specialists in their fields, suppliers know the factors governing quality and price.

■Tell the buyers if they should be ordering different quantities or whether a standard part can substitute for a special part.

■Show advantages of their suggestions in terms of lower prices, longer life, use of readily available materials, etc.

Be sure suppliers who make solid suggestions reap some benefit.

Source: Somerby R. Dowst, *More Basics for Buyers,* CBI Publishing Co., Boston.

Setting Up Systems Contracts With Suppliers

Systems contracts* can cut inventories, paperwork, and other related costs. But they often misfire.

When setting up workable systems contracts with the company's vendors, start with clear, quantifiable objectives. Decide how much inventory the company's going to cut. Set a dollar and a unit goal. Also set a dollar goal for savings in expediting and order processing. Measure performance.

Don't bastardize the concept. The aim is to negotiate lower costs (not prices) by getting the vendor to do some of your work. The company isn't trying to get him to give it a volume discount on a bunch of items. Stress to suppliers that reliability and speed will be the criteria for selection.

Propose systems arrangements only to vendors with known track records for performance. Stress that competitive—not necessarily the lowest—prices are required.

Systems contracts mean that the company will be dealing with fewer vendors. If this is unacceptable, then forget the systems idea.

Make sure adequate volume exists. Unless the company can deliver good volume for the vendor, there's no way he can cover his costs and deliver the kind of service the company is seeking.

*Vendor agrees, for guaranteed annual volume, to stock supplies until the customer needs them, and delivers quickly upon request.

Don't spread a contract over too many items. A large number of small orders can't be handled efficiently by anyone.

Get a commitment from top management. Systems contracts wipe out vast amounts of paperwork that often is near and dear to accounting, stores, production, and finance. Unless the top boss understands that old procedures will have to be modified and is willing to accept these changes, the idea won't work.

Make sure the company's buyers know and understand systems contracts. Their aim is to cut inventory, paperwork, and expediting. Simple release systems have to be set up, and order matching eliminated.

Audit the purchasing department periodically. Look for: 1. Instances of continued expediting, and 2. Continuation of old work procedures. Unless there is a marked reduction in both, something is wrong.

Watch out for squirrels. Normal tendency for production people is to set up sub-inventories. This undermines the systems approach completely. Find out from production what items they are worried about. Make sure vendors know about these worries. Then check regularly to make sure vendors know from the start that you are going to level with them on needs.

Excuses Purchasing Agents Give For Not Getting Competitive Bids

Explanations that don't hold water:

■Earlier bids are already on file. Weakness: Those bids may be too old. Or the order quantity may be different and now qualify for a lower price.

■Quality and delivery are more important than competitive pricing. Weakness: The statement that the chosen vendor gives better service must be substantiated with specific benefits.

■All standard items are priced alike. Weakness: There is price competition on most standard items. Also consider service, terms, size of orders.

■The product is patented. Weakness: Engineers may not have been queried or presented with alternatives in some time. Also likely: Engineers have not kept abreast of alternatives.

■Customer specifications. Weakness: The customer may no longer care for the detail.

Source: *Purchasing,* Boston.

To increase competition among suppliers, let rival salespeople bunch up in the reception room or suggest that the order will be split between sellers if the price is not right. Or carry on negotiations with two different companies in different rooms at the same time.

Source: Dr. Chester L. Karrass, Center for Effective Negotiating, Santa Monica, CA.

Bribe, Kickback Signals

■The purchasing agent takes no vacations.

■The list of suppliers and vendors never changes. (Most firms change 20%–25% of their suppliers every year.)

■The lifestyle of the purchasing agent is better than what would be expected from his salary.

■Only one person decides what to purchase; little or no assistance is given by technical staff people.

■Large purchases are "chopped up" into small and misleading elements (such as add-ons and changes) instead of being taken care of by one single order.

■The scales on the company loading dock are never working properly.

■The cost of suppliers has increased faster than inflation in the supplier's industry.

■Vendors complain to top management that they can't get an appointment with the purchasing agent.

Some ways to prevent bribes of purchasing agents:

■Rotate agents to different areas regularly.

■Make it clear that purchasing isn't a dead-end job.

■Pay purchasing agents better. Encourage them with incentives and bonuses based on performance.

New Opportunities In Equipment Leasing

Two big tax incentives for equipment leasing were lost in 1988—investment tax credit and accelerated depreciation. However, leasing still has powerful tax and other financial advantages for many companies.

Example: Some companies—especially those that pay the Alternative Minimum Tax—may not benefit from the depreciation deductions if they bought the equipment outright. On the other hand, they can lease the equipment from a company that can make use of the deductions. In return, the leasing company passes on its tax benefit through lower lease payments.

That's an advantage in almost any economic environment. But it especially makes sense today, when financing a purchase is increasingly difficult due to tight bank regulations and escalating interest rates.

Example: Many U.S. airlines are heavily in debt today, just when they need to replace their aging fleets. But since they don't have the cash and are leveraged to the limit, more and more are relying on lease arrangements rather than purchases.

The same option is available to companies of any size, whether they need one piece of equipment or entire plants.

Example: Energy project developers completing construction of qualified property with special tax benefits that they will be unable to utilize can essentially refinance their projects by selling them to tax-benefit-hungry lessors and leasing them back (the transaction must close on or before December 31, 1990 for transition property).

The Cash Advantage

Leasing can also be a financial boon to companies that have already bought equipment but which now are short of cash. They can sell the equipment to a leasing company and lease it back. Airlines have been using this technique for many years. Energy project developers frequently engage in sale/leaseback transactions of their projects to obtain cash needed to fund development of their next project, while maintaining operating control of the leased project.

The changed tax laws don't eliminate the major advantages of...

■The immediate cash infusion from the sale.

■The ability to expense the lease payments.

■The relief from the concern of how to dispose of the equipment when its life-time ends.

Caution: Lease-back arrangements aren't generally available to financially unstable businesses without credit enhancement. Leasing companies enter into the deals with the anticipation of being able to lease and depreciate the equipment for a certain number of years. They can't take a chance that the lessee will go bankrupt.

New International Deals

Changes in national tax codes have created unique new opportunities in cross-border equipment leasing. Though the specific differences are usually complex, the advantage boils down to this...in different countries, both the lessee and lessor may be considered owners and therefore get the depreciation benefit of an equipment purchase (the so-called double-dip).

Example: In France, a company can buy equipment and lease it to an American company with an option to buy at a nominal price. French tax law considers the company in France to be the owner, while US law considers the American company to be the owner because of the nominal purchase price.

Result: Both the French and American company can take the tax benefits of their respective countries on 100% of the purchase price of the equipment. Moreover, part of the French company's depreciation benefit is passed on to the US company in terms of lower lease payments.

Investment bankers in Hong Kong, Ireland, Japan and Sweden have also become active in this type of cross-border lease.

Caution: Just as the company would consult a domestic tax expert to review a conventional lease deal, it's essential to have an international leasing expert counsel you on cross-border leasing. Among other points, the agreement can be structured to shield the company from losses related to currency fluctuations.

Thinking Twice

Despite the edge that can go with leasing, it isn't for every business. Companies should be cautious about leasing if they...

■Must retain complete control over the equipment, such as a computer that they may eventually want to customize.

■Are already leasing a large amount of equipment and/or are heavily in debt. In those situations, leasing companies may charge a premium to cover the added financial risk they perceive.

■Want to retain control over their own equipment insurance and maintenance. Lessors—and, more important, their lenders—usually have their own insurance and maintenance requirements, and these may conflict with a lessee's financial abilities.

■Suspect that the lessor isn't in top financial condition. Unless lease agreements are very carefully written, a business can have its leased equipment taken away if the lessor gets into financial difficulty.

To find a leasing company, consult an investment banker, the company's attorney or tax adviser, a commercial bank, or a company in your industry that has had extensive experience in the area of leasing. Increasingly, financial subsidiaries of utilities and large industrial corporations have gone into the leasing business.

Examples: AT&T, Chrysler, Florida Power & Light, Ford and GE.

Source: Joseph Halliday, Jeanine Rosen, Pamela Olson and Eduardo Vidal, members of the Lease Financing Group, Skadden, Arps, Slate, Meagher & Flom, 919 Third Ave., New York 10022.

Energy Cost-Cutting Secrets

In contrast to the 1980s when energy prices declined, the 1990s is be a decade of rising fuel costs, due to limited production capacity and growing worldwide demand.

Important: Shrewd management of energy costs will be a key factor that differentiates successful companies from those that are less competitive.

Start planning now for more energy-efficient operations. This will mean different things for different types of companies. But, since most companies have already taken the easy steps of insulating buildings and replacing inefficient lighting, what's needed now is a more strategic analysis of the company's energy usage. Examples:

■Manufacturing companies: Measure energy consumption levels of all manufacturing processes to make sure they're not using too much oil or natural gas. This is also the time to examine all of the possible options for using alternative sources of energy. Even if it's not appropriate to shift right now, you'll be ahead of the game if you've done all the necessary cost analyses in advance.

■Companies about to expand: Add operations with energy costs in mind. Favor plant sites where the climate is temperate, or where energy or electricity are plentiful and relatively cheap—such as the Plains states. Shut down inefficient facilities that can't be upgraded. Reconsider manufacturing some energy-intensive products.

■Companies that rely on raw commodities: Consider sourcing raw materials from countries where energy costs are cheaper or energy supplies are abundant. Such an edge in costs will become more critical in the future.

Smart Steps for All Companies

Begin hedging to protect the company from energy price increases that almost certainly lie ahead as worldwide demand for oil approaches OPEC's capacity to produce crude. Gas prices have already moved up sharply and will continue to rise since the so-called surplus is now over. In some areas, there could be severe shortages of natural gas due to supply or transportation problems. Steps to take…

■Negotiate long-term contracts to lock in current prices as long as possible.

■Buy oil or natural gas reserves and store them against the time when prices rise sharply. If you don't actually buy the reserves now, at least line up future supplies.

■Invest only in energy-efficient equipment. At the least, take potential future energy problems into account when purchasing new equipment or facilities. Buying smarter today heads off future energy cost problems.

■Consider cogeneration. If the company's industrial processes can, say, use steam recaptured from a cogeneration plant and sell excess electricity to a neighboring company or the local utility, it might make sense to add the company's own capacity. Caution: Gas-fired cogeneration could become less attractive as gas prices rise and profits shrink. Coal-fired cogeneration could run into environmental problems. The Clean Air Act will limit emissions from all big coal-powered plants.

Cogeneration no longer looks as promising as it once did, but it can be appropriate for certain companies.

Get Expert Help

If the company doesn't have its own engineers and energy experts, seek help from local utilities. Many utilities now have sophisticated programs to encourage companies to become more energy-efficient.

Source: John Sawhill, The Nature Conservancy, 1815 N. Lynn St., Arlington, VA 22209.

Chapter 49
Purchasing And The Law

When Buyers Can Be Held To Unsigned Order

Buyers don't have to sign a purchase contract for it to be valid under the Uniform Commercial Code.

Example: Buyer and seller work out a "rough" agreement; the seller writes out the details and sends a copy to the buyer. That is binding upon the buyer, unless he objects within ten days.

Exceptions: The rule applies to "merchants" and other businesspeople, but not to consumers. The dividing line can be hazy. Some state courts have ruled that farmers and unsophisticated "ma & pa" organizations are exempt, too.

Oral Sales Contract Update

Oral contracts for more than $500 are no longer valid under the Uniform Commercial Code. There must be a written order and a written acceptance. But the new ruling says that once buyer and seller have agreed on the terms of a deal, a purchase order standing alone constitutes an enforceable contract if there is an indication on the order that it follows an oral agreement and the seller does not object in writing.

Source: *Bazak International v. Mast Industries,* CA NY, 2/16.

Arbitration—Alternative To A Lawsuit

When a business deal turns sour, a lawsuit is not the only answer. If both sides are willing, an impartial arbitrator that they choose can decide who's right. The award will be legally enforceable in most states.

Advantages of arbitration:

1. It's not necessary to retain a lawyer. However, attorneys' costs for an arbitration hearing are much lower than they would be for a court proceeding.

2. The arbitrator can be a person particularly familiar with the industry. This can be important if the issue is the quality of merchandise.

3. An arbitration hearing can usually be arranged within weeks.

4. Because arbitration is private, neither the public nor government regulatory bodies are alerted to facts about trade practices or credit standing.

There are disadvantages as well. Arbitration may not be the answer where a very large sum of money is involved. The finality of arbitration is great for the winner, but bad for the loser if an appeal is blocked.

Also, if important legal issues are involved, court proceedings may be better in the long run. In a patent infringement issue, for example, the patent owner may want a court decision to stand as a warning against other potential violators.

The fact that commercial arbitration awards are not routinely published thus becomes a disadvantage to the patent holder.

The first step toward arbitration is to contact the local bar association or the American Arbitration Association, 140 W. 51 St., New York 10020.

Protecting Inspection Rights

A buyer can take a reasonable time to examine a shipment and still reject it if the merchandise is unsatisfactory. What's a reasonable time? As little as a few hours or as much as several months for complex equipment that takes repeated adjustment to get it working.

Signing the trucker's receipt does not constitute acceptance of the goods as satisfactory. It merely acknowledges that something was received. The buyer can decide after inspection whether to accept or reject the shipment.

What buyers should do to protect their rights:

■Be sure not to use the item if it doesn't meet the specs. Using it can constitute acceptance and the buyer would then have to pay for it. If part of the shipment is acceptable, notify the seller before use that part of the shipment if acceptable but part is being rejected.

■Don't delay informing the seller of rejection. A buyer who fails to give notice of rejection, within a reasonable time, is deemed to have accepted the shipment and will have to pay the seller for it.

■Don't pay if the goods are unsatisfactory. It's still possible to reject after payment in some cases. (For example, C.O.D., where the buyer is required to pay before inspecting.) But many buyers who paid before learning of the defect have lost when they sued to get money back.

The buyer also must act in good faith. If the goods are perishable, the buyer must take steps to avoid spoilage. But, if time is crucial, he may cover his needs by buying replacement goods elsewhere. The buyer can then sue for the extra costs.

Source: Dr. Russell Decker, *Purchasing*, Boston.

Warning Signs Of Purchasing Fraud

Be suspicious of collusion between company supplier and purchasing representative when:

■Buyer's working files are not readily accessible or so disorganized that a given transaction can't be tracked.

■Buyer consistently uses verbal bids instead of formal, signed bids, always pleading lack of time.

■Orders are smaller than they should be for no logical reasons. (The buyer's logic is that small orders command less attention.)

■Purchase-order amendments authorizing changes in price do not have supporting explanations or approval signature higher than the buyer's. (Price renegotiation is one of the most fertile areas of fraud.)

Source: Robert N. Huntoon, *The Challenge of Profitable Procurement,* Redding, CA.

Chapter 50
Environmental Issues

Business And The Environment

To protect the environment—and cut costs at the same time...

■Cooperate with the company's suppliers and customers by shipping back returnable containers and packaging.

■Ask suppliers to help identify better packaging alternatives.

■Set up a recycling program for wood, paper, plastic and other materials. If the business is small, look into joining forces with others in the area.

■Consider recycling materials for the company's use. Use plastic totes for storage and make wood chips from damaged pallets to use for landscaping.

■Save plastic loose fill. Use it in company shipping department and offer it to employees for their personal use.

■Lengthen the life of pallets and containers through more careful use and preventive maintenance. Salvage good components of damaged pallets and containers and use those parts in the repair operation.

Source: *Modern Materials Handling*, 275 Washington St., Newton, MA 02158.

Cutting Paper Usage

Transmit documents using electronic mail or a fax board installed in a PC, rather than by normal fax machine. When documents are composed on a computer, edit them on the computer, instead of on a printed copy. Recycle photocopier paper by using both sides for most documents.

Source: *Home-Office Computing*, 730 Broadway, New York 10003. For more information, call the Environmental Defense Fund, 800-CALL-EDF.

Environmental Respect

Concern for the environment has become a prominent part of today's business world. And, because the news about world pollution is so frightening, the importance of environmental concern will continue to increase in coming years. Important lesson: Businesses that face up to the environmental challenge fast stand to gain an edge over the competition.

How business can profit from managing environmental issues...

Avoid surprises: This is probably the most valuable advantage to becoming environmentally aware.

Example: With a multitude of new environmental laws—federal, state and local—all too many violators don't even know they're running afoul of the rules. As many companies have learned, that can be a particularly nasty surprise—since fines can amount to millions of dollars.

Trap: Complying with existing environmental laws won't be enough. Laws on this subject are changing constantly, and unless companies make themselves aware of developments, they risk being caught with big costs.

Example: Some businesses will need to make substantial expenditures to comply with the new federal Clean Air Act, passed by Congress in October. Some environmentally aware companies are prepared for the heavy cost of compliance, having set funds aside beginning two years ago when debate on the law was becoming serious. Other, less-prudent companies may have to scramble to find money for compliance.

Another type of surprise hits those businesses that fail to thoroughly investigate the environmental condition of a property before they buy or lease it. They get stuck with huge clean-up bills after they discover the site is considered an environmental threat.

Safeguard: Retain an environmental specialist with a strong track record of inspecting sites and spotting problems, not just doing "paperwork studies." To find one: Ask companies in your industry for referrals or contact trade associations and regulatory agencies for names of specialists.

Polish the image: Because consumers have been key instigators of environmental consciousness in recent years, companies have an opportunity to gain consumer loyalty by demonstrating their environmental concern. Or, at the very least, they can head off criticism from an environmentally aware public.

Example: McDonald's, which was once criticized for dumping mountains of non-biodegradable waste, recently announced the phase-out of plastic foam sandwich containers. McDonald's was quite certain that it would not lose large numbers of customers by doing this. In fact, the move is almost certain to win McDonald's new customers since it's already winning praise from environmental groups.

Reaching green markets: Don't overlook the important fact that the environmental movement also includes groups concerned with health and animal rights. Many companies are making changes which they hope will attract consumers who are sensitive to these issues as well. Examples:

■Starkist and Chicken of the Sea Tuna have been persuaded to make costly changes to fishing technology to prevent dolphin killing.

■Body Shop Cosmetics, a British company, has made inroads in Europe and the U.S. by using natural rather than synthetic ingredients, and by not testing products on live animals.

Progressive environmental policies will give a substantial edge to U.S. companies that want to market in Europe. There, the green movement is larger and stronger. American companies that make the effort to understand environmental politics there will have an advantage in analyzing European markets and developing products for them.

Environmental product technology: Of course, there are also huge opportunities to develop environmental technology and to take advantage of technologies that others develop. There will be a growing demand for products and technologies that solve major environmental problems.

Examples: Technology to lower fuel consumption, remove pollutants, increase crop yields...products that use solar energy, components for light-weight cars, appliances that use less electricity.

Taking the high ground: When a company shows concern for the environment, it demonstrates a type of altruism that can only help it.

Example: Wal-Mart now requires suppliers to document that their products are environmentally acceptable. The move may not trigger a new spurt of sales for Wal-Mart, but it will certainly attract some environmentally aware customers. And it will head off the possibility of an environmental backlash like the one that plagued McDonald's.

How To Boost Awareness

Whenever possible, screen out job applicants who are openly hostile to environmental issues. Give key employees periodic training in environmental issues.

Most major consulting companies offer training programs in environmental issues, just as they do in law, employment practice, finance, etc. Essential: Follow up the initial training course with periodic sessions to keep key employees up-to-date on changes in environmental law and other aspects of the issue.

Source: S. Noble Robinson, director, Arthur D. Little's Environmental, Health and Safety practice, Acorn Park, Cambridge, MA 02140.

Chapter 51
Inventory Management

Inventory Management For Tougher Times

Cutting inventory costs should involve more than simply cutting the sheer number of widgets stored in the warehouse. To get real savings in inventory management, businesses must make changes throughout their operations. Aim: To actually eliminate inventory, rather than just reduce it.

Shrewder Strategies

Inventory managers can start by figuring out which items or stockkeeping units (SKUs) are obsolete and can be discontinued...and devising ways to eliminate or postpone the cost of stocks and supplies while still having them physically available for use. Inventory elimination techniques...

■Standardization (simplification). Have the design, engineering and purchasing people conduct ongoing reviews of active inventory items to see which might be combined with others of similar specifications for materials, width, tensile strength, color, etc. Look at all the hinge sizes, screws, bearings and pumps that are carried with only slight modifications, for example, and settle on the few that can perform most flexibly. Eliminate the rest, except for a selected few items that must be custom-made.

■Commonality analysis. A variation of standardization, this entails analyzing items by what they do.

Example: A screw, bolt and nut, tack welding, clamp, cotter pins and bonding materials such as glue all fulfill the same function—fastening. Reduce the numbers of such items that now exist in inventory down to a few by redesigning products.

This doesn't mean an overzealous one-size-fits-all approach. But without some standardization and commonality analysis, the company will miss many valuable opportunities for inventory cost reduction.

■Vendor and consignment stocking. When purchasing people have gone as far as they can in price negotiations, instruct them to try for non-cost stocking—the vendor stocks the company's needs on either their premises or the company's, but the goods are not actually paid for until they're used in production. Remember, the cost of inventory is related to the time of ownership. The meter doesn't start until the bill is paid. Suppliers who are anxious to get the business will usually agree to these kinds of arrangements.

■Contractor maintenance. In many industries, maintenance has become a huge cost item. If the company can move maintenance responsibility to an outside contractor, expensive maintenance inventories can be moved out of the facility or at least out of the carrying cost of inventory. Many airlines are now doing this, so they incur no maintenance inventory costs until the contractor submits a bill for the completed job.

■Make-or-buy decisions. Never base make-or-buy decisions on fixed costs only, which will remain the same no matter how the item is sourced. The main thing that should guide the decision is the cost of money—a variable cost. Make the best possible estimates about future interest rates and prices, but if these aren't clear, it's usually best to buy rather than make. The same kind of logic applies to buying huge stockpiles. Usually, it turns out that carrying a big excess inventory costs more than taking chances in the marketplace.

■Shrinkage program. This is an accounting exercise designed to bring the company's Accounts Payable into the closest possible alignment with its Accounts Receivable. Thus, if the company is on a 30-day payment cycle, try to arrange for line items to be paid for at the same time as receivables. Point: This reduces the need for borrowing.

Getting Started

To start eliminating inventories and get away from using so much energy on procuring, storage and moving materials:

■Pick a sample situation to improve, such as a costly part or assembly operation. Try the techniques listed above on this pilot situation. Involve all of the required personnel skills, including design, operations and purchasing. If necessary, bring in talent from other divisions or hire objective consultants.

■Extrapolate these gains to other operations. Use any gains achieved in the sample to sell a broader program of inventory elimination throughout the company.

■Establish a continuing program with set priorities and goals. Determine how much money the company wants to save on inventory six months, nine months, twelve months hence. Then, budget for the expenditures needed to make constant progress toward better inventory management.

Source: Norman Kobert, Kobert & Associates, Drawer 21396, Ft. Lauderdale, FL 33335. He is an international management consultant on asset management and the author of *Inventory Strategies* (Boardroom Books) and *Inventory Management for Cost Reduction* (Prentice-Hall).

Signs Of Inventory Problems

■Competitors' prices are lower.
■Slow-moving items are reducing cash available for new inventory.
■Odd and nonstandard sizes are overstocked.
■Too many seasonal items are carried over.
Inventory aids:

■Arrange for quick delivery from suppliers for seldom ordered goods. (This can mean an extra charge.) An alternative is an informal borrowing system with friendly competitors.

■Grade inventory according to profitability. Ensure 100% availability of biggest profit-earners. Stock down or out on all slow-selling items.

■Color-code bin or package labels to indicate month of receipt. This provides visual identification of slow-moving merchandise.

■Establish a monthly schedule of returns of excess inventory. Hit minor suppliers once or twice a year, major ones on a more frequent schedule.

Source: Bruce M. Bradway and Robert R. Pritchard, *Protecting Profits During Inflation and Recession,* Addison-Wesley Publishing Co., Reading, MA.

Reducing Excess Stocks

First identify specific excessive stocks. Next, determine the cause of overstocking. Excessive inventories and imbalances between what is purchased and what is used, what is manufactured and what is shipped, what is put on distributors' shelves and what they are actually able to sell to retailers or end-users. Imbalances can also arise where, say, three components go into a product. If supply runs short on one component, supplies of the other two are useless at that time.

Common causes of imbalance:

■Engineers and design people insist on having immediate access to many components they use or might use. If the company has a large engineering and design department, or is technologically oriented, look here first.

■Irregular demand. Assumed inability to forecast precise demand encourages larger-than-necessary initial orders.

■Lead time is out of whack. Because delivery times in recession tend to grow shorter, chances are the company is purchasing and receiving in advance of actual need. Revise purchase orders on basis of current lead-time experience.

■Usable supplies may be low, relative to the total amount stocked. This often happens with a new product when tolerances have not been fully worked out.

■Supplies in the pipeline are not being taken into consideration before reordering. As a result, reorders are placed too soon.

■Excess sitting time. If the components for 1,000 products come in each week and 1,000 finished products are shipped out, it is not necessary to maintain inventory levels of 5,000. Cutting to 4,000 would leave an adequate cushion.

■Decisions made in affluent times may not be appropriate in recession. For example, "We will never again run out of this item." "Let's keep several suppliers on this component." "We'll sell more typewriters if we also offer a full line of cases and supplies."

Reexamine these premises. Now is the time to reconsider the benefits of working very closely with a single source. Have the sales department reevaluate how important a full line is.

■Too-specialized components. If standardization of parts has never been tired, consider the idea. Do a commonality analysis to identify product applications where various functions could be performed by the same component. Also, discourage all special-order items.

It's a good idea to make materials lists available to engineers and designers before they write up specifications. Get purchasing people and engineering department to cooperate in cutting manufacturing costs without hurting product quality

Source: Norman Kobert, Kobert & Associates, Fort Lauderdale, FL.

Chapter 52
Transportation

Shipping Alternatives

Licensed freight transportation brokers now book nearly 20% of the nation's total truck traffic. In addition to acting as middlemen between shippers and trucking companies, the brokers can...

■Locate specialized trailers for highway use.

■Furnish extra equipment to help out during peak shipping periods.

■Set up a private fleet operation.

■Help lower less-than-truckload shipment costs by combining freight from several shippers for lower truckload costs.

■Supply customers with computer reports on inbound and outbound shipments.

Source: Transportation Brokers Conference of America, 14508 John Humphrey Dr., Orland Park, IL 60462.

Holding Down Freight Costs

Ideas to put a lid on industrial freight costs, which are rising a lot faster than the general price level:

■Standardize shipping instructions based on urgency. When the lack of an item threatens a production shutdown, specify small-package or priority airfreight. When the lack could cause a stock outage, specify nonpriority (two to three days) airfreight or LTL (less-than-full-truckload). Specify a truckload or rail shipment for items for regular stock resupply or normal reorder.

■Consolidate inbound freight. Have the carrier consolidate two or more shipments from a single vendor (or even from several vendors) into one. Advantages are weight breaks and minimal delivery charges.

■Think total cost. Direct shipping charges (rates, packing, crating, insurance) aren't all. The final cost decision on mode must include indirect shipping costs such as capital that is invested in inventories, carrying charges, warehousing, cost of damage, theft, pilferage, etc. In addition, intangible considerations, such as system flexibility, competitive advantage, and customer goodwill.

Source: *Purchasing World,* Barrington, IL.

Avoiding Unnecessary Charges

When the company uses regulated common carriers, watch for extra charges that are legal but avoidable:

■Single-shipment charges. Assessed when only one shipment is picked up. Therefore always contract for more than one load, or use carriers that do not charge for this service.

■Pickup and delivery charges. Assessed to cover unusual or difficult situations, usually in big cities (particularly New York). Instead use companies that specialize in serving congested areas at regular rates.

■Arbitrary charges for freight tonnage imbalances when a truck returns empty from a trip. Use carriers that regularly service the delivery area and do not make an arbitrary charge.

Handle as many shipping chores as possible in-house. For example, provide return bills of lading, use proper labels, and do necessary repackaging. The freight firm will charge extra for these services.

Source: Donna Behme, Behme Assoc., *Sounding Board,* Cherry Hill, NJ.

When Air Freight Is Essential

■Shipment time eats up selling days (seasonal merchandise) and cuts turnover of expensive merchandise.

■Transportation delays discourage orders and reorders.

■Speed is required to beat or meet competition.

■Important markets are long distances from vendors.

■Inventories must be lean because of cash or space limitations.

Truck Leases: Which To Use And When

■The capital lease. It's generally long-term. The accumulated payments nearly equal the truck's purchase price. Companies can use the capital lease as a substitute for a loan to purchase. If a fleet is being leased, the interest charges may be well below the prime rate. But the lessee must be willing to maintain, operate, and dispose of the trucks involved.

■The operating lease. The lessee pays only for the use of the truck when he needs it. The lessor provides the maintenance and insurance and disposes of the truck when the lease expires. However, the truck is not counted on the lessee's books as an asset, although this may be negotiable. Operating leases are generally more expensive than capital leases because of the services provided.

A lessee should always shop around and bargain for the best price. Successful leasing is based on negotiation.

Trucking Challenges

Trucking challenge #1: Tougher environmental requirements. Solution: Companies will begin using two fleets, one that meets standards for highly polluted areas and a second for lower-density areas. Challenge #2: Higher operating costs. Solution: Trucking rates will change to reflect peak and off-peak prices. Industry lobbyists will work to extend highway financing beyond user tolls. Challenge #3: Shortage of long-haul drivers. Solution: Cross-country relay systems that allow drivers to get home every two days.

Source: Thomas C. Schumacher, executive vice-president, California Trucking Association, writing in *Diesel Equipment Superintendent,* 50 Day St., Norwalk, CT 06856.

Chapter 53
Company Cars

Buy Versus Lease Company Car

Leasing a car costs an average 15% more than buying, but it pays off in some situations. You should lease if you: Keep a car for only two or three years. Don't like to deal with auto maintenance. Want to use the auto down-payment money for other investments. Are a high-mileage driver. Prefer a medium- or high-priced vehicle.

Restocking The Company Auto Fleet

Instead of standardizing on a single new model, consider a fleet of various sizes of models, in different fuel-economy categories.

With demand rising for smaller cars, delivery time for them is running longer. Adding some larger vehicles to the mix will assure a steadier flow of replacement cars through the year.

If the smaller-car trend reverses, a mix of models will provide a hedge against any steep decline in fleet value on the resale market.

Gradually stepping back down to smaller cars each time the fleet turns over will ensure continued annual improvement in overall fuel economy well into the future.

Source: Peterson, Howell & Heather, Baltimore.

Basics In Fleet Cost Cutting

■Reward employees who achieve the largest cuts in gasoline usage.
■Switch to smaller cars. They are cheaper to buy and operate.
■Consolidate sales territories.
■Encourage telephone sales for customers whose business doesn't justify face-to-face visits.

Source: Robert H. Kastengren, Runzheimer & Co., *Sales & Marketing Management,* New York.

How To Design A Car Reimbursement Plan

Reimbursing employees who regularly use their own cars for business travel requires a system that's fair and efficient. Built it around these five elements:

1. Keep the plan simple. Once the plan is set, the only thing the employee must report is actual mileage driven.

2. Reimburse on a formula based on fixed costs for the vehicle, as well as the per-mile cost of driving.

3. Weigh the formula to recognize important cost differences in different drivers' territories (weather conditions, for example).

4. The cost formula should assume that everyone is driving the same car, however, regardless of which cars the drivers may actually choose to drive. This allows employees to choose their own (more expensive) cars if they choose to while the company's low-cost fleet operation is preserved.

5. Update the allowances and reexamine the formula regularly.

Source: *Survey and Analysis of Business Car Policies and Costs,* Runzheimer and Co., Inc., Rochester, WI.

Part V

**THE GREAT BOOK
OF BUSINESS SECRETS**

Personnel Administration & Labor Relations

Chapter 54
Successful Interviewing

Better Interviewing—Better Hiring

Two out of three employees are either underqualified or overqualified for their jobs. The situation not only leads to rapid employee turnover but is costly in terms of an interviewer's time, agency fees, preemployment physicals, possible relocation costs as well as training time.

To address this problem, interviews should:

Clarify any confusion in the application, for instance, years not accounted for.

■Test the truthfulness of the applicant to the extent possible. (Do oral responses coincide with the information that is written on the job application or resume?)

■Evaluate the personality of the candidate in terms of the job to be filled.

■Explain the job's requirements. Include any conditions of employment.

■Make the applicant eager to work for the company.

Some interviews fail because the person conducting them does not:

■Establish rapport with the applicant.

■Question the responsibilities of the applicant's past and present jobs enough.

■Adequately explain the prospective job to the applicant, including skills, work environment, and responsibilities.

■Determine what the applicant has been paid to do and is capable of doing.

■Maintain objectivity whether or not the candidate is likable.

A realistic assessment distinguishes what is ideally desired from what is in fact required. For example, does the candidate really need a college degree in order to do the job?

Interviewing basics:

■Make the applicant feel comfortable. Establish trust. Interview in an informal atmosphere where the interviewer devotes full attention to the applicant and is not distracted by phone calls or other interruptions.

■Use nondirective questioning. After an applicant has answered a question, the interviewer should pause to give the applicant time to fill the silence vacuum. The interviewer can then observe when the candidate is not giving a pat answer to an expected question.

■Ask why the candidate is seeking the job. Encourage the applicant to ask questions about the company, future advancement, colleagues, etc.

■Tell the applicant to expect feedback within a given time, whether hired or not.

References:

A previous employer is required only to answer questions about an applicant's work record. A company that catches an employee stealing cannot legally divulge that information if it does not prosecute the worker. Since the company will often give the employee the choice of being prosecuted or resigning, the application may show the person left a previous job voluntarily. And a reference check will only confirm it. The interviewer must then follow up by asking if the company would rehire the former employee.

To get qualitative information from a previous employer, interviewers must establish a friendly, nonthreatening conversational tone. Next, seek confirmation of observations rather than answers to specific questions

Use Résumés To Ask Better Interview Questions

Résumés are the best sources of questions to ask job applicants during an interview. Instead of asking a series of stock questions that may or may not elicit substantive answers, carefully review a candidate's resume to find guidance in framing questions that can yield important information.

Highlight parts of the resume you wish to explore further. Read a part of the résumé to the applicant, and then ask the pertinent questions. Focus on the applicant's achievements when using the résumé as a questioning guide. These are areas candidates should be most comfortable about expanding on.

Added opportunity: Many candidates have more than one résumé. Each is tailored to the kind of job the candidate is considered for. This is not necessarily deceptive. It's done to enable the interviewer to more easily focus on attributes being sought for the particular job. However, valuable qualities are often left out when writing new versions of a résumé. Simply ask the candidate if he/she has another résumé which reveals attributes not included in the one you received. By reviewing other versions, you might learn that the candidate really is the right person. Or, you might find that there's simply too much irrelevant experience in his/her background.

Source: Robert Half, Robert Half International, 111 Pine St., San Francisco 94111.

Mistakes People Make Interviewing People

Even managers with years of experience in interviewing sometimes make terrible hiring mistakes. Reason: They haven't focused on all of the many common interviewing mistakes.

■Mistake: Not taking notes at each interview. Taking notes reduces the risk that the interviewer will overlook the best candidate, who may have been one of the first ones interviewed.

■Mistake: Overlooking either ability or willingness to do the job. These are the two most important attributes of job candidates. No matter how qualified people are, if they're lazy, what good will they be? On the other hand, a person may be willing to work, but may lack the ability.

■Mistake: Giving interviewees answers to key questions. Example: In interviewing an accountant, the interviewer says, "Budgets are very important in this job. Do you have a good background in budgets?" It's a rare applicant who would not answer, "Yes." Better: Ask the candidate to tell what he/she knows about budgets.

■Mistake: Losing control of the interview. An interview often becomes a maneuver for control between the candidate and the interviewer—since all the books on interviewing teach job candidates how to take control. Interviewers must keep control by digging into the candidate's answers to questions. Probe for answers of greater depth. An interviewer should not move on until the question has been satisfactorily answered.

Useful: Before the interview, review the candidate's résumé once more. Prepare questions to ask about points in the résumé. Aim: To make sure the candidate understands what he/she wrote in the résumé.

■Mistake: Not testing the candidate's communication skills. The ability to communicate well is an important aspect of most jobs. One way to test is to ask candidates to explain some technical jargon from their current jobs that they use during the interview.

■Mistake: Hiring a person who is not interested in some parts of his/her current job, or company. Measure the level of job interest by asking the interviewee questions such as, "What excites you most about your job?" or, "Tell me something about your best client." Look for insight and enthusiasm in the answers.

■Mistake: Prehiring. All too often, a candidate is hired before sitting down. The applicant looks right, and the résumé and references are perfect. At this point, interviewers should take a step back and force themselves to make the candidate prove that he/she is perfect for the job.

Don't base hiring decisions on stereotypes. Just because a person looks like a good accountant, doesn't mean the candidate actually is. To avoid hiring based on stereotypes, do a first brief interview over the telephone.

■Mistake: Having departing employees conduct the interviews for their replacements. This is almost always a mistake. The departing employees will tend to want to hire candidates not quite as strong as they are. And, their hidden agenda is to keep the door wide open in case their new job doesn't work out.

■Mistake: Failing to check references. It's important to check references no matter how highly recommended a candidate is. In an independent survey we commissioned, 40% of the respondents said they would lie to their friends to help someone get a job. Former employers may feel sorry for an employee they fired and will cover up the reasons for termination to help that person get a new job.

One of the best ways to check references is to network. Ask the person whose name has been given by the candidate to give the name of another person who might give a reference.

The higher up in the organization the reference is, the more candid the reference will be. The chairman of the board is less likely to be nervous about giving a reference than an assistant in the personnel department.

In checking references, look for enthusiastic responses.

Point: Tell candidates that their references will be thoroughly checked. This will eliminate some people who have shaky references—they'll generally call to say they've found another job.

Source: Robert Half, Robert Half International, Inc. He is the author of *Robert Half on Hiring*, New American Library, 1633 Broadway, New York 10019.

Questions You Can't Ask A Job Candidate —And How To Get The Answers

Five questions to avoid: 1. What is your religion? 2. Do you have school-age children? 3. How long have you been living at your current address? 4) Are you married? 5. Were you ever arrested?

What to ask instead: 1. Will there be any problems, if you have work on a weekend? 2. Are there any reasons why you might not be able to make an overnight business trip? 3. What is your address? 4. Defer questions on marital status until after the employee has been hired. Then they are completely proper if asked in connection with such purposes as insurance, etc. 5. Were you ever convicted of a felony? (Ask only if the question is job-related.)

Source: Hunt Personnel, Ltd., New York.

The Art Of Checking References

Fear of lawsuits now makes former employers extremely wary of saying anything critical of ex-employees. Result: Reference checks reveal little more than where the applicant was employed, for how long and job title.

Recommended: Arrange face-to-face meetings with references when filling senior-management jobs. Reason: The facial expression and tone of voice give important clues. Plus: As rapport builds, answers become more truthful.

Trap: Phony references can easily be arranged. One common ploy: A believable story is told about how the previous boss is always traveling, but the applicant suggests phoning him away from the office and gives a number. Result: A glowing recommendation from an impersonator. Rule to follow: The reference must be called at the office of the company.

Fail-safe measure: Verify educational credentials, professional memberships and honors. Someone who lies in these areas is probably not telling the truth about more important matters. It takes time and often must be done in writing on firm's letterhead.

Protection: A preemployment investigation by a private firm. It is essential for anyone handling company funds.

Safeguards: Hire everyone contingent on a full reference check. State on the application form that falsifying information is grounds for dismissal.

Source: Robert Half, president, Robert Half, Inc., executive recruiters, New York.

■Ask a candidate for at least six references. Check the three at the bottom of the list. These are more likely to offer a balanced assessment of the person than the top three names.

Source: *Recruiting and Selecting Profitable Sales Personnel*, by Edgar S. Ellman, CBI Publishing Co.

■Avoid vague questions that can be met with equally vague answers. Example: What kind of guy is Ed? Instead, ask for concrete instances of what Ed did. Example: For a marketing director applicant, ask: What was Ed's contribution to any new products put out during his tenure?

■Listen carefully to the former supervisor's tone of voice over the phone. Hesitations or false heartiness may be warning signs, but do not jump to this conclusion. Many managers are unused to giving recommendations and they respond awkwardly.

■Do not settle for a reference from the personnel department. It knows almost nothing about the applicant's day-to-day performance.

■For key positions: Take the reference source to lunch, if possible. Frankness is likelier in a face-to-face situation. Do not solicit references by letter or request written responses.

■Double-check an overly negative response to a reference call. Reason: The supervisor may personally dislike the applicant.

Source: Harry Daviod, principal, H. D. Associates, recruiters, Washington, DC.

Chapter 55
Hiring And Firing Wisdom

Employee Referrals

Use incentives to get the company's work force to become a good source of new personnel. Give a referring employee a bonus of 5% of what the newly hired employee earns during the first 13 weeks on the job.

Some guidelines may be necessary to make the program feasible. Job applicants must show up for the first interview with a note of introduction from the employee (the personnel department can prepare cards for the purpose). No bonus is paid unless the new worker proves satisfactory and stays on the job at least 13 weeks. Consider restricting the plan to a limited number of hard-to-fill jobs, for maximum cost-effectiveness, with minimum fuss.

Take note that the Equal Employment Opportunity Commission has said that filling jobs by employee referrals tends to perpetuate the existing racial balance of the work force. But there should be no problem where minorities and women are already employed and where employee referrals are the exclusive way to recruit.

How To Avoid Errors In Hiring

Many mistakes in hiring employees are obvious and can be avoided easily, specifically: failing to describe jobs adequately to prospective candidates, hiring overly qualified people. Other mistakes, however, are often difficult to avoid.

■Too little information in help wanted ads. Include required skills, duties, type of business and location, benefits, advancement opportunities and name of specific person to contact.

■Failure to prescreen applicants before scheduling interviews can result in time wasted interviewing unsuitable candidates, while good prospects are overlooked.

■Inadequate interviewing. This is a task for someone with plenty of skill and time. Interviewers should explain the interview purpose and company policies and encourage applicants to ask questions. They should not ask for information which may be negative without first allowing the applicants to establish their strengths.

■Unchecked references. This applies especially to those who claim success in previous jobs.

■Rejection because the applicant might not stay a long time. Good employees benefit the company even in short stays.

■Delays in making the hiring decision. If an applicant is going to be rejected anyway, the company should use its time to find other prospects. If the applicant is going to be hired, delay cuts productivity.

■Hiring friends or relatives who are not qualified. A uniform hiring policy boosts morale among those employed.

Source: Alan Leighton, vice-president, Cole Associates, management consultants, Short Hills, NJ.

How To Hire The Right People ...And Keep Them

Turnover is very expensive to a company, particularly fast turnover. The best way to keep turnover costs down is to hire the right people in the first place. Smart hiring techniques act as a kind of insurance...

■Hire from within the company—whenever you can. It's safer to promote people you know than to hire people you don't know. Current employees have known qualities—you don't have to check their references. You know they're loyal, reliable and honest. These qualities can more than make up for any lack of experience that an employee may have. Extra benefit: Hiring from within encourages other employees to stay with the firm. It shows them that there are opportunities for advancement.

■Pay enough. You get better people if you pay just a little bit more for the job than the prevailing salary. People who are being paid relatively well are reluctant to quit, and they often give even more work than the extra pay calls for.

■Look for loyalty. You want an employee who will give you consistently honest time and effort. The last thing you want is employees who take trade secrets with them when they leave, or raid a department for other employees. When you interview job candidates, look for signs of potential disloyalty. Never hire a person who is willing to divulge confidential information about his present company. Never hire people who are eager to leave without giving proper notice. Never hire people who promise to bring their whole department with them. People who are willing to be disloyal to their past employers could just as easily make you the victim of their disloyalty.

■Find nice people. It's always best to hire someone who will have no trouble getting along with other employees. (You're not likely to fire someone you really like.) If you bring a difficult person into the company, you'll immediately have an adverse reaction from current employees. Sooner or later, one or the other will go, either the disruptive newcomer or loyal, long-time employees. Take your pick.

■Don't clone yourself. It's tempting to hire a person with the same education and training as you have, but you're generally better off getting someone with a different background. If you hire for diversity, you'll get more creative thinking and a cross-section of ideas. When you hire people who look alike and think alike, you'll ultimately find yourself with too many voids, and a need to hire more people.

■Find out what you need to know at the interview. If the interviewer isn't capable of asking the technical questions that must be asked of job candidates, get the department head involved in the hiring process. Be persistent in questioning candidates. If you're looking for hard workers, be sure to find out whether the candidates fit that description. Pump them. Ask them to describe instances that required them to work late. Ask for details. How late? When did you get home? How often did it happen? Find out what you need to know.

■Careful reference-checking. It's imperative to check references, even those of job candidates who come to you highly recommended. The son or daughter of a friend might be under indictment for securities fraud. The friend won't tell you. You won't find out until its too late—unless you check the candidate's references.

Source: Robert Half, Robert Half International, Inc. Mr. Half is author of *Robert Half on Hiring*, Crown Publishers, 225 Park Ave. South, New York 10003.

Secrets Of Much Better Firing

Most managers, sooner or later, must fire an employee, either because of performance problems, organizational downsizing or for another reason. It's important to carefully think through a termination before proceeding.

Most firings are emotionally charged for all parties and, if not handled sensitively, they can produce intense anger and anxiety.

The best way: Handle firings just like any other business decision. Plan them carefully and carry them out methodically.

Planning Ahead

When planning a large staff reduction, start to plan for it three to six months in advance. Make sure you have a solid performance appraisal system in place that will help you identify the weakest performers.

Always consider the possible effects of a firing on the remaining employees. Whenever you terminate one person, the rest of the staff's morale is affected. It's a big problem if the staff feels the firing was unfair.

Prepare to meet with remaining staff and discuss their future with the company. Otherwise, rumors will spread and valued employees will lose confidence in the organization…and start sending their resumes out.

On The Day Of Termination

■Plan a 10–15 minute meeting—at most. Use a prepared statement that explains to the individual exactly what is happening and why. Avoid restating the same points. This can be very damaging to the employee.

■Avoid prefacing a firing with small talk. Don't ask, "How was the football game this weekend?" Don't even say, "Good morning." Prolonging the task simply worsens the awkwardness. Best: "Please sit down. I have some bad news for you." Then get right into it. Example: "I'm going to have to let you go from the company," or, "I'm going to have to terminate your services."

■Avoid ambiguity. Flawed statements: "This doesn't seem to be working out…I think we might have to think about terminating you." Stick to your statement. It may sound cold and calculating, but it's much better than rambling or making mistakes.

■Don't make promises you can't keep. Don't say, "I can help you get a new job, I know some people." If you do know of some opportunity within or outside the organization, hold back with the information until you have made absolutely sure that you can deliver.

■Prepare for attempts to go over your head. Make sure the employee understands that the decision has been reviewed by management, and that there's no recourse.

■Prepare for a variety of responses. Don't become defensive if the employee becomes angry. Anger begins the healing process.

Of greater concern is the controlled response. For example, the employee says, "No problem. I expected it to happen. I'll live." That may be a false front or simple denial. Probe to make sure the person really understands what's happening, that he has so many days left of employment, that there is a severance package, etc.

The shocked response may be the most difficult to deal with. The person looks at you, but doesn't really respond—or cries a little. This employee needs to be watched closely, and the company should be prepared to help him get further counseling.

Source: William Morin, chairman and chief executive officer, Drake Beam Morin, Inc., a leading outplacement firm, 100 Park Ave., New York 10017, and co-author of *Dismissal*, available from DBM Publishing.

How To Fire People

Firing does not get easier with practice. Some consolation: Employees usually expect it by the time it is necessary. Most will understand your position. Basics:

■Do it in person. The person being fired deserves to hear the painful news from the highest-ranking person he or she reports to. This is a situation where a surrogate just does not do. Pink slips or other impersonal notification leave a backwash of trouble.

■Do not drag it out. Start off by stating the facts with an air of finality: "John, I have to tell you we won't be needing your services any more."

■Be supertactful. Give the employee some truthful explanation that he or she can live with: "This department has been losing money for two years."

■Have separation material at hand. Be prepared to tell the employee exactly what benefits are due. If there is separation pay or a final check have it ready to hand over on the spot. Be as generous as possible, but be firm and final. Where the company would be willing to pay for executive outplacement, offer the alternative or cash instead.

■Move the person out fast. A departing employee becomes a disturbance to the ongoing business.

■Watch your comments to other employees. If you cannot say something nice about the person, do not say anything at all. Chances are there will still be social contacts between current and dismissed employees.

■Analyze what went wrong. Surveys show that top executives think the supervisor is to blame when someone has to be fired. Ask what led to hiring the wrong person in the first place and what can be done to prevent the same thing from happening again.

Source: Robert Half, president, Robert Half International, New York, and author of *The Robert Half Way to Get Hired in Today's Job Market*, Rawson Wade Publishers.

■Friday has always been a convenient day to fire an employee. But over the weekend, when little can be done about the situation, an employees thoughts may turn to retaliation. Instead: Fire employees early in the week. Then the individual can immediately begin looking for another job.

What To Ask Yourself Before Firing Anyone

■In what ways has the employee failed?

■Is part of the failure the company's fault? Has management tried hard enough to help the worker overcome problems?

■Has the company given enough credit to the employee when tasks were well done?

■Is a replacement likely to do much better?

■What will be the reaction of employees who have been associated with the worker? How will that reaction affect the company?

■Has the worker shown interest in another area?

■Could the investment in the employee be salvaged by transfer to other work?

■Will it be troublesome if a talented and trained person winds up working for a competitor?

Legal Perils To Avoid When Firing

Businesses are in the midst of a genuine revolution, as far as employment laws are concerned. At no time in our history have employees had so many opportunities to challenge management for alleged abuses...and at no time have they been more willing to take advantage of their rights.

The new climate is especially turbulent in the area of termination. There are dozens of traps waiting to spring shut on companies that think they can tell just any worker to clean out his desk by five o'clock.

The Biggest Pitfalls

Almost all courts now take the view that it's unlawful to fire an employee solely for exercising his legal rights. Examples:

■Asking for time to serve on a jury.

■Filing a workers compensation claim or a complaint with the state wage and hour board.

■Refusing to commit an impropriety, such as falsifying documentation that will be submitted to a court or regulatory agency.

Some courts have gone even further: They now hold that in some cases it's unlawful to fire a worker who refuses to commit an act that may be perfectly legal, but which nevertheless goes against public policy, at least in the eyes of the court.

Example: A hospital worker protested that there wasn't enough staff on duty for a particular shift, and to dramatize his protest he eventually walked off the job. The hospital discharged him. A court later ruled that the discharge was illegal, reasoning that the worker acted in the interest of public policy to protect hospital patients.

Compounding the problem for companies: Public policy hasn't yet been clearly defined, and courts in each of the 50 states have their own interpretations.

The no-win reality: A company can, for example, be fined millions of dollars in punitive damages for unlawfully firing a worker who makes only $25,000 a year. Even if the company wins, the cost of litigation can be immense.

Though public policy cases create a legal minefield for companies, there are safeguards to reduce the chances of being hurt. Recommended:

■Prevent any manager, even the CEO, from having the unilateral power to fire an employee.

■When a manager decides someone must be fired, the decision should be reviewed by the company's labor counsel and human resources director. These professionals must make sure that there's adequate documentation to justify the discharge. The last thing they should have to do is hunt for documentation after the fired worker has sued for unlawful discharge.

Further Preventive Measures

■Require the company's lawyers to keep the human resources department abreast of court decisions in states where the business operates. In general, courts are extending protection to workers, and without knowledge of new precedents, companies are increasingly vulnerable.

■Pay special attention to performance reviews. They're usually the first line of defense in a termination case. But supervisors typically fall into two traps. They either...1. include remarks in the performance reviews that can be used as evidence of prejudice, or 2. write only glowing reviews about less-than-glowing workers who, when fired, cite the documentation of their good performance review as evidence of their unlawful dismissal.

Helpful: Let the company's labor lawyer spot-check performance reviews.

■Provide managers with courses in termination law...then periodically offer sessions to update them with the latest court decisions. These sessions don't have to be formal. They can be lunch meetings with an attorney or human resources consultant.

And The Traps Continue...

■Discrimination. I've never met a supervisor who says he wants to fire someone because the worker is Hispanic or pregnant or over 50. But companies get into trouble in this area because they don't apply their discharge procedures consistently.

The issue is important because the 1964 Civil Rights Act outlaws firing on the basis of color, national origin, race, religion or sex. A later law adds age to the list. In addition, companies are now vulnerable to a suit if a worker has reason to believe he was discharged because he was close to having his pension vested.

Safeguard: Be prepared to demonstrate—in writing—that company policy was followed...and that the company has acted consistently in firing both workers protected by federal law and those not protected. Example: There should be no difference between procedures used to fire a young white male and a 60-year-old black woman...or between company procedures in firing those near pension vesting and those who are years away.

Detailed documentation is the company's key protection here. Record each step of the termination process, to prove consistency in the firing policy.

■Defamation. In firing a worker, companies often make accusations they can't prove, such as, "He was a chronic liar." The accusations can come up during the discharge, in statements made in front of other employees...or later, when a prospective employer calls for references. Safeguards:

■Be able to prove everything said or written about the termination...and periodically remind supervisors of the need for documented proof.

■If you're called for a reference, either decline to give details of a termination, or phone the person back after checking with a lawyer.

■Consider asking discharged employees for a release that permits you to talk freely with his prospective employers.

■Handbooks. Typical mistakes: The handbook says workers are subject to dismissal for any of, say, 10 reasons. But if an employee is fired for any other reason, he may have a good unlawful discharge case against the company. Or, the handbook may say that discharge is preceded by an oral warning, written warning and suspension. If a worker is then fired on the spot for gross insubordination, he may also have a good case.

Safeguard: In addition to the preventive steps mentioned earlier, ask lawyers acquainted with the latest discharge decisions to review company handbooks, manuals and disciplinary procedures. Attorneys should also make sure the procedures are consistent with actions the company has actually taken.

Source: Michael Lotito, labor law specialist, Jackson, Lewis, Schnitzler & Krupman, 525 Market St., San Francisco 94105.

Chapter 56

Discrimination Traps

Legal Traps In Saying "No"

■Don't confuse job experience with personal qualifications. For example, the requisites for a receptionist don't have to be previous work experience, or any work at all. But the person should have the right personality traits, such as neatness, a friendly manner, clear speech, and so on, to deal with the public.

Don't tell a rejected applicant for an unskilled job that you need someone with more job experience. A women rejected by a department store because of "lack of experience" as a clerk sued the store after they hired a woman who had no more job experience. Court testimony revealed that the claimant was turned down because she seemed immature and made a poor impression during the interview. The judge awarded damages. A better course would be to tell the applicant that another candidate has personal qualifications more suited to the job.

If the circumstances are not favorable for a pleasant interview, ask the applicant to come back another time. One Hispanic applicant, who showed up late in the day, tired from job-hunting, was interviewed by a person who was distracted with other business. A court held that, in this unfavorable atmosphere, race may have been a contributing factor in the decision not to hire her.

Persons applying for entrance-level jobs usually have little experience in being interviewed. Make allowances for this.

Source: 21FEP Cases 1664.

The Law And Hiring Former Drug Addicts

The pervasive use of drugs in today's society means that most companies will have to deal with drug use among current or former employees and job applicants. The laws governing the management of these individuals are stringent...

Reformed drug addicts, including those who are still under treatment, are legally considered to be handicapped, or disabled, under both federal law and the laws of most states. This means that they are protected, by law, against discrimination. They're in the same category as minorities, women and other protected classes.

Employers can't refuse to hire former drug addicts solely on the grounds of their disability. Nor can employers discriminate against former drug addicts in any way once they are hired.

Examples of practices that would be considered discriminatory...

■Imposing special security clearance requirements on former drug addicts.

■Barring them access to classified documents.

■Singling them out for drug testing.

Former drug addicts must be treated like other employees unless the company has a reason for restricting their activities other than the fact that they were drug users.

Where past drug use is suspected, employers should be careful to document any problems they have with the employee. Detailed records should be kept of disciplinary action.

Purpose: To show, if a discrimination suit is ever brought, that the company had a good business reason for taking action against the employee and treated the employee in a way consistent with company policy and practice.

Job Interview Trap

It is unlawful, in many states, for an employer to ask prospective employees if they have ever had a drug problem. Employers are prohibited from asking, either directly or indirectly, about an applicant's disabilities, except where the disability has a direct effect on the applicant's ability to perform the job in question.

Notes referring to an employee's former drug problem should not be part of the employee's personnel file. If notes are left in the file, a court could infer that the information was used to affect an employment decision. That would be discriminatory.

Drug Testing

While it would be legally risky to test only former drug addicts for drug use, absent a state statute to the contrary, in most instances, private employers are not prohibited from giving all employees pre-employment or random on-the-job drug tests.

However, some states—New York, for example—take the position that requiring pre-employment physicals of any kind, including drug testing, is prohibited except where there is a bona fide occupational qualification, such as driving ability for applicants for jobs as school bus drivers. New York's position is currently in litigation and may not hold.

Source: Stuart H. Bompey, partner, Baer, Marks & Upham, specialists in employment litigation, 805 Third Ave., New York 10022.

New Age Discrimination Law

The Older Workers Benefit Protection Act (OWBPA), which was signed into law in late 1990, amends the 1967 Age Discrimination in Employment Act (ADEA).

Main purpose of the new act: To eliminate confusion in the ADEA legislation concerning older workers' rights to the same benefits as younger workers.

Additionally, OWBPA contains important new provisions governing management's conduct in asking employees to waive their rights under ADEA to sue their employers on grounds of age discrimination. Most courts applying the ADEA decided that companies could ask employees to waive their rights in exchange for receiving additional compensation, such as severance pay or an early retirement incentive. But the conditions under which such waivers could be signed by employees were unclear, and many lawsuits arose concerning whether the agreement waiving the employees' rights was a "knowing and voluntary" one. OWBPA now clears up the confusion by spelling out the minimum requirements for a valid waiver.

To avoid the risk of future litigation, companies that ask their employees to sign such voluntary waivers must be sure that they use a procedure that adheres to these new minimum standards. The waiver must...

■Be part of a written agreement.

■Be written in a manner calculated to be understood by the individual waiving his/her rights.

■Specifically refer to rights arising under the ADEA and only release rights or claims in existence at the time of signing.

■Be signed after the employer has advised the employee in writing to consult with an attorney before signing the agreement.

■Be given in exchange for some consideration in addition to anything of value to which the employee is otherwise entitled.

■Have been signed only if the employee had been expressly given at least 21 days to consider the waiver.

■Provide that the employee may revoke the agreement up to seven days after signing.

In addition, when the waiver is part of an exit incentive or group termination program, the employee must be given 45 days to consider the agreement. The employee must also be given information concerning program requirements, time limits, job titles and ages of all eligible individuals and the ages of all individuals in the same job classification who are ineligible.

Source: John P. Furfaro, special counsel, and Maury B. Josephson, associate, Skadden, Arps, Slate, Meagher & Flom, 919 Third Ave., New York 10022.

Avoiding Discrimination Problems

Good intentions and affirmative action programs notwithstanding, it's easy to fall into traps that can lead to government investigations, lawsuits, and big settlements to "wronged" employees for back pay.

Biggest pitfalls: Outmoded job descriptions, discriminatory pay scales, and hiring/promotion standards that stem from them. Government investigators looking into alleged equal pay law violations don't go by company descriptions.

You should be sure to take the following steps:

■Update descriptions (and adjust pay scales) at least once a year. Spell out each job individually as it's actually being done, focusing on functions, percentage of working time spent on each, quantitative and qualitative output and performance requirements (units produced, documents typed, employees supervised, etc.).

■Avoid lumping "similar" but different jobs in a single category. Machine jobs vary substantially depending on equipment used. Secretaries don't just "handle" correspondence; they type form letters, take dictation, or answer routine correspondence themselves.

■Test hiring and promotion qualifications for relevance to the job as it's now being done.

■If a promotion is offered and it is declined, thank the employee in writing and invite the worker to reconsider. Reason: This proves the employer made an affirmative effort.

Chapter 57
Hiring And Firing Executives

Mistakes To Avoid In Hiring Key Executives

Most companies spend too little time defining what they want in a new key executive and preparing the way for the recruited executive's entry and smooth integration into the firm.

The first essential step is to assess the existing management's strengths and weaknesses honestly. Define what aspects of top management the newcomer should either complement or counterpoint.

Common mistakes to avoid:

■Failing to inform employees that a search is going on to fill a top slot. Instead, prepare people on the inside when someone new is coming. That defuses jealousies and the sense of being passed over. The danger of secrecy is that some good key employees may become apprehensive or discontented enough to leave. Before beginning a search, tell inside executives that they are not quite ready for the higher position, but top management is keeping an open mind and, quite possibly, after looking at outside candidates the company may conclude that the choice should be made from within.

■Failing to spend enough social time with the outside prospect before hiring. Top managers must get beyond superficial good chemistry with a candidate. That can only be done over time. Arrange a weekend breakfast with a prospect, play tennis, go sailing, have dinner a number of times. Meet the prospect's spouse over dinner and determine how he or she feels about the move to another company, or a relocation.

■Propelling a new executive straight into a division or even corporate presidency without a period of testing and adjustment. The ideal situation would be to bring a new key executive aboard for six months in a visible but understudy position. Natural leaders and high-caliber managers will be recognized as such and their skills will be sought out by others in the company. It's not easy to get a top-notch executive to leave a company for a situation where he will be offered a top job only after he proves out. One way to do it is to make the contract terms especially attractive.

■Failing to check references carefully. Most people at the top tend to give positive references. It's important to be alert to anything less. Watch for neutral remarks, they are an important warning signal. Probe further.

■Promoting a new executive into a higher-level position than he had at the former company. The new executive must learn a great deal, besides having to adjust to the new company. This makes the risk of failure higher. Incoming key executives should have more experience than is actually required for the immediate job.

■Not being willing to pay the market price for the best person. Excellent executives are never available at bargain prices. You get what you pay for.

Source: Millington McCoy, Gould & McCoy, executive search consultants, New York.

Objectively Evaluating Top-Management Candidates

Bringing in an outsider to fill a top-management position in the company is always a delicate task. The most common mistake companies make in such recruiting is to select the manager too hurriedly from three or four candidates introduced by a recruiter or identified as prospects by company managers.

Consider using a professional consultant or other person familiar with the company and its top managers to help match the job with a prospect.

The most important task for the consultant is to assess the duties of the job and the important relationships in the company with which the newcomer will have to deal. Against that assessment, evaluate each candidate in terms of those requirements developed by the job analysis.

Let the consultant know why the position is available, and also tell the consultant what happened to the last person who held the position.

Source: David Goodrich, Ph.D., consultant, Rohrer, Hibler & Replogle, Inc., Stamford, CT.

How To Fire A Key Executive

If the firing of high-level executives isn't handled correctly, the consequences can be troublesome—with the fired executive taking customers with him. And, a bad departure will disrupt other managers.

Prepare for the departure—well in advance of the firing—by using other employees to back up the manager in his dealings with important customers.

Example: If the manager is the only person dealing with a key customer, start sending a lower-ranked employee out to assist the executive. In reality this assistant is there to develop his own relationship with the client.

If the executive who is being fired has a mentor, it's a good idea to discuss the situation with him before the firing. The mentor may know facts about customers or even about the executive's personal life that will make the termination easier.

Severance Guidelines

A termination shouldn't be designed as punishment. An adequate termination package will support the person until he finds a new position. An unfairly low severance package simply gives the fired manager a reason to hurt the company if he ever has a chance. Guidelines:

■Six month's to one year's salary. That may seem too liberal, but it can well take that long for a senior executive to find a new position.

■Continuation of health insurance until a new job is found, up to one year.

■Professional outplacement assistance.

■Use of office space, secretarial services and a short-term travel allowance.

Keep the termination interview short—no more that 10–15 minutes—and to the point. Explain to the executive:

■That the decision is final.

■What he'll get in benefits and reemployment assistance. It's useful to follow up an oral explanation with a letter that spells out the details.

■That it's best to clean out his desk after business hours.

Then introduce the outplacement consultant. Turning the terminated executive over to the person who will assist him in developing his next situation ends the interview on a positive note.

Firing Myths

■It's wrong to fire on Friday. This supposedly avoids giving the terminated executive a weekend to brood over the firing. Reality: There are no weekends until a new position is found.

■Letting the manager work for a few more weeks makes the termination less painful. In reality, it's foolish to squeeze a few extra weeks of work from a person whose mind ought to be on finding another job. It also gives him false hope that the decision will be reconsidered.

■A termination is always the executive's fault. In reality, only 17% of top managers are fired because they are no longer productive. In most cases, the company is equally at fault. Blaming the individual only makes the executive more bitter toward the company.

Source: E. Donald Davis, senior vice-president, Right Associates, Inc. outplacement consultants, 640 Fifth Ave., New York 10019.

One Way To Replace Veteran Managers

Problem: A company has a long-time employee whose work is as good as it ever was, but now falls below standard because the rest of the company has moved ahead. The company wants to replace the manager in his job. But there's no obvious place to transfer him. And there are no clear grounds to fire him.

Solution: Offer the manager a consulting job for three or four years at half his previous pay. The company thereby lives up to its obligations to the veteran, while replacing him, and still gets the benefits of his long experience with the company. The veteran gets some work and a base from which he can pick up other consulting clients.

Source: Sherman Lurie, director of marketing, Cadence Industries, West Caldwell, NJ.

Compulsory Retirement At 65 Is Possible

Executives and high policy-making employees with retirement plan benefits of $27,000 a year or more can be forced to retire at age 65 (instead of age 70) under federal law.

New EEOC regulations, under Sections 12(c) and 12(d) of the Age Discrimination in Employment Act, limit the exemption to top-level executives and to high-policy-making employees who play a significant role in the development and implementation of corporate policy. They must be in such a position at least two years immediately before retirement.

The $27,000-or-more pension has to be made available within 60 days of retirement and be unconditional during retirement. Retirement income from Social Security, employee contributions, and prior employers cannot be included in the $27,000. But plan payments in lump sum or in some other form, whose value equals the cost of a single life annuity yielding at least $27,000, qualify.

A legal alternative to forced retirement may be a lesser, or part-time, position, if accepted by the employee.

Source: David L. Hewitt, vice-president, Hay Huggins, Philadelphia.

Tax-Free Severance Pay

In times when top executives can lose their jobs any day, it is more important than ever that any severance or termination payments receive the most favorable tax treatment possible. Key: Severance pay is taxable as ordinary salary. But payments made to compensate the ex-employee for damages are tax-free.

The dismissed employee can bring suit against his former company in court, or before a federal agency (such as the Equal Employment Opportunity Commission), alleging that he suffered damages as a result of his wrongful dismissal. (The dismissal may have harmed his business or personal reputation, caused embarrassment or resulted in physical or emotional harm.)

The objective: A settlement can be reached with the company that allocates part of the termination payment as compensation for harm. What would have been *taxable severance pay* is converted into *tax-free damages*. Extra benefit: The company can profit from this sort of agreement as well. Since it is paying its former employee in tax-free dollars, it may be able to negotiate a smaller settlement that gives the employee more in the end.

Chapter 58
Handling Layoffs

Reducing The Work Force In Hard Times

Periods of economic downturn provide a good opportunity to eliminate over-staffing that has crept into company operations during good times. In many cases, companies find they can cut staffing by 20% more than required by scaling back of operations and still maintain the same production level.

To do it, don't make seniority the exclusive determinant of who is kept on and who is laid off or fired. Instead, use rules violation records and poor-performance evaluations to weed out ineffective workers. Make exceptions for very talented younger employees who are likely to become major assets to the company in the future. (Many union contracts allow management to exempt about 10% of the work force from seniority-based protocol for layoffs.)

Don't scrap seniority considerations completely, even where possible. Such a policy will weaken morale. Employees expect the company to show loyalty to veteran workers. Any indication that their future may be in jeopardy will cause some good employees to desert the company at the first opportunity.

Other considerations in implementing a cutback include moving swiftly and making the cutback criteria clear. Uncertainty breeds rumors that the worst is yet to come, and erodes productivity as employees spend time worrying—or looking for other jobs. Tell laid-off workers approximately when they'll be rehired.

The Importance Of Minimizing Layoffs

Management has traditionally seen layoffs as the quickest way to cut costs in a recession. That can now be considered a partially counterproductive strategy, especially in view of antidiscrimination laws and the existence of the Equal Employment Opportunity Commission.

Firings should actually be viewed as a last resort. In fact, laying off large numbers of employees is often more expensive than carrying them along for a few months.

Real layoff costs:
- Severance pay, typically a week's wages for each year of service.
- Accrued vacation time.
- Pension vesting.
- Higher unemployment insurance in the future.
- Programs to help fired employees to relocate or adjust.
- Antidiscrimination-suit liability.
- Future recruiting and training.

■Delays in gearing up for the upcoming cycle.

After adding up these costs, companies will realize that there are many options:

■Cut staff by attrition.

■Extend plant shutdowns.

■Reschedule vacations to coincide with the slowdown.

■Postpone pay increases and reduce fringe benefits.

■Cut salaries.

■Share the work load.

■Retire employees early.

A company that's willing to invest time in analyzing its financial position may hit on a cost-cutting system that leaves personnel virtually unscathed.

Best strategies to improve the company's financial position:

■Improve the cash flow by establishing tighter controls, collecting receivables faster, and slowing down payables.

■Improve inventory levels. Stall on purchases and speed up deliveries.

■Consolidate activities by selling off some facilities and reducing fixed charges.

■Revise marketing strategies, perhaps by making short-term cuts in advertising budgets or adopting a new pricing policy.

■Cut overhead items such as training and management programs.

■Monitor expense accounts more closely. Reduce allowances, too.

The potential for a company's success at cost reduction, using these tactics, will depend largely on how well managed it was before. But for nearly all companies, tighter controls and cash management will forestall layoffs for some months.

Capital-intensive companies are, of course, better positioned to trim costs because they can cancel or defer major projects. For labor-intensive companies, the day of reckoning may come much sooner.

After deciding what volume of expenses should be cut, determine how much of it can be accomplished through attrition and encouraging early retirement.

Nonunion companies should zero in on the least-productive and highest-paid employees. Unionized companies should be communicating the problems to union leaders now. This may pave the way for options such as work-sharing. Some states offer partial unemployment benefits to workers on reduced schedules.

Consult lawyers on ways to avoid violating the Equal Employment Opportunity Commission's regulations. Seniority considerations, for instance, may be mandated in union contracts, but using them for layoffs may violate government regulations if women and minorities have been the last hired. Courts now tend to consider the result of layoffs, not the method used to implement them. Regardless of how fair a company's layoff policy might seem, it may be in violation of EEOC regulations if women or minorities are hurt more than others.

Public-relations problems. A company almost always loses some prestige in the community after mass layoffs. The loss may even make it hard to hire workers when times improve.

Make a clear explanation that the survival of the majority of jobs is at stake. On the other hand, a company can chalk up a public relations victory by keeping people on and using them for slack-time projects. Jobs such as reorganizing a warehouse and overhauling files rarely get done when business is booming. Also, use downtime to explore new markets and to develop mid- and long-range plans.

Source: Donald Law, partner, Arthur Young & Co.; James A. Giardina, principal in Arthur Young & Co.

Taking Steps To Retain Skilled Workers

Hiring back skilled workers after a recession layoff is difficult and expensive. The right strategy is to take steps now to keep them on the payroll through the next downturn.

■Promote highly trained employees into the more senior job categories that aren't immediately affected by economic downturns.

■Make plans to move skilled workers into standby jobs or even jobs that aren't essential. Rather than lay off highly skilled employees in its plastics machine-tool division, Cincinnati Milacron recently moved them to its regular machine-tool operation. As a result, it incurred the slight expense of overstaffing, but key workers were still on the payroll when orders revived for the plastics tool division.

■Temporarily transfer some key workers to company branches in areas less affected by recessions. Most workers prefer temporary relocation to being laid off.

■Seek union cooperation to avoid having to lay off apprentices in highly skilled categories.

■Plan a public relations program to cushion the impact of layoffs when they must be made. Bendix Corporation paid for newspaper ads to publicize its efforts to find other jobs for laid-off workers at its Kansas City plant. Workers remained in the area, and when the recession was over, many were eager to go back to work for Bendix.

By keeping skilled workers on the payroll during a downturn, companies help them to maintain seniority. The effort goes a long way toward solving the problem of having to lay off skilled employees with little seniority. In general, companies should work with unions toward a personnel structure where skill and seniority are both important.

Chapter 59
Personnel Policies

Smarter Personnel Policies

Broad statements of company policy and goals are often found in the first few pages of the company's employee manual. When properly worded, these statements can be a useful tool for both the employee and the company. But improperly worded policy statements can be very dangerous.

Trap: Many states hold that an employee manual can be enforced as if it were a contract. Sloppy wording can thus give disgruntled employees powerful ammunition in a lawsuit.

Biggest mistakes companies make in their personnel manuals…

■Using virtuous statements of ethical policy—without realizing such policies may be inappropriate in future cases.

Example: Company A has a written policy stating that it honors the privacy of its employees and will not get involved in their personal lives. Then the company runs into this problem…An employee becomes romantically involved with an official of a competitor. The employee's supervisor, afraid that company secrets will be divulged, tells the employee to end the relationship or quit the job. The employee is fired, sues the company for wrongful discharge and wins. One of her legal arguments is that the company broke its contractual promise to honor her privacy.

Privacy statements can also cause problems if the company wants to search the office or locker of an employee who is suspected of theft—or drug use.

Self-defense: Make it clear in the personnel manual that the company maintains the right to inspect lockers and offices. Also, give employees notice not to store things they would prefer not to be revealed.

Also risky: Stating that employees will be entitled to "fair treatment." Fired employees can use this in court, letting the judge or jury decide whether the company has treated them fairly.

Better: Avoid making well-meaning statements that can be interpreted as giving employees rights. Let policies develop on the job, as situations arise.

■Including statements that can be taken to mean a promise of lifetime employment. Statements about joining the company "family," or statements that imply that employees will be "taken care of" as long as they do their job well can be used as a basis for wrongful-discharge suits. The introductory remarks in a personnel manual should focus on the company's goals, not the security of employees. Key phrase: Use the term "at will" to describe the term of employment—meaning that the term of employment is up to the company.

■Failing to define the employee group that the manual covers. Top executives are generally covered by a different set of policies than rank-and-file workers. But companies often forget to specifically exclude top management from their general employee manuals. Trap: An executive who is fired for political reasons can argue in court that the company didn't follow the progressive discipline procedure laid down in the employee policy manual.

Self-defense: Make it clear that the general manual is for employees up to a certain level and that people above that rank are covered by a different set of rules.

■Committing the company to a policy of progressive discipline. Some offenses are so serious that the company will want to fire an employee on the spot. But if the company has a written policy of progressive discipline, including a warning and a chance to correct the problem, it may not be able to fire an employee outright. It may have to adhere to its announced disciplinary process or face a lawsuit brought by the employee.

■Over-particularizing work rules. It's better to write broad work rules and then develop specific procedures on a case-by-case basis as problems come up. For instance, on the subject of absenteeism, it's best to have a rule that says, "those who are excessively absent can be disciplined, up to and including discharge." A very detailed statement of procedure can lead to trouble. The problem with giving details—such as, "absent X times and you'll be warned, absent X more times and you'll be suspended, etc."—is that some employees will push the policy right up to the limit. They'll be absent all right, but not enough to get fired. With a more general policy, the company has flexibility to deal with the worst first, until it has an absentee rate that's acceptable.

■Carelessly worded severance-pay policies. Trap: The company can be forced to pay severance to an employee who hasn't lost a day's work. This can be triggered when the company is bought out and the employee stays on with the new company. Severance-pay policies must be worded to prevent this from happening.

■Committing the company to give raises every year. It's a mistake to say "your salary will be reviewed once a year for an increase." There may be a time when the company can't give raises. Employees who don't get raises may try to hold the company to the commitment it made in the manual.

Self-defense: Say, "Your salary may be increased" or say, "We will review performance periodically and, when appropriate, offer increases in accordance with your performance and the needs of the company." This gives the company an out when times are bad.

■Failing to include the right to amend written policies. It may be necessary for the company to change the conditions of employment, especially if the economy takes a downturn. There may be no raises, for example. To avoid problems, the company should clearly reserve the right to change its employee policies. This should prevent employees from saying, "I've worked for it and I must get it."

A rule that should be in all personnel manuals...The right to discharge an employee who fails to cooperate with a company investigation.

This gives the company an independent basis for terminating an employee who refuses to cooperate in the investigation of an infraction that could lead to discharge. Employees are not entitled to "plead the fifth" unless an employer gives them that right by inference, or a carelessly worded personnel manual.

Source: Peter M. Panken, chair of the labor and employment law department of Parker Chapin, Flattau & Klimpl, 1211 Ave. of the Americas, New York 10036.

Fair Pregnancy Policies

Many companies still lack a formal policy pertaining to leave for pregnancy.

The federal rule on fair treatment for a pregnant employee has been clear for some time. A pregnant woman is entitled to the same treatment the company offers to any other temporarily disabled employee.

Result: If the company's policy is to hold a job open for two months, or four months for an employee recovering from a heart attack, a back problem or any other disability, a pregnant employee who is disabled is entitled to leave for the same length of time, either paid or unpaid, depending on the company's policy— and with the same job guarantee upon returning.

In addition, federal court decisions have established that pregnant women are entitled to the same or a similar job when they return in some cases. The company can escape from that requirement only if it can demonstrate that it underwent major changes during the employee's leave. This is hard to prove when the woman was away for only two to four months.

State laws may require more leniency toward pregnant employees and the Supreme Court has held that it is not unfair to male employees for women employees to benefit from such laws.

In California, for instance, women who are disabled due to their pregnancy must be offered at least four months unpaid leave.

Congress now has under consideration a parental leave law that would prohibit larger companies in all states from terminating employees who are on disability leave because of pregnancy even when that is their practice for other disabilities.

Overcoming Hardship

Holding a job open for a key employee even for only two months can create big problems for companies with sparse backup resources. They must do it, however, or face the threat of a discrimination suit. About 3,600 pregnancy-related complaints are filed with the Federal Equal Employment Opportunity Commission each year and more with state-level agencies. Options:

■Hire a consultant to take over on a per diem basis—or on a lump sum basis— for the amount of time a pregnant employee will be absent.

■Fill in with retired employees.

■Temporarily rehire former employees.

Source: Cheryl Fells, principal and technical consultant, Towers, Perrin, Forster & Crosby, management consultants, 245 Park Ave., New York 10167.

Corporate Child-Care Strategies

Many companies recognize that they can no longer afford to be without child-care benefits. To remain competitive in today's tight labor market, the company must have a child-care program of some kind. It helps draw new employees to the company and it increases the productivity of working mothers already on staff.

"But what are our options?" That's the question CEOs and human resource professionals ask when the subject of child care comes up. Here are the main options:

■On-site day-care centers. These are employer-owned and independently managed. The cost to the employer is greater than other options because of high start-up and maintenance costs.

Employees are typically charged a weekly rate competitive with other child-care facilities. Employers choose this option when there aren't enough local day-care centers to accommodate employees, or the company wants to carve out a clear competitive edge over other employers.

■Off-site centers in conjunction with other employers. The company gets together with other firms to provide day care for employees at an off-site center. Benefit: Costs are shared, so the cost to an individual employer is reduced.

■Contracting with a local child-care center to buy open slots for employees' children. This can sometimes be done by making a contribution to the center.

■Provide financial assistance through a voucher or reimbursement program. Reimbursements might be a flat dollar amount per week, or a percentage of expenses. The employer reimburses the employees for a portion of their child-care costs.

■Company-sponsored sick-child services. This provides employees with alternatives to missing work to care for sick children. Some programs use sick-child programs at local hospitals or day-care centers, others use organizations that send care workers to the employee's home to look after sick children. Costs can run as high as $10/hour.

Salary reduction programs. These are very popular, in part because they don't cost the employer much. Under Section 129 of the Tax Code, up to $5,000 of dependent-care assistance payments paid by an employer under a written plan are excluded from an employee's gross income. With a salary-reduction plan, up to $5,000 of an employee's salary is devoted to child care. That salary is not subject to income tax or Social Security tax. In a way, this is the least an employer can do, since it is the employee's own salary that goes to child care. The company pays the cost of developing and administering the plan.

How To Choose

Besides the cost, employers must consider the needs of specific employees in a particular area. For example, in some areas, a reimbursement program isn't much help because there aren't adequate child-care facilities in the community. All an employer can do is help develop a child-care center either on-site or off.

In other areas, where there are adequate facilities, what the employees need is financial support.

A growing number of outside organizations help companies set up child-care centers. They'll shield the employer from liability for on-site facilities. Kinder Care* is a national organization. In the Northeast, Bright Horizons** and Workplace Connections*** do this kind of work.

The question of fairness. Helping with day care does favor employees with children over childless employees. But other benefit programs also favor particular groups of employees. Companies typically spend more on health-care benefits for employees with families. And they pay more in retirement benefits for people who are older. Also, tuition-benefit programs favor a special group of employees.

Sensible solution: A cafeteria plan for company benefits, where employees choose from a menu of benefits up to a fixed dollar limit.

*Kinder Care Learning Center, Inc., 764 Main St., Waltham, MA 02154.

**Bright Horizons Children's Centers, Inc., One Kendall Square, Cambridge, MA 02139.

***Workplace Connections, 200 Fifth Ave., Waltham, MA 02154.

Source: Susan J. Velleman, managing director, William M. Mercer Meidinger Hansen, 200 Clarendon St., Boston 02116.

Jury Duty Pay Policies

Deduct jury fees if workers are paid for jury duty. Require workers to report for work when excused from court duty early in the day.

Special problems may occur on grand juries: In some states these juries use volunteers, or jurors are nominated by organizations. Pay arrangements must be different. These jurors were not summoned and not required to serve; service may be much longer than on trial juries.

One company's solution to grand-jury problems:

1. Hourly workers who are called are paid regular wages.

2. Those who volunteer to serve must ask for unpaid leaves of absence. Leaves may be denied if their absence would require the hiring of temporary replacements, or the scheduling of excessive overtime.

3. Managerial employees who volunteer for grand juries are paid regular wages. They are expected to perform as much work as they can. As grand juries often function in afternoon or evening hours, managers are usually able to keep an eye on things at work.

Job-Elimination Policy

Employees whose jobs are to be eliminated should be given up to three months' notice of the elimination, and in no case less than one month's notice. Best: Put notice in writing, including the possibility of termination if an alternative position can't be found. Help the employee find another job by looking within the company and, if necessary, with other employers. Allow generous time off from work during the notice period for the employee to interview with other companies. Notify other businesses in the area about qualified employees' availability.

Source: *Personnel Policy Briefs,* 817 Broadway, New York 10003.

Is Your Vacation Policy Too Generous?

Check the following table to see how the company's vacation policy stacks up with what other companies are doing:

	Industrial (%)	Financial (%)	Utilities (%)
Two weeks			
Immediately	15	20	13
After 1 yr.	79	70	75
Three weeks			
Under 5 yrs.	11	14	4
5–9 yrs.	80	62	88
After 10 yrs.	9	24	8
Four weeks			
Under 10 yrs.	6	3	—
10–14 yrs.	41	9	25
15–19 yrs.	44	61	75
After 20 yrs.	7	26	—

Source: Robert Einhorn, director of benefit information services, Towers, Perrin, Forster & Crosby, New York.

Sick-Leave Plans That Discourage Malingering

Paid sick leave should be thought of as income maintenance during occasional periods of illness. Long-term absence due to chronic conditions or serious physical disorders should be covered by insured plans that begin when paid sick leave is no longer available.

Recommendation: Eligibility should accumulate at the rate of about a day a month. The employee should be permitted to carry over unused sick leave from year to year, until 30 days are "in the bank." If accumulation is not permitted, workers will be tempted to call in sick whether ill or not, just to prevent the time from going to waste. And accumulation is a reward for long service.

Absences due to industrial accidents usually do not count against allowable sick leave. They're covered by Workmen's Compensation and other insured plans.

No matter how the plan is designed, some employees will use an occasional day of "sick leave" to take care of personal business. It may be better to permit limited use of sick leave for such personal business than to try to forbid it altogether. One way: After an employee has accumulated ten sick leave days, he may be permitted to use up to three for personal business when cleared in advance with supervisor.

Advantages: Coordination of sick leave with personal leave rewards the employee with a good record. Moreover, it helps overcome the inclination of foremen and supervisors to overlook dissembling when they think the sick leave policy is too harsh. Limited use of sick leave for personal business may also help curb absenteeism. Reason: Leave is accumulated only during a month of perfect attendance on all perfect workdays. However: Personal leave time drawn from the sick leave bank cannot be added to vacations.

Verification is always a problem. It's not feasible to expect an employee to furnish proof of a one- or two-day illness. But a sick leave plan might contain a statement reserving the right of the management to ask for documentation after an employee has been out sick ten days in any calendar year. Note: Employers have the right to request verification at any point, with or without explicit warning. But a statement expressing an intention to question heavy use of sick leave sets a proper tone. It may also serve to dissuade would-be malingerers.

Record-keeping is important, too, not only to make sure employees are credited with allowable sick leave, but to pinpoint problems. Employees who never have sick leave to carry over from one year to the next may need counseling or prodding. The formal sick leave plan should allow room for special consideration, on a case-by-case basis, if a long-service employee needs help after using up accumulated paid leave.

Source: Morris Stone, retired vice-president, American Arbitration Association.

Controlling Absenteeism

A no-fault absenteeism policy can eliminate many headaches for operations that require regular attendance.

Chief benefits:

■Rewards the workers with good attendance.

■Discourages one-day absences, especially on Mondays and Fridays.

■Curbs lateness and early leaving.

■Motivates absent workers to call.

■Ends need for supervisors to differentiate between unacceptable and acceptable reasons for an absence.

How no-fault absenteeism works:

■Each absence, regardless of length, counts as one point. Goal: Not to penalize those truly ill.

■Tardiness or early departure counts as one-half or one-quarter point, depending on the time lost.

■Not calling if out sick counts as two points.

■Each month of perfect attendance erases one point.

■Unavoidable absences (funerals, military or jury duty) do not count.

Use the points to work out a system of progressive discipline: X number of points means $X loss of pay. Final penalty: Dismissal for excessive absenteeism.

Source: Frank E. Kuzmits, assistant professor, University of Louisville School of Business.

Cure Monday absenteeism. Change payday from Friday to Monday.

Source: Dr. Marilyn Machlowitz, organizational psychologist, New York.

When Absenteeism Is Company's Fault

While worker absenteeism is one of the costs of doing business, many organizations accept a level that is intolerably high.

Prime causes:

■Employee's preoccupation with leisure-time activities.

■Fringe benefits, such as paid sick days. At many companies, the policy about sick days is "use 'em or lose 'em." This means that employees must take sick days during a given time period or be denied them.

■Overtrained workers. They find little satisfaction and stay away out of boredom.

■Undertrained workers. They experience high levels of anxiety about their incompetence. Staying home is often safer than risking exposure on the job.

■Poor physical environment. Dangerous jobs conducted under hot, unventilated conditions, for example.

How to help matters:

■Make the plant pleasant.

■Give incentives and rewards, such as an occasional day off. The bonus time will cost less than a high rate of absenteeism.

■Establish clear attendance standards.

■Try a flexible schedule to break the routine. Examples: Long hours one day, short hours another. Or, four ten-hour work days a week.

■Abandon the mandatory paid-sick-days policy. Pay employees for sick days not used every year. Or permit them to carry the days over.

■Involve employees in the decision-making process concerning work schedules. Instruct supervisors to make time available for constructive give-and-take.

■Concentrate on the 10% of employees who account for half of all absent days. Place chronic cases under attendance-control programs. Steps: Warnings, suspension from work, probation, then discharge.

Source: *The Effective Supervisor's Handbook* by Louis V. Imundo, AMACOM.

How Company Handbooks Protect The Company

A written employee handbook can minimize potential liabilities. It can eliminate confusion and misunderstanding about corporate policies. Employers can apply these office policies consistently to minimize the likelihood of legal liability problems that could otherwise result.

Example: Your company has two employees who are both late for work every day. Employee A has consistently performed below company standards and Employee B is a model employee in all respects except the tardiness. You decide to fire Employee A, and keep Employee B. Without a properly written handbook that contains disclaimer language and an at-will statement, Employee A can take the case to court with the potential of winning a lawsuit for improper termination. With a properly written employee handbook that contains disclaimers and reserves the right of management to fire anyone with or without cause (at-will statements), the likelihood of marginal success of a lawsuit is greatly reduced.

The wording of the employee handbook is of critical importance. Specific conditions and stipulations may negate any disclaimers and at-will statements. Flexibility is advised so the employer can deal with individual situations.

Example: A clause stating that "employees will receive a written warning before termination." Once you've written a clause like this, you've restricted yourself to the written warning.

By printing the company's policies for complying with various government rules and regulations, the company protects itself when an employee is dismissed for not complying with these written policies. When an employee is terminated or leaves the company, it's difficult for him to say he never knew about the policies if he had signed a release stating he'd read and understood the handbook when he received it.

Handbooks can also help boost morale. Small companies often ask employees to give their input when putting a handbook together. Most employees feel good about contributing to the company this way.

Source: Michael Berke, president, Business Resource Group, Inc., a personnel administration and benefits company, 35 E. Wacker Dr., Chicago 60601.

Chapter 60
Evaluating Employees

Performance Appraisals That Work

Informal appraisals of employees go on all the time, but they often seem unfair to many workers. Reason: There is usually no balance between criticism, praise and inquiry into the employee's ideas of how to do the job better.

The advantage of formal appraisals: Employees recognize that their work is being evaluated by standards that they themselves can understand. Formal appraisal systems, however, don't always succeed because management sees them as a one-time effort instead of an ongoing process.

To use the appraisal system as a way to achieve greater productivity, link appraisals to compensation in a way that is clear and fair to employees. How to do it:

■Clear up the basis for salary ranges (skills, experience, responsibility, marketplace for the worker's skills, etc.).

■Set specific criteria for promotions, demotions, terminations.

■Make clear how often performance appraisals will be done and salaries reviewed. (Semiannually or annually is best.)

Useful guidelines for raises:

■When appraisal is commendable, raise salaries up to 20% more than average.

■When appraisal is adequate, make the raise average.

■When appraisal is unsatisfactory, give no raise. Instead, issue a warning that a second unsatisfactory review will result in dismissal or demotion.

Top management must take the performance-appraisal system seriously for it to have any impact on worker performance. Instruct managers to:

■Keep the appraisal sessions free of interruptions.

■Listen to employees. Allow them to give a self-appraisal first.

■Tell employees what they are doing well and ways they can improve.

■Assume employees are creative and want to contribute. Ask them for suggestions.

There should be no surprises for an employee during an appraisal session. Don't appraise too much. Set two or three primary objectives at most. Once primary objectives are consistently met, add new objectives—but only one at a time.

Source: Norman Auslander, group vice-president and general manager, Miracle Food Mart, a division of Steinberg, Inc., Rexdale, Ontario.

A Peer-Review Survey

A peer review survey is an effective means of learning about an employee's strengths and weaknesses as perceived by others. The results can be surprising to both employees and supervisors. How a successful survey works: Each year, employees are asked to evaluate co-workers on leadership, organization, communication and interpersonal skills. Results are tabulated by an outside firm (not supervisors) and are reported directly to the person evaluated. Survey results are then discussed at the annual performance review. Weaknesses pointed out by co-workers are addressed for improvement. Strengths which a supervisor may have overlooked or undervalued are targeted for further use.

Source: Bernard L. Jennings, vice-president of sales training, Maritz Motivation Co., St. Louis, quoted about his company's experience in *Sales & Marketing Management,* 633 Third Ave., New York 10017.

Mistakes To Avoid

How to make fewer errors in evaluating employees:

■Avoid judging an employee without knowing the details of the job. Your concept of the job may differ from the employee's.

■Measure performance against what was done by others in the position rather than against a mythical perfect standard.

■Recognize that an employee's performance reflects his reaction to many situations. Some of these are beyond his control.

■Don't let personal feelings color your judgment.

Source: *Office Administration Handbook,* Dartnell Corp., Chicago.

Surveys That Evaluate Executives

Don't put an executive on the spot simply because his subordinates rate him harshly on a survey. He may be the victim of politically motivated underlings. To check the accuracy of a negative response:

■Go over survey answers with the manager's subordinates. Can they support their contentions with specifics?

■Focus on questions that reveal whether some people are stirring up resentment against the boss to strengthen their own power base.

■Ask the executive who he feels are potential rivals or manipulators. Whom does he distrust? Why?

Think of survey results as a first step, not as the last word.

Source: *The Levinson Letter,* Cambridge, MA.

Chapter 61
Compensation/Wage Policies

Setting A Wage Policy

The advantages of operating without a formal policy on salaries:

■Individuals can be rewarded with merit increases without setting precedents.

■The annual raise does not become automatic. Instead, employees know they must demonstrate that they deserve more.

■There are no rules to break.

Advantages of a written policy:

■Salary costs are protected from overinflation. Easier budgeting.

■Employee turnover is lessened because compensation levels stay competitive and rewards for advancement are known.

■Legal problems over discrimination are less likely.

Source: Stanley B. Henrici, *Salary Management for the Nonspecialist*, AMACOM, New York.

How Compensation Can Boost Productivity

Inflation-inspired pressures for sizable pay hikes, even in the face of declining (or flat) productivity, is a continuing problem. To break out of this cycle, managers must alter their approach to compensation strategies. Specific suggestions:

■Put teeth into merit programs by giving merit raises and bonuses only to the best performers. By giving fewer but bigger bonuses, management encourages continued high performance of recipients, and makes clear to other workers what their stake is in increasing output. This step requires tight control over the company's definitions of performance. It demands that managers rate their subordinates' performance accurately.

■Change the pattern of raises by granting fewer routine increases. Instead, keep workers on the same base salaries longer, and reward outstanding performance via bonuses.

■Emphasize current rather than deferred dollars. Pay workers higher salaries but offer them fewer deferred benefits. This takes some of the sting out of inflation, and makes sense given the fact that inflation will erode the value of deferred benefits anyway.

■Be flexible in offering non-cash benefits. Without increasing the cost to the company of worker fringe benefits, management can increase the value of those benefits by letting workers choose their own fringes.

For example, a worker with young children wants maximum medical coverage, while another with college-age children prefers a maximum tuition-support program. Workers allowed to choose these benefits cafeteria-style will feel better compensated. But cafeteria-style benefits increase administration costs and, in some cases, insurance premiums.

■Reward workers most who use costly fringe benefits the least. Example: A company covers all its workers with the same medical insurance. One worker costs the company $1,000 in medical expenses over a year. Another worker costs the company nothing in medical expenses. If the company rewards the worker with no medical bill by giving him a small cash bonus, this will encourage other workers to use the company's medical plan more sparingly.

Source: Robert S. Nadel, partner, Hay Associates, New York.

Who's Exempt From Overtime

A bona fide executive administrator, professional, or outside salesman is exempt from the wages and hours provisions of federal law, which defines who can get overtime.

■Executive: According to Labor Department regulations, an executive is one whose primary duty is management; regularly directs two or more employees; has authority or the right to make recommendations on hiring, firing, promotions; regularly exercises discretionary powers; doesn't spend more than 20% of his time on non-executive functions, and is paid a weekly salary of not less than $155. If his salary isn't less then $250, he's an executive employee if he satisfies only the first two.

■Administrator: Defined in terms of doing office work directly related to management policies or general business; exercises discretion; regularly assists an owner or executive; does work requiring special training or knowledge; doesn't spend more than 20% of his time on nonadministrative work, and whose salary isn't less than $250, he is an administrative employee if he satisfies only the first two.

■Professional: Goes beyond lawyer and doctor—includes artist, musician; salary level placed at $170 per week. Again, if the salary isn't less than $250, he may still be classified as a professional if his work requires advanced knowledge, discretion, invention, imagination, or artistic talent.

■Outside salesman: Defined as a salesman regularly and customarily engaged away from employer's place of business. No earnings level.

For further details: Department of Labor, Employment Standards Administration, Washington, DC 20210. Ask for publication WH 1281.

Making Overtime Policies Fair

Prime dispute concerns whether employees are obligated to accept a reasonable amount of overtime. When a plant is nonunion, or when union contracts omit this point, the assumption is that employees can avoid overtime only for good cause (just as they might be excused from regular work because of illness, urgent family problems, etc.).

An exception would be in unionized plants, where there's been a history of leniency or where companies have tried unsuccessfully to add compulsory overtime provisions to union contracts.

Distinguish between scheduled overtime and extra hours that suddenly become necessary. If overtime is scheduled a day ahead, employees may have to work unless their excuse is persuasive. On short-notice overtime, lesser excuses (or no excuses at all) may be considered acceptable.

Chapter 62
Executive Compensation

The Corporate Owner's Salary

The head of a closely held corporation must be careful in setting his own salary.

The problem lies in determining what salary will keep personal and corporate tax liabilities to a minimum.

There are hidden dangers. Salary payments considered unreasonably large by the Internal Revenue Service will be deemed dividends from profits. They will be subject to double taxation, first as corporate income, then as personal income. If too little salary is taken, the corporation may accumulate excessive earnings and face an accumulated earnings tax penalty.

In favor of a low salary:

■The company may be able to afford greater fringe benefits (for example, insurance), which are deductible to the firm and excluded from the individual's income.

■Retention of earnings will increase the value of the firm and maximize the capital gain available if it's sold or liquidated.

You can show a salary is reasonable by comparing it with the salaries of individuals performing similar duties for other firms. The Bureau of Labor Statistics is an excellent source of compensation figures. One way to justify an unusually high salary is to show that the owner took a correspondingly low salary in earlier years to help the firm get established.

How to avoid trouble with the IRS:

■Don't be greedy. A salary that impinges on cash flow will be questioned by the IRS.

■Separate salaries from stock. If salaries are paid in proportion to stockholdings, the IRS may call them dividend distributions instead. It's helpful to have all working shareholders receive raises at the same time other employees do.

■Avoid bonuses. A bonus paid out at the end of a good year might be considered a distribution of profits (taxable to the company and to the recipient).

■Pay dividends regularly. When the IRS doesn't find declared dividends, it looks for hidden ones.

The specific tax effects of various distribution schemes must be worked out on a trial-and-error basis. Consider the different investment opportunities available to corporations and individuals, as well as the differences between the corporate and personal tax rates.

A repayment agreement might prove useful. This calls for the employee to repay the firm any amount of his salary that might later be deemed excessive. The repayment is deductible by the employee. Repayment agreements can be dangerous, and must be carefully considered and drafted by an expert. the repayment of a large amount of salary could result in a firm's having to pay taxes on excessive accumulated earnings.

Compensating Key Executives

A company learns that one of its key executives has received an offer from a competitor that would boost the executive's salary 30%. The company doesn't want to lose the executive. But it doesn't want to match the outside offer either.

One solution is to offer the executive a deferred compensation program that guarantees him income on top of the ERISA-approved pension plan.

There are advantages for both the executive and the company. A deferred compensation program will provide the executive with retirement income when he needs it and avoid a salary boost that will put him in a higher tax bracket.

A deferred compensation program in lieu of a raise keeps the company from getting caught in a salary war. Properly structured, these programs for key executives are self-financing and not subject to ERISA requirements.

The company takes out dividend-bearing whole life insurance policies on its key executives. Initially, the company pays the premiums with money it borrows against the policies at the standard rate charged by insurers.

Eventually, through the maturing face value of the policies and the benefits that accrue as retired executives die, the company builds up a fund that:

■Finances the extra retirement income promised.

■Covers both the current and start-up costs of running the deferred compensation program. The program can be structured so the company also gets a return on the use of the money it invests in it.

These deferred compensation programs now exist for companies with payrolls ranging from 200 to 15,000 employees, and from 1 to 50 key executives. The benefits offered range from 50% to 90% of the executives' salaries at the time of retirement. The start-up costs vary widely. Each situation requires its own calculations.

Source: Paul A. Fierstein, C.L.U., benefits and compensation consultant, New York.

How Cash-Poor Executives Can Exercise Stock Options

Finding the cash to exercise a nonstatutory stock option is a common problem, even for high-salaried executives. One technique is to exchange stock already owned for the new share options.

An executive wants to purchase 1,000 shares of the company stock. The option price is $20 a share when the market price is $40 a share. The executive already owns company stock bought for $10 a share. The executive exchanges 500 of the old shares at their market value of $40 each ($20,000) for the 1,000 shares (also $20,000).

As a result, the employee must treat the difference between the new shares' option price and their market value ($20,000) as compensation. The maximum tax is 50%, so the executive's net cash outlay is $10,000.

In comparison, an employee who purchases the new stock for cash has the same taxable gain. But $20,000 also has to be paid for the stock. Thus, net cash outlay is $30,000. That's three times the cash needed in a stock exchange.

The Internal Revenue Service has approved option stock exchanges. And the Securities and Exchange Commission has said exchanges may be undertaken by corporate insiders. Special rules apply if you exchange stock already owned for incentive stock options (ISOs).

Source: Francis M. Gaffney, national director of tax services, Main, Hurdman & Cranstoun, CPAs, New York.

Chapter 63
Employee Benefits

Trimming Benefit Costs

As benefit costs continue to rise, companies should look harder than ever for ways to cut outlays without reducing services.

Recommended:

■Keep medical, dental, and eye-care plans separate from life insurance. This allows easier price comparisons and more room to negotiate.

■Before renegotiating a benefit plan, figure the cost-benefit ratios offered by prospective carriers. Use the data to win lower prices.

■When a company expands to more than 35 employees, it should renegotiate insurance, since nearly all insurers reduce rates around this level.

Source: Jack O. Remp, benefits consultant, Jack O. Remp Co., Palos Verdes Estates, CA, quoted in *Business Insurance*.

Flexible Spending Accounts To Cut Benefit Costs

Flexible spending accounts (FSAs) are an effective way for companies to save money by making cuts in benefits more palatable to employees. The accounts let employees set aside part of their salary tax free so they can pay medical, legal and dependent-care expenses not covered by the company's benefit plan. Fortunately, flexible spending accounts have survived Tax Reform nearly unscathed.

How They Work

In the fall the company offers employees the opportunity to put as much of their salary as they want in a tax-free account for the next calendar year. The employees must decide then how much of the salary to earmark for healthcare and dependent-care benefits in the company's plan.

These amounts can't be changed during the year except when there's a change in family status that also affects the employee's eligibility for benefits.

Examples: A birth, death, divorce, etc. As employees pay for expenses not covered by the benefit plan, they submit claims and are reimbursed.

Though there's still some uncertainty about how the IRS treats funds not used during the year, companies have the right to use them to defray administrative costs of the FSA. Rulings later this year should clarify other ways in which companies can use the excess funds.

FSA Advantages

When companies lower healthcare costs by increasing deductibles or introducing coinsurance or other methods that force employees to assume more of their own expenses, morale can drop quickly. Some workers may even leave the company. And in unionized companies, contract talks often break down because of benefit reductions. FSAs can soften the impact.

Example: If the company has increased deductibles from $100 to $300, it might set up flexible spending accounts to stifle employee opposition to the change. When employees earmark money for an FSA, the funds are tax deductible to the company and tax free to the recipient.

Necessary prerequisite: Before it can offer FSAs, the company must meet the requirements of Section 125 of the Internal Revenue Code, which governs benefits.

The company benefits because funds earmarked for FSAs aren't spent right away. The company can invest those funds for its own income in the interim.

Moreover, these funds aren't subject to Social Security taxes, to either the company or the employee. And in most states FSAs are ignored for purposes of state income tax. Exceptions: Alabama, Arkansas, New Jersey and Pennsylvania.

Traps For Employees

The fact that the IRS requires employees to stick to their commitment of funds frightens some workers who fear they may need that money for something else as the year progresses. Solution: The company or its insurance consultant can offer guidelines as to appropriate amounts.

Some companies set maximum limits of, say, $2,000 for medical care. The amount depends on the company's insurance plan and how complete it is.

To make sure that employees aren't left with big balances at the end of the year, the company or its insurance agent should send out statements as early as September, notifying employees how much balance remains in their account. Then they have several months in which to figure out how to spend it.

There are other IRS rules that the company must explain to employees. To use the funds for dependent care, for example, an employee must claim that dependent on his own tax form, not his spouse's. The dependent must be under 15 or incapable of caring for himself. Whether the funds go for a housekeeper or an approved day care center, the IRS sets an annual cap of $5,000. The company should provide a forum where employees can learn about these rules.

Tax traps: Two-income couples making $40,000–$45,000 a year are probably better off taking advantage of flexible spending accounts, but for lower-paid individuals it may be more advantageous simply to use the dependent-care deduction on their income taxes. Important: The company bears some responsibility for offering employees guidance on these tax nuances.

Source: John J. Rzasa, assistant director of flexible compensation, Aetna Life Insurance Co., 151 Farmington Ave., Hartford, CT 06156.

Chapter 64
Pension Plans

Integrated Retirement Plans

The big mistake management makes with retirement plans is to think about them simply as a way to provide income to retired company officers and employees. The best retirement plans are integrated into company financial and tax planning, and into estate planning for a manager-owner.

A defined-benefit plan provides annual retirement benefits in fixed dollar amounts to retired employees.

For this type of plan, the annual retirement benefit cannot exceed 100% of the average of an employee's compensation in the three highest-paid years, or $124,500 per year, whichever is less. The maximum benefit limitation increases each year with the cost of living. But the maximum benefit is 10% less for each year the employee has worked less than 10 years.

A major advantage is that the company can make a deductible contribution of any size that is necessary to fund the benefit. An older owner-manager can reduce the company's taxes while adding significantly to his own retirement income. However, this type of plan is usually less useful for a company with many employees who would have to be covered.

With a defined-contribution plan each year the company contributes to the plan an amount equal to a percentage of the employee's income.

The company's annual contribution to the plan for one employee cannot exceed 25% of the employee's compensation, or $41,500, whichever is less. (The dollar limit rises with the cost of living.) The contribution limit applies to each year separately. One year's contribution cannot exceed the limit because a prior year's was under it. There is no limit, however, to the size of the employee's ultimate benefit. The totaled contributions and investment income set the retirement income.

One drawback is that contributions tied to employee compensation can burden a firm in a cyclical business, where profits may be up one year and down the next. Alternatively, the company can adopt a profit-sharing plan that ties contributions to profitability. The same contribution limits apply.

There are special ways to use a retirement plan.

■Reduce excess accumulated earnings to avoid an IRS penalty tax by adopting a defined-benefit plan. The benefits can be funded all at once by removing a large amount from accumulated earnings and placing it in the plan. Accumulated earnings are thereby reduced to an acceptable amount. And the company gets a deduction in the amount of the contribution, further reducing taxes.

■Reduce employee turnover. Benefits under a defined-contribution plan can be made to vest over a period of years. A contribution need not vest for a period of four years, unless the employer wants to be more liberal. If an employee leaves, the invested benefits are forfeited.

■Provide employee incentives, as in a profit-sharing plan. This ties benefits to profitability, encouraging employees to provide their best efforts.

■Facilitate estate planning. In a small, closely held firm, the top employees are able to direct the plan's investments and arrange its payout procedures so as to reduce their estate taxes. They are not taxed on their retirement plan accounts in the meantime.

Retirement plans are not without problems. For example, the company's contribution to an executive's account in a retirement plan is part of the executive's total compensation. This must be considered if the executive's salary is already large enough to be challenged by the IRS as unreasonable.

Source: Gerald Reich, partner, Shore & Reich, New York.

New Ways To Use Your IRA

Once upon a time, long-term capital gains were favored under the tax law, and, once upon a time, you could claim a deduction for your contributions to your individual retirement account (IRA), and let it garner income without the imposition of current taxation. Your level of income didn't matter, and it didn't matter if you were covered by any other retirement plan. Now, if you are in another retirement plan and your income is too high, you may not get a deduction for your IRA contribution.

The old rules were great, but this is now, and now you should not discount the value of your old IRA, especially with regard to its investments.

When capital gains were taxed at lower rates than ordinary income, it was not advisable to produce long-term gains in your tax-sheltered retirement account. The benefit was wasted. The thing to do then was to invest the IRA for lots of ordinary untaxed current income.

Now that all income, long-term gain or not, is taxed at the same rate, you should consider investing in assets that can produce big gains as well as assets that yield current dividends or interest.

You may continue to make a contribution to an individual retirement account each year within the familiar $2,000 limits (expanded to a total of $2,250 if a spousal IRA is included), but your contribution will be deductible only if: a) you (include your spouse if you file jointly) are not an active participant at any time during the tax year in a retirement plan maintained by an employer, or b) if your income is below a certain level. The level depends on your status. If your adjusted gross income is between $40,000 and $50,000 and you're an active participant in a plan, the deductible part of your contribution is phased out on a joint return. On individual returns, the deduction phases out on income between $25,000 and $35,000. For married couples filing separately, the phase out starts at zero and is completed at $10,000.

As under prior law, once a tax year begins, a contribution to an IRA may be made at any time before the due date of that year's return. Don't wait until the last minute; the sooner you fund your IRA, the more growth there will be.

Regardless of whether your contribution to your individual retirement account will be deductible, its earnings will not be subject to tax until they are withdrawn. Now is the time to consider setting aside $2,000 to grow tax free, and that investment might, if you like, be in an asset that will increase in value over the long term and produce capital gains.

Under prior law, IRAs were not permitted to invest in collectibles or precious metals. That rule has been relaxed, and now your IRA can hold silver or gold coins issued by the United States. No jewelry, though—you can't wear your IRA.

Source: *New Tax Loopholes For Investors*, Robert Garber, Boardroom Special Report, Springfield, NJ 07081.

Your IRA—After Tax Reform

■Taxpayers who are not "active participants" (see below) in a qualified pension plan can continue to make deductible contributions of up to $2,000, as before.

■Taxpayers who are "active participants" in qualified pension plans can continue to make deductible contributions of up to $2,000, provided their adjusted gross income (AGI) is no more than $40,000 (joint filers) or $25,000 (individual filers).

■Joint filers with income between $40,000 and $50,000 and individual filers between $25,000 and $35,000 can make deductible contributions. But, the deductible amount is reduced by 20% of AGI in excess of $40,000 (joint) or $25,000 (individual).

Example: Brown, a joint filer, has AGI of $44,000. He can make deductible contributions of $1,200–$2,000, less $800 (20% X $4,000), the excess over $40,000. Brown can contribute up to $2,000, but only $1,200 will be tax deductible.

■Joint filers with incomes over $50,000 and individual filers over $35,000 can make no deductible contributions. They can, however, make nondeductible contributions up to $2,000, and the earnings from their contributions will accumulate tax free.

Note: For taxpayers who qualify for spousal IRAs, the maximum is $2,250, rather than $2,000.

Nondeductible contributions can be withdrawn at any time without tax or penalty; but earnings on the contributions are taxable and are subject to early withdrawal penalties. And if you do withdraw nondeductible contributions, a pro rata part of the withdrawal will be allocated to earnings.

"Active participants" in qualified plans. Anyone covered by a qualified pension plan is a participant, even if he/she has no vested rights. However, employees who have not met the eligibility requirements (e.g., they haven't worked long enough) are not active participants.

A self-employed person who has a Keogh plan for himself is considered a participant in a qualified plan.

Trap: If your spouse is a participant in a qualified plan, the "participant" rules apply to you, even if you yourself are not covered by any plan.

Early withdrawal penalties. Starting as of 1987, taxpayers under age $59^{1/2}$ will not be penalized if the withdrawal is to be paid out in equal installments over a lifetime (e.g., an annuity). Other rules on early withdrawals remain unchanged, with one exception. If the amount withdrawn is more than $112,500, the excess is penalized 15%, rather than 10% (does not apply to withdrawals of contributions made before August 1986).

Source: Deborah Walker, Peat Marwick Main & Co., 1990 K St. NW, Washington, DC 20006.

How Safe Is Your Pension?

How to check on the safety of your retirement income:

For employees of public companies: Basic information is included in the firm's annual report. Usually the size of a firm's unfunded pension liability and the size of its past service liability are disclosed in footnotes. More detailed information is available in the financial section of the firm's 10K report, filed with the Securities & Exchange Commission.

For employees of private companies: Everyone who is in a qualified plan (one approved by the IRS under the Code) has the right to obtain information about his pension from the trustees of the plan. They may be either internal or external trustees. The average person may not be able to decipher the information. If you can't, then take it to a pension expert, actuary, lawyer, or accountant for an analysis. Cost: $500–$800. Whether you are examining pension information of public or of private firms, you are seeking the same sort of basic information.

Principle: The size of a company's liability for retirement payouts is not as important as the assumptions about funding these liabilities. Like a mortgage, these obligations don't exist 100% in the present. Concern yourself with how the company expects to fund its liabilities.

Types Of Liabilities

Unfunded pension liabilities. The amount a firm expects to need over the next 20–30 years to supply vested workers with promised pension benefits. These figures are derived from various actuarial assumptions.

Past service liabilities. Created when a company raises its pension compensation. For instance, a company may have been planning to provide 40% of compensation as a pension. One year it may raise that to 45% and treat it retroactively.

Trouble Signs

A poor record on investing. Compare the market value of the assets in the pension with their book value. If book value is more than market value, the trustees have not been investing wisely. If the fund had to sell those assets today, there would be a loss. You might also get a bit nervous if the fund is still holding some obscure bonds or other fixed-income obligations issued at low rates years ago.

Funding assumptions are overstated. Actuaries have myriad estimates on how long it takes to fund pension plans and what rate of return a company will get. What to look at:

■Time frame: This should not be long. If the firm is funding over 40 years, you will want to know why and how, since 10–20 years is more customary. The investment world will be different in as little as 10 years from now; assumptions made on 40 years may not hold up at all.

■Rate of return: If a company assumes a conservative 6%–7% or less right now, you can be comfortable. If the assumed rate is 10% or more, you will want to know how it is going to meet that expectation for the entire fund over the long run.

■Salary and wage scales: The company should be assuming an increase in compensation over years. Most plans have such provisions. They must start funding now for future salary increases.

■Assumptions about the employee turnover rate: These should be consistent with the historically documented turnover of the company. If a firm has a very low turnover rate and assumes a 4% turnover, the plan will be underfunded at some time. Estimates should be conservative.

To assess your own status in a corporate pension plan, see how many years you have been vested. Many people have the illusion that they are fully vested for maximum pensions after only five years or so. In truth, companies couldn't afford to fully vest people with such short service. They may offer some token pension for such service, but most people are not fully vested until they have worked for the firm for 10 or even 20 years. Even then, they might be vested only to the extent of their accrued pension to date, not the full pension expected at normal retirement. With so much job-hopping in the past two decades, an individual's pension-fund status may be much less than imagined.

Employees of troubled or even bankrupt companies need not panic. Trustees of the plan have an obligation to the vested employees. The assets of the plan are segregated, and no creditor can reach them. In fact, as a creditor, the corporate pension plan can grab some corporate assets under certain circumstances. And if there has been gross mismanagement of pension funds, stockholders of a closely held company can be held personally liable.

Source: James E. Conway, president of Ayco Corporation, a consulting firm specializing in executive finances, 1 Wall St., Albany, NY 12205.

Insurance After Retirement

Getting life insurance coverage for one's later years can be a problem, since most company group policies end at retirement. Premiums are astronomical if the executive buys an individual policy at age 65 or 70. One solution is for the company to make tax-deductible payments on behalf of executives into a fund held by the insurance company (or a trustee). When the executive retires, the fund buys him a paid-up policy. It's called Retired Lives Reserve. The company may buy coverage for executives only, and not for other employees, without losing the tax-deductible feature. (If the company has ten employees or fewer, it most cover all of them, but it can provide more liberally for officers.)

Working After Retirement

Many retirees would like to keep working after retirement, at least part-time. But those who want to work for financial reasons should be aware of these drawbacks:

■You can work and still collect full Social Security benefits, but if you're under age 65, for every $2 earned above a government-determined ceiling you lose $1 in benefits. If you're older than 64 but younger than 70, you'll lose $1 for every $3 in excess earnings. When you add your commuting costs, job-related expenses, and payroll deductions, you may find part-time work doesn't pay off.

■If you continue working part-time for the same company, you may not be eligible to collect your pension. One way around this, if the company will go along, is to retire as an employee and return as a consultant or freelancer. Since you're now self-employed, your pension won't be affected.

■Although most employees can't legally be compelled to retire before age 70, companies still set up retirement ages of 65 or under. You can work past that age, but you won't earn further pension credits. And you lose Social Security and pension benefits while you continue to work.

A very attractive alternative to working part-time is to start your own business. Professionals such as lawyers can often set up a practice, setting their own hours. Or you might turn a hobby into a business.

Source: William W. Parrott, a chartered financial consultant at Merrill, Lynch, Pierce, Fenner & Smith, Inc., 1185 Ave. of the Americas, New York 10036.

Chapter 65
Dealing With Unionized Workers

Freedom From Union Time

Organized labor is in such disarray these days that management can hope for more than wage givebacks and other concessions. It may finally be able to kiss the union good-bye.

Getting rid of an entrenched union through decertification is a complex technical process governed by stiff federal rules. Among other requirements, the move must be initiated by employees. Despite the difficulties, more and more decertification elections have been taking place—and in more than three-quarters of them, the union has lost.

Signs Of Weakness

How to tell if your union is vulnerable:

■Employees are unwilling to attend union meetings.

■The union has trouble getting people to serve as stewards or members of bargaining teams.

■Employees express dissatisfaction over the union's handling of contract negotiations or other dealings with the company.

■The union's visibility diminishes in the plant or office.

■Workers begin coming directly to company management to express grievances.

■Employees start asking more questions about dues, fees and other assessments charged by the union.

Proceed With Caution

Exciting as it may be for management to hear rumblings of discontent with the union, companies should proceed with caution. Almost every natural management reaction runs the risk of violating one of the National Labor Relations Board's many governing rules.

Example #1: Starting decertification proceedings requires a petition signed by 30% of the workers covered under the union contract. The petition can't be either initiated or circulated by the company or its supervisors. However, the company is allowed to tell employees what the petition form should say if they request that information.

Example #2: It's illegal to allow employees paid time off to solicit signatures for their NLRB petition.

Because rules can get so tricky, companies need special help. Look for a management law firm with specialties in labor disputes. Start the search by 1. Talking to other companies that have made decertification attempts, 2. Contacting your industry trade association or 3. Requesting a referral from the company's regular law firm. Important: Experience in several dozen union campaigns and specific experience in decertification.

Don't call in lawyers until you have evidence of employee unrest. Typical scenario: Dissident employees come to management asking if there's any way they can get out from under their union.

If management doesn't know what to say or, worse, says something illegal, the opportunity could be lost. Best response: "We'll consult our lawyers and then get back to you."

How Union Busters Work

Despite what the unions say about union busters, they can't create antiunion feelings that aren't already there. The first thing these legal specialists typically do is evaluate whether a decertification election can be won. There's a big difference between the normal grumbling about the union and the kind of deep, pervasive dissatisfaction that leads to a successful decertification election.

When decertification looks like a real possibility and the company decides to support it, be prepared to slug it out. The union will probably start a campaign of fear, warning employees that without union representation their jobs won't be secure and wages will be at risk.

Management can't legally ask employees how they plan to vote or suggest that they'll get better wages once the union is gone.

What management can do: Inform employees of better benefits or working conditions at other, nonunion divisions. However, it shouldn't make any promises. Management may tell employees that, in its opinion, a union isn't in the workers' best interests.

At an early stage, the labor specialist/consultant will meet with managers and first-line supervisors to make it very clear what they can and can't do and say under the law. It's crucial, particularly in the early stages, that management doesn't break an NLRB rule. That could serve as grounds for the board to dismiss the petition for an election.

If that happens, the company would have to go ahead and negotiate a new contract with the union because in most cases another election can't be petitioned for until 60-90 days before that contract ends...perhaps three years from now.

The lawyer/consultant then helps lay out the strategy and tactics for the campaign. Examples: Speeches by top management, newsletters, fliers, posters, payroll stuffers and letters to employees' homes. The success of the campaign often depends on management's ability to communicate its side of the story, reminding employees of things the company has done for them without union prodding, and answering specific union charges.

Expect a decertification campaign to take several months and require a team of at least two lawyers. Cost: About $25,000 for a complex case.

Source: Alfred T. DeMaria, a management-only labor lawyer with the firm Clifton, Budd, Burke & DeMaria, 420 Lexington Ave., New York 10170. He's the author of *The Process of Deunionization,* Executive Enterprises, 33 W. 60 St., New York 10021.

Watch The Bylaws In A Union Agreement

A company's agreement with union officers to disregard a contract provision may be worthless if it isn't ratified by the rank and file. The basic question is "Does the union constitution or bylaws require membership ratification of the contract?"

For example, a company and union agreed that, despite a just-cause-for-discharge provision in the contract, drivers could be fired if they became uninsurable. A driver was later dismissed under this sidebar pact, but an arbitrator reinstated him because the new understanding had not been ratified.

The sidebar agreement approach is worth trying, especially if it relieves economic hardship. But be sure safeguards are taken to make the new deal stick. Be sure to get them in writing.

Source: *Piggly Wiggly Warehouse,* 103 LRRM 2646.

How To Defuse Workplace Problems

Before putting money, hours, and fringe benefits on the bargaining table, listen to and do something about employee complaints. Workers who think management is being fair are less likely to strike.

Set up interviews with employees, hourly workers up through middle managers, in randomly selected and mixed groups. Select an upper-management representative who is not well known to the employees to conduct the session. Or choose an outside consultant. Have the office or plant manager sit in to answer questions and respond positively to complaints.

Do not permit any discussion of negotiable items such as pay or benefits. Instead, ask employees about safety, comfort, security, workflow, supervision, and absenteeism. Typical complaints include dirty rest rooms, poor ventilation and heating, lack of communication between foremen, work stoppages, inefficient scheduling, not being listened to.

Be aware that strong evidence of us-against-them feelings about supervisors and management means a strike attitude. Appropriate action should be taken to correct deficiencies that are important to workers, even if they seem trivial to management. The cost of rectifying complaints is small compared to a strike.

Source: *Letting the Employee Speak His Mind,* Imberman & DeForest, managemen consultants, Chicago.

Firing Troublemakers.

If union rules say that nobody with the authority to hire and fire may belong to the company union, pay special attention to troublemakers who are union members. Do this for a few months, then promote the troublemaker to a hire-and-fire position. That requires the troublemaker to resign from the union.

Frequently, this redirection of energies works well for both the company and the individual. If not, the troublemaker can be fired.

Meeting Union's Discrimination Claims

Workers in a nonunion shop who are fired for misconduct somtimes run to the appropriate union and claim they were fired for their pro-union activities in violation of the Taft-Hartley Act. But even if management knows the workers are union activists, it can still fire them provided it proves just cause.

An important National Labor Relations Board citation* states: "The mere fact that an employer may desire to terminate an employee because he engages in protected activity [being allowed to try to organize union] does not, of itself, establish the unlawfulness of a subsequent discharge. If an employee provides an employer with sufficient cause for his dismissal by engaging in conduct for which he could have been terminated in any event, and the employer discharges him for that reason, the circumstance that the employer welcomed the opportunity to discharge does not make it discriminatory and therefore unlawful."

The key words are "sufficient cause for his dismissal." The NLRB isn't likely to look favorably upon a company that discharges a union activist when a lesser form of discipline would be more appropriate.

*Fiske Bros. (98 LRRM 1411).

Benefits During A Strike

When a company and a union settle a strike, they usually backdate the new contract to the day the old one expired, but the problem of how to handle employee benefits retroactively remains. Should workers be paid for holidays during the strike? Should they be able to collect for disabilities that began while they were out?

In general, labor laws say a strike does not terminate the employer-employee relationship. But companies can attempt to negotiate contract terms that hold down retroactive benefits.

Problem areas:

■Holidays. Companies that commonly give holiday pay to workers on layoff may be vulnerable to pressure for holiday pay during strikes. To avoid this, make holiday pay dependent on working the days before and after the holiday unless excused by management. (This allows the workers on layoff to collect, but not the strikers.)

■Vacations. Time of is usually based on years of service. Similarly, vacation pay may increase according to yearly incremental schedules. As a result, in a long strike, employees may make significant gains for time spent walking a picket line. To prevent this, base vacation pay on the previous year's work.

■Salary increases. State clearly whether strikes stop the clock for merit and regular salary reviews. The union will usually demand automatic increases. The company should relate raises to time on the job.

■Disability benefits. A worker will expect uninterrupted coverage from a backdated contract unless an exclusion is written into the new contract. An option is to exclude accident and sickness benefits for a disability that begins during the strike.

What A Strike Costs The Company

The net earnings loss during the stoppage is a poor measure. Just the threat of a strike cuts productivity 2%–12% and causes customers to split orders or demand extra production.

Post-strike costs include loss of trained employees, catch-up overtime, customer defections, and reduced sales effectiveness. Average gross losses during a stoppage: $200 (if there are fewer than 100 production workers) to $300 (500–1,000 production workers) per man-day.

Source: Woodruff Imberman, Imberman and DeForest, Chicago.

Part VI

THE GREAT BOOK OF BUSINESS SECRETS

Executive Life

Chapter 66
Executive Secrets

New Tricks For The Shrewd Traveler

When you arrive at the hotel, check your bags. Then go to the pay telephone in the lobby and call the hotel. Ask to have your reservation confirmed, give them your charge card number and go on your way. In this way you sidestep convention check-in lines.

To avoid the long line after the convention, go down to the desk very early in the morning, before official checkout time, and check out. You won't have to turn in your room key, and you can still use your room until official checkout time (usually around 1 p.m.).

Don't stay glued to your hotel room if you're waiting for a call. If notified, the hotel operator will transfer your calls to another room, interrupt the call you're on for a more important one or hold any calls while you run out for a soda.

Save money by not paying for things you didn't order. Don't charge anything to your hotel room. It's too confusing when you're checking out to verify the list of room charges. And it's only too easy for the hotel to make a mistake. Most travelers just sign and pay without looking at the list. If you don't charge anything at all, you'll know that extra items on your bill can't be yours. How to do it: Pay cash for room service, laundry, etc. Use your credit card for food.

And don't depend only on the hotel for information. If you need a service in a strange city (typing, film developing, etc.), call the local convention bureau. It's specifically set up to help out-of-town businesspeople, and every city has one.

Source: Dr. Barbara A. Pletcher, National Association for Professional Saleswomen, Box 255708, Sacramento, CA 95865.

Safe Way To Fly On Commuter Airlines

Even seasoned travelers often don't realize that commuter airline passengers have much more control over flight operations than do passengers on the big trunk carriers. Strategy: Assume that you and the pilot are the only ones on the plane...even if you're surrounded by other passengers. Commuter pilots have more leeway than you'd think and, according to our sources, are often willing to act on passenger suggestions...as long as they're reasonable and don't jeopardize safety.

Whether you're flying in a 20-seat jet or a two-seat air taxi, there are a few things you can do to increase your personal safety. Some of these steps might cost you time or money, but they can save your life.

■Watch that the pilot checks the plane thoroughly before takeoff. For example, does the pilot take fuel samples?

■Ask about weather conditions. If the skies are cloudy, ask whether the pilot is instrument-rated, whether he is up-to-date on the navigation equipment and whether a flight plan has been filed to allow the plane to be navigated based on instrument readings rather than on visual information. If the answer to any of these questions is no, you are in great peril…especially at night. If at all possible, skip this flight.

■If every seat is full, ask if the plane is too heavy for takeoff…especially on a warm day or when you're taking off from a short runway. Many smaller planes are dangerous if every seat is full.

■Once in the plane, watch the pilot closely while he gets ready for departure. He should be using a checklist and checking everything methodically. Don't trust anything to his memory.

■Once aloft, watch weather. If you hear the pilot talking about thunderstorms with an air traffic controller and the plane's not equipped with radar or a Storm-scope, tell the pilot that you're in no hurry. He can take a longer—and safer—route.

■If you see ice forming on the plane, suggest that the pilot take a rest room stop. (It sounds odd, but it's more common than most people think.)

■If the pilot is flying visually (by sight, not instruments), and it appears that he can't see a good distance, tell the pilot that you'd prefer to discontinue this flight. Other reasons to discontinue: Clouds below the plane…rain…snow…flying low.

■If the pilot tries to entertain you by flying low, making steep bank turns or pulling the plane in for a closer look at something on the ground, insist calmly that he take you back to the airport.

■If an approach and landing are being tried in bad weather, tell the pilot that it's OK with you to land at another airport.

■If fuel gauges appear low or the pilot says he's stretching it, suggest a refueling stop…sooner, not later.

Warning: Commuter airplanes are not governed by the same stringent rules as the large trunk carriers. If your trip requires a change of plane, the second leg of your journey could be on a commuter plane. Option: Consider renting a car or taking a train or bus.

Source: Conversations with pilots, air traffic controllers, consumer protectionists, and government officials.

Stress-Free Flying

Myth: The safest seats on commercial aircraft are those next to emergency exits.

Reality: Aisle seats close to the over-wing emergency exists are safer. These seats are commonly in the mid-front section of the plane. If you sit in the window seat next to an emergency exit, you may be worse off in the event of a crash that jams the exit. Aisle seats near several exits give you more escape options in the event of a crash.

Lifesaving precaution: When you take your seat in the plane, count and memorize the number of rows to the nearest exits. Reason: If smoke fills the cabin after a crash, you may have to feel your way in the dark to an exit. This precaution is based on the tactics that crash survivors actually have used to get out of a plane.

Lifesavers

■For some protection against fire, wear full-length clothing, suits or dresses, made of wool or cotton, sturdy shoes and eyeglasses with an attachable lanyard. Avoid wearing shorts or clothing made of synthetics like polyester which can melt to your body in a fire.

■Women should not wear high-heeled shoes on a plane. They can cause you to trip, and they can snag on the emergency exit slide.

■If the plane fills with smoke, stay low, even if you have to crawl. Two or three breaths of toxic smoke can kill you. If there's enough warning before a crash, place a damp cloth over your mouth in order to breathe through smoke.

■Get as far away from the plane as possible if you're lucky enough to escape it after a crash. People on the ground are often killed when a downed plane explodes.

■Learn how to open the exits by reading the emergency instructions soon after you get on the plane. That's something you don't want to learn as the aircraft bursts into flames.

*800 Independence Ave. SW, Washington, DC 20594. Phone: 202-382-6600.

Source: Chris Witkowski, director, Aviation Consumer Action Project, an advocacy group for airline safety and passenger rights, 2000 P St. NW, Washington, DC 20036. The organization also publishes *Facts and Advice for Airline Passengers*, a booklet that gives more information on safety and consumer rights, ACAP, Box 19029, Washington, DC 20036.

What The Airlines Don't Tell You

■Never accept the first fare quoted. Half the time, some other airline's flight within hours of the one you booked has a special, less expensive deal.

■Take advantage of "illegal" connections. These are connecting flights usually less then 45 minutes apart—that usually do not even show up on the computer when your trip is being routed. Solution: Have your agent write up your flight in two separate tickets. The second is for the illegal connection that originates at your transfer point. To make fast transfers, travel with carry on luggage.

■Use do-it-yourself searches with a CRT. Plug into the Official Airlines Guide data base and search out the flights available at the desired time. Using another code, find out what fares are available on each airline for the time period. If no asterisk is shown, it's possible to book the flight up to the last minute. If there is an asterisk next to the airline flight number, ask the system what the restrictions are.

Source: Harold Seligman, president, Management Alternatives, New York.

How To Cancel Non-Cancellable Tickets

Problem: "Super Saver" tickets cost as little as 30% of regular airfares, but airlines say you can't get a refund if you change travel plans.

Solution: A cooperative travel agent. When you buy a ticket from an agent, the agent makes your reservation immediately. But he doesn't forward your money to the airline for a few days—in some cases not until a week later. That's because agents pay airlines only once a week. During the time gap a friendly travel agent will let you cancel the reservation and get your money back.

■Caution: Travel agents don't have to accommodate you. But if you're a good customer and the agent wants to keep your business, chances are good that you can get a refund.

■Helpful: Check with your agent to see if two round trip, non-cancelable discount fares cost less than one full round trip ticket. Even if you use only half of each of the discount tickets, the cost for both may be less than a full fare ticket.

Source: Harold Seligman, president of Management Alternatives, travel management consultants, Stamford, CT.

Traveler Beware

■Don't fly within 12 hours after dental work. The change in atmospheric pressure can cause severe pain.

■First-class air travel. Not worth the 30% premium unless the flight lasts more than four hours.

■You shouldn't pay the 8% federal tax on airfare if you're flying from one U.S. city to another U.S. city in order to catch a flight to another country. You may have to show the agent the foreign ticket.

■Carry your medical history. Fold a one-page summary of health data into your passport. What it should include: Blood type, allergies, eyeglass prescription, medications currently being taken, any preexisting health condition.

■Don't buy travel insurance at airports. Coverage is much more expensive and rates vary from city to city. Better: Buy directly from insurance company.

■Confirm airlines reservations when the small box in the center of the airline ticket is marked "RO." It indicates that the travel agent has only requested a seat, and wait-listing status is a possibility. A confirmed reservation is indicated by an "OK" on your ticket.

■Avoid consuming all the food and drink offered on airplanes. Alcohol, nuts, soft drinks, and other foods that have empty calories can cause a swing from high to low blood sugar. You go from feeling great to feeling tired, cramped, and headachy.

■Alcohol has more punch during an airplane flight than on the ground. Reason: Body fluids evaporate quickly in the pressurized dry cabin. And, under pressure, the alcohol absorbs more fluids in the intestinal tract, thus making itself felt more quickly. Alternative: To reduce the dehydration of a long flight (six hours or more), drink three or four pints of water.

Reduce Airline Luggage Losses

Buy extra baggage insurance when you check in at the airport. It's called excess valuation. Estimate the value of your bags and their contents. For 50¢–$1.00 per $100 of value, you're insured in case of total loss. You must provide receipts of the contents to collect on a loss. However, the chances of loss are reduced because airlines take extra care in handling bags covered by excess valuation.

Source: *Travel Smart,* 40 Beechdale Rd., Dobbs Ferry, NY 10522.

Smart Alternatives To Traveler's Checks

Credit cards are now better than traveler's checks for most trips overseas. Aside from the cards' convenience, they save as much as 6% on exchange costs. Best bet: Visa and MasterCard, with conversion markups only 1% or less above the wholesale bank currency rate. Other major cards carry a 1% markup—still far better than the 3% or more you'd pay for retail markups on traveler's checks.

Exceptions: Poorer European countries such as Spain, and Third World countries, where dollar-hungry bankers often give a break on traveler's checks or cash.

Recommendation: Check expiration dates of credit cards before you leave on your trip. An unexpected expiration would be a very troublesome surprise. (Leave unnecessary cards—such as those for local department stores—at home

Source: *Forbes,* New York.

Saving On Hotel Bills

Ask hotels for their corporate rate. All chain motels, and many individual hotels, have them. And business people on personal trips can use the corporate rate, too.

As an example, if the range of rates if $45 to $70, the corporate rate might be $50. That means $50 or less, never more, even if the hotel assigns a deluxe room.

Make arrangements in advance, not at check-in time. To be eligible for corporate rates, a few hotels require a minimum number of visits per year. But many give them to any travelers who write for reservations on their companies' letterheads.

Source: *Business Traveler's Report,* New York.

Catch Errors In Your Hotel Bill

Pick a number, from one to nine, when you check in. On all hotel charges, add a tip so that the total comes up with that digit at the end. Example: Using the number 3 as your "control" digit, add a tip of $1.24 to a $7.59 room-service bill. When checking out, anything on your bill not ending with a 3 is an error. If the cashier can't produce a signed charge slip, you don't have to pay.

Source: *California Business Traveler's Bulletin,* 1 Colby Court, Sacramento 95825.

Credit Card Calling

When you have more than one phone call to make from a hotel or pay phone, don't hang up after each call. Push the # button between calls. This will allow you to stay connected with your chosen long-distance carrier. Added benefit: Most hotel computers will register several calls made this way as a single local call, saving you surcharges.

Source: *Travel and Leisure,* 1120 Ave. of the Americas, New York 10036.

How To Get Great Service At Great Restaurants

The best way to get great service at a restaurant is to go there often. Restaurants pay close attention to the customers they see frequently. Recommended: Choose four to six restaurants you really like and develop a relationship with them.

To Start A Great Restaurant Relationship

■Call and speak with the maître d' or owner when you make your first reservation. Tell him/her, "I'm making this reservation because I've heard so much about your restaurant. It's a special occasion, so I'd like to be sure of a good table and good service."

■Dress appropriately. Even if diners wearing torn jeans and sneakers are admitted, they're probably hidden in the back—restaurants like to keep the better-dressed clientele up front.

■Arrive early—especially if you are meeting guests. You want to make sure you like your table. If not, explain, "I don't want to be near the kitchen door. Could we have a nicer table?"

■Be very pleasant, yet firm, about what you want. If something isn't right, ask to see the manager or owner immediately. Then quietly and politely, air your complaint..."We've been waiting quite a long time and no one has taken our order."

Don't let the waiter rush you or talk you into ordering a dish you don't want. Tell him, "We would like to study the menu. If we have any questions, we'll ask."

The same is true of the wine list. If you don't know what to order, ask for suggestions, but be cautious about taking the first one—it will probably be expensive.

■Write a short note of confirmation if you've had to make a reservation far in advance. Say something like, "We are coming on January 20 and are truly looking forward to our meal. I hope we will have one of your better tables." This will help you stand out from the crowd and will also show that you truly care about your dining experience.

What Not To Do

■Don't tip in advance. If you have very good service, you should, of course, tip after the meal...perhaps generously so they remember you. But never walk into a restaurant flashing money—it encourages the wrong attitude. Good service should be natural and forthcoming...you should not have to do anything special to get it.

■Don't feel you have to learn about the cuisine to understand the menu. You shouldn't have to work that hard for a meal.

■Don't be shy about asking prices of off-menu specials. They are usually at the high end of the price range.

The final word on good service: If you don't get it...don't go back.

Source: Mimi Sheraton, the famed restaurant critic and publisher of our favorite restaurant-review newsletter *Mimi Sheraton's Taste*, Box 1396, Old Chelsea Station, New York 10011.

How To Negotiate A Big Raise

The best way to get a sizable raise is to start campaigning for it on the day you're hired. Don't talk dollars then, of course, but it's important to set up standards of performance that will be the basis for future wage negotiations with your new boss. If possible, find out if there are ways you can influence the standards so that your strongest qualities are rewarded.

In gauging the company's position, find out:

■Pattern of raises for your type of job.

■Extent to which pay is part of a fixed budget process.

■How much autonomy your boss has in granting raises.

■Business conditions in the company and in the industry.

Don't let your request be treated in an offhand manner. Make a date with your boss to talk just about money, and if he puts it off, persist.

Key to successful negotiation: Narrow down obstacles until the supervisor is holding back because of one major factor ("Things are tough this year"). Let him cling to that, but in the process make sure he assures you that your performance has been excellent. Then attack the main obstacle ("Are things really that bad?"), pointing out that your capabilities should be rewarded in any case.

Unless you're quite sure of your ground, don't threaten to quit. Even if you are a ball of fire, the boss may welcome your departure because he's scared of you.

Source: *How to Negotiate a Raise* by John J. Tarrant, Pocket Books, New York.

Better Than A Raise

Employee business expenses, along with the cost of investment advice, tax preparation fees, and other miscellaneous items (such as the cost of subscribing to business or investment publications) are deductible, under tax reform, only to the extent that their total exceeds 2% of adjusted gross income. Thus, a person with adjusted gross income of $50,000 can get no deduction for the first $1,000 worth of such items.

When executives have large unreimbursed business expenses, they may do better by negotiating with their employers for an increase in their reimbursements instead of a raise. If the executive gets a raise, it will be taxed, while the executive will lose at least part of the deduction for the unreimbursed expenses. On the other hand, an increase in reimbursements will be tax-free and completely cover the cost of expenses.

Negotiating Your Salary

Guidelines for salary negotiations when job discussions get down to the nitty-gritty:

■Try not to specify a figure. (It will inevitably be lowered.) Get the other person to mention one first.

■Evade the question. If you are asked what you made at your last job, say: "That salary is not especially relevant because the job I was doing was very different from what I'll be doing now. Perhaps if you could tell me what the salary range is, I could say whether it seems appropriate."

■Ask the salary range of workers reporting to you if the company has no established salary range.

■Establish the value of benefits before agreeing on a salary figure.

■Ask for a performance and salary review in six months.

What To Leave Out Of Your Résumé

The style used for writing résumés has changed over the last few years to make them more persuasive and concise. Ultimately, each résumé entry should convince readers that they should hire the writer. What to omit:

■Photos. A picture may let employers form misleading impressions.

■Salary requirements. Why should applicants price themselves out of a job or show that they are a bargain?

■Reasons for leaving jobs. These are better explained in interviews.

■Date of résumé preparation or date available to begin work. Both indicate how long you have been looking for a job. Exception: when looking for seasonal work.

■References or a statement that references are available on request. Instead: List them on a separate sheet and adapt them to each individual employment situation.

■Empty assurances. All applicants think they are good, honest, loyal and healthy workers. Demonstrate these qualities through concrete examples during interviews.

■Vague references to time gaps. Employers look for holes. Explain them in terms of accomplishments. Example: Travel to improve a language capability or research a specific project. Caution: Never claim to have been a consultant without proof.

■Hobbies and outside interests. Exception: Those that relate to professional interest or show traits that an employer wants. Avoid listing any dangerous or time-consuming activities.

Source: *Résumés: The Nitty Gritty* by Joyce Lain Kennedy, Cardiff, CA.

Best Days To Job Hunt

Most job-seekers think Monday is the best day to look for a job because there are more jobs advertised in the papers on Sunday. But jobs advertised on Sunday actually become available the previous Wednesday.

Recommendations:

■Look every day of the week.

■If you have to skip one day, Monday is the best choice. You will not be slowed down by the same hordes of competition on other days.

■The best job-hunting may be when the weather is bad. Again, there are fewer competitors. Management may well believe that the bad-weather candidate is more interested in employment and will work harder with less absenteeism. However, interviewers may be depressed and executives busy filling in for absent staff when the weather is poor.

Source: Robert Half, president, Robert Half International, Inc., New York.

Ways To Take Money Out Of The Company

The tax law creates ways for business owners and top executives to be paid by the company in tax-advantageous ways.

■Interest free loans can be made from the company to owners and top executives. Loans that have been properly drawn up have repeatedly withstood IRS challenges. Key: You must be able to show that the loan is legitimate. So agree to a reasonable repayment schedule, and observe all the legal formalities.

■ Pension pay-outs. The new tax law provides that pensions need not be taken right after retirement. The first pension payments can safely be delayed until at least age 70. Point: Many executives remain active for some years after they retire. They may continue to do special tasks for the company, or act as paid consultants for other businesses. These executives may not need their pension benefits right away. Advantage of waiting: The pension plan account continues to accrue earnings tax-free. So you receive greater benefits when you choose to take them. Review the company's pension plan to be sure it allows a delay in drawing benefits.

■Deferred compensation. The company may not be able to afford a pension plan that covers all employees. But it may still want to provide retirement benefits for top executives. To do it: Set up a deferred compensation plan. This takes the form of a contractual commitment to pay top executives a certain amount after retirement. The payments are deductible by the company when made.

■Stock appreciation rights. Rights may be suitable for some closely held companies. How they work: The executive is treated as if he owned company stock. If the value of the stock goes up by a certain date, the executive receives a payment determined under a pre-arranged formula. The payment may be deducted by the company. Advantages: Managers get an incentive interest in the company that is similar to ownership. But the company avoids increasing the number of its shareholders. Drawback: Incentive amounts that accrue under the plan must be charged against corporate earnings even before they are paid out. So reported earnings are reduced. If the company is sensitive about its reported earnings, this type of plan may be disadvantageous.

Source: Richard Reichler, principal, Ernst & Young, New York.

If You Have To Go To Court

Selecting counsel: The best trial lawyers don't necessarily work for the biggest firms. Many of them are with smaller ones where chances for broad experience are greater. Choose the lawyer, not the firm. Trial law is a specialty. Seek out counsel with trial experience in the field. A local trial attorney who's familiar with the court where the case will be tried is usually best. If represented by a lawyer from out of town, most courts usually require local counsel, too.

Negotiating the fee: Avoid contingency arrangements. A fee based on time spent is safest, but get assurance that rates won't change during period of litigation without prior discussion. Costs quoted can be deceiving. A $40-per-hour fee for a lawyer fresh out of law school is no bargain. Better to pay much more for experienced senior partner who knows how to get work done in one-tenth the time. An hourly rate of $25 for law firm's paralegals is too high if they perform file clerk's job.

Questions to ask: Many law firms have more than one rate for attorney. Are you getting best price? Travel time: How much is charged for day spent away from office? How many hours count as a day? Are you charged for whole day if only part is used for your case? What if the trip is for more than one client? Is there a charge for weekends and holidays if lawyer doesn't work? Tourist or first-class travel? Disbursements: Are secretarial and messenger work handled as disbursement or overhead? How is duplicating of documents in law office charged?

Client's rights: Law firms are a business like any other. It's proper to demand good service, protest excessive costs, keep lawyers on their toes without compromising their professionalism. Ask for litigation plan in advance: Who will do what and when. Hold law firm to it. Counsel in charge of your case should stay with it from beginning to end, supervise internal administration (including billing) as well as represent your company in court.

■Get itemized monthly record of charges with duplicates of all papers drawn up. Record should contain name of everyone in law office working on case, hourly rate, and time spent.

Watch for signs that people already familiar with your company's business are being rotated out and replaced by staff who must be educated at your expense.

■Question overtime closely. Someone's work is being done during regular office hours; why not yours?

Costly delays can pile up when trial lawyers on opposing sides exchange "professional courtesies" to accommodate personal or vacation schedules. Don't accept postponements unless they will clearly help the case.

■Be sure counsel knows enough about your business to handle any questions that may arise in the courtroom.

Trial lawyers tend to be cynical, need to be sold on merits of client's case. The more confident an attorney is that the client's right, the better his performance.

Source: Milton R. Wessel, Esq., New York University.

Lawsuit Guidelines

There are many exceptions, but as a rule: 1. Don't sue for less than $25,000. A lawsuit will cost so much that even if you win, you can only break even. 2. Keep in mind that the legal bills may cripple or kill your company. 3. Remember that if your company is sued by a determined one that's much bigger than yours, your company doesn't stand much of a chance. The legal help your company receives depends on the size of its bankroll—the facts of the case are only incidental. 4. Don't be the first to suggest a settlement. The unreasonable party usually wins.

Source: David W. Swanson, president, Daavlin Co., Box 626, Bryan, OH 43506.

How To Really Read Financial Reports

The growing complexity of corporate finance and recent changes in accounting standards can make it difficult for even the most sophisticated investor to accurately judge a company's health from its financial reports.

However, we have come up with simple ways to translate the increasingly garbled language of financial reports. What we watch:

■Annual reports. Compare the latest report with the two previous ones. Though the chairman's letter usually portrays the company in a positive way, the best way to measure management integrity is to watch what was promised in years past and see how those promises turned out.

If the chairman's letter is so optimistic that he would be better suited to work as a Florida sunny-weather forecaster, beware. Coleco was like this. Management projected nonstop optimism all the way to bankruptcy. Now the company is in Chapter 11. Tipoff: Any glossing-over of obvious negatives.

■Annual and quarterly SEC filings. Study the latest 10K and 10Q reports that are submitted to the SEC. They contain more information than many companies report to shareholders. They're available from the company itself or from the SEC. They're worth reading. The 10Qs, for example, offer the only way to be sure of getting a complete income statement and balance sheet 45 days after the end of a quarter. The SEC documents also contain much more expansive discussion of legal problems, competitive problems and other important developments.

■Proxy statements. They provide information on the salaries, bonuses and stock holdings of the company's officers. Proxy statements also spell out special relationships between, say, company officers and their suppliers. And, intercompany transactions involving financial, operating and other arrangements are often financial red flags.

Example: If the company is leasing warehouse space from one of its officers, we check to see if the rent is out-of-line. In fact, the whole deal may be out-of-line.

■Income statements. Helpful: Pay close attention to income statements in the company's financial reports. Aim: To see how clear the earnings statement is of non-operating items such as deferred income tax credits, sale of assets and interest income. Such earnings are real, but they're not the same as operating earnings. They may not occur again.

Example: A recent accounting change that distorts earnings...the Financial Accounting Standards Board's Statement 96 holds that because corporate tax rates were reduced, companies have to reduce the deferred tax liabilities reported on their balance sheets. This results in deferred income tax credits, which appear on the income statement.

Result: A quick, one-time boost to earnings. Of course this is only a paper entry. It doesn't add to the company's cash flow. But it can create a big bulge in reported earnings for the year.

■Balance sheets. A key element: Debt. How much debt is short-term (due within a year) and how much is long-term? Too much short-term debt can squeeze the company's operating flexibility by hurting cash flow.

For most industrial companies, a balance of 40% debt and 60% shareholders' equity is about right. Above 40% of total capital debt can become worrisome.

In tough times, the interest payments on that debt loom larger in relation to income and the company may have to cut its dividends and/or reduce capital expenditures. That would be bad for the company's future. Top-heavy debt can lead to violations of loan covenants and lower its credit rating.

Under the "Current Assets" column, the two critical items are accounts receivable and inventories. If either or both are rising faster than sales, it's a serious warning.

Important: The trend of inventory levels. If, for example, inventories suddenly jump 15%–20% over the trend line...beware! Watching these signs would have saved investors from big losses in Gap Stores and Crazy Eddie. Latest examples: Reebok and Seagate Technologies, where receivables and inventories are now rising faster than sales.

■Footnotes to financial statements. These tie in with, and further explain, the income statement and the balance sheet. Sometimes, there can be as many as 30 footnotes. And they can be very complex. Always read them, however, because they often contain information you can't get anywhere else. Example: Details about lawsuits against the company which could represent big future liabilities.

Source: Ted O'glove, whose *The Quality of Earnings Report*, is published by Reporting Research Corp., 560 Sylvan Ave., Englewood Cliffs, NJ 07632. The report assists institutional investors in their financial evaluations of corporations.

How To Buy a House With No Money Down

As hard as it is to believe, it's not only possible to buy property with no money down, it's not even that hard to do—provided you have the right information.

Note: No money down doesn't mean the seller receives no down payment. It means the down payment doesn't come from your pocket.

■Paying the real estate agent. If a seller uses a real estate agent on the sale, he's obligated to pay the agent's commission. At the average commission of 6%, that can involve a substantial sum of money. The sale of a $100,000 home, for example, would return to the agent at least $6,000.

Strategy: You, the buyer, pay the commission, but not up front. You approach the agent and offer a deal. Instead of immediate payment, suggest that the agent lend you part of the commission. In return, you offer a personal note guaranteeing to pay the money at some future date, with interest. If you make it clear that the sale depends on such an arrangement, the agent will probably go along with the plan. If he balks, be flexible. Negotiate a small monthly amount, perhaps with a balloon payment at the end. You then subtract the agent's commission from the expected down payment.

■Assuming the seller's debts. Let's say, as so often happens, that the seller is under financial pressure with overwhelming outstanding obligations.

Strategy: With the seller's cooperation, contact all his creditors and explain that you, not the seller, are going to make good on the outstanding debts. In some cases, the relieved creditors will either extend the due dates, or, if you can come up with some cash, they'll likely agree to a discount. Deduct the face amount of the debts you'll be assuming, pocketing any discounts from the down payment.

■Prepaid rent. Sometimes you, the buyer, are in no rush to move in and the seller would like more time to find a new place to live—but you'd both like to close as soon as possible. Or, if it's a multi-apartment building and the seller lives there, he may want more time in the apartment.

Strategy: Offer to let the seller remain in the house or apartment, setting a fixed date for vacating. Then, instead of the seller paying the buyer a monthly rent, you subtract from the down payment the full amount of the rent for the entire time the seller will be living there.

■Satisfying the seller's needs. During conversations with the seller, you learn that he must buy some appliances and furniture for a home he's moving into.

Strategy: Offer to buy those things—using credit cards or store credit to delay payment—and deduct the lump sum from the down payment.

■Using rent and deposits. If it's a multi-apartment building, you can use the rent from tenants to cover part of the down payment.

Strategy: Generally, if you close on the first of the month, you are entitled to all rent normally due from tenants for that month. Therefore, you can collect the rent and apply the sum toward the down payment.

■Using balloon down payments. Arrange to give part of the down payment immediately and the rest in one or several balloon payments at later, fixed dates.

Strategy: This technique gives you breathing room to: 1. Search for the rest of the down payment; and/or 2. Improve the property and put it back on the market for a quick profit.

Caution: This move can be risky if you don't make sure you have a fall-back source of cash in the event that time runs out.

■Using talent, not cash. In some cases you may be able to trade some of your personal resources if you are in a business or have a hobby through which you can provide services useful to the seller in lieu of cash.

Strategy: Trading services for cash is, among other things, very tax-wise. Many working people can provide services in exchange for down payment cash. Most obvious: Doctors, dentists, lawyers, accountants. Less obvious: Carpenters, artists, wholesalers, entertainers, gardeners. Note, however, that bartering produces taxable income, and taxes have to be paid on the value of such services.

■Raising the price, lowering the terms. Best applied when the seller is more interested in the price than in the terms of the deal.

Strategy: By playing with the numbers, you might find that you save a considerable sum of money if you agree to a higher price in return for a lower—or even no—down payment.

■High monthly down payments. If you have high cash flow, this could be a persuasive tactic to delay immediate payment.

Strategy: It's not unusual for a seller to be more anxious for steady cash flow after the sale than for immediate cash in hand. An anxious seller might bite at this offer because it gives him the full price. It also offers you the prospect of turning around and quickly selling the property—since you aren't tying up ready cash.

■Splitting the property. If the property contains a separate sellable element, plan to sell off that element and apply the proceeds to the down payment.

Strategy: Perhaps a portion of the land can be sold separately. Or there may be antiques that are sellable...the proceeds of which can be applied to the down payment.

Source: Robert G. Allen, a real estate insider and author of the bestseller, *Nothing Down*. He's also publisher of the monthly newsletter, *The Real Estate Advisor*.

What To Read Twice In A Real Estate Sales Contract

1. "Mother Hubbard" clause. It is important to have a true description of the property being conveyed. Sometimes there is more than one description of the property because it consists of several tracts of land. There may also be rights to travel over and use adjoining property. To cover this situation a clause may be added to the effect that the seller is conveying any and all property rights owned at a particular location.

2. Certificate of occupancy. The buyer may ask for a current certificate of occupancy to be sure the buildings are in compliance with local laws.

3. Flood areas. If there is any doubt have the seller warrant that the property is not located in a flood-prone area. (If it is in a flood-prone area, don't buy it.)

4. Brokerage fees. It is not cast in stone that either party to a sale must pay the cost of brokerage. This sum can be a wide-open topic for negotiation, and the contract can specify any division of responsibility for payment.

5. Inspection clause. The purchaser may obtain the right to inspect the property at specified times. Often, the purchaser will negotiate the right to inspect 48 or fewer hours before closing, to be sure all is in proper order as indicated in the contract of sale.

6. Condition precedent. The purchaser or seller may want a specific event to occur before the obligation becomes fixed. For example, a purchaser may want the town to approve the building of a new road before the contract binds him to the purchase. Likewise, a seller may require that before the purchaser's rights become fixed there must be a third-party guarantee of the purchaser's payments under the contract.

7. Authorization. If the purchaser is a corporation, partnership, or a representative, the seller may want proof of his authority to close the transaction. The form of such a proof should be determined by counsel.

8. Survey. An accurate survey can be very expensive and either party can be forced to absorb this expense. It is a point of negotiation.

9. Building permits. The seller may be asked to make the sale conditional on the purchaser obtaining necessary building permits within a specified period of time. The buyer may also pay a set sum to have the seller put the sale at risk during that period.

10. Guarantee. The seller may desire the purchaser to obtain a guarantee of payment by a financially sound and acceptable third party.

11. Risk of loss. Damage to the property after signing the contract but prior to the closing can be borne by either party. The seller can be obligated to restore the property or may be able to subtract its loss of value from the purchase price.

12. Title report. Who pays for the title report is another item that is open for negotiation. The name of the title company that performs the work is also a matter for discussion.

13. Assignment. A buyer may want the contract of sale to be assignable. The seller will have to agree that such a substitution can be made.

14. "As is" clause. The seller may allow the purchaser ample time to inspect the property to determine whether it meets his investment needs. At that point, the seller may wish an "as is" clause, stating that he is not making any representations or warranties of any kind.

15. Zoning. The seller may be asked to warrant the zoning applicable to the property. Proof of zoning may be in the form of a letter from the local zoning board showing the present zoning classification.

16. Encumbrances. The title report will examine all the encumbrances on the property, such as mortgages, leases, easements, and restrictions of use. How these items affect value is a matter for negotiation.

17. Title insurance. The cost of title insurance is often a major cash expense at closing. Who pays for this insurance is an appropriate item to bargain for.

18. Time of essence. Unless the contract states that time is of the essence, delays of the closing date by the buyer or the seller may be excused. This clause removes all doubt that the closing must be held on a specified date.

19. Purchaser or seller action. Where either part allows the contract to be contingent on something the seller or purchaser must perform, there should be a clause to assure compliance. Such a clause appears where zoning must be changed, plans must be drawn, tests must be made, inspections must be done, or some other matter affecting the property needs to be taken care of before both parties are satisfied. Sometimes such actions can be on a "best efforts" basis.

20. Mortgage assumption. If the purchaser is assuming an assignable mortgage on the property, the specifics should be detailed. The seller may want more money because the purchaser is obtaining financing below the rates currently available in the marketplace.

21. Property taxes. Most contracts provide for the buyer and seller to divide property taxes and certain other items so that each pays what is owed during his period

of ownership. This process is called proration and will be discussed below. The seller pays property taxes up to the point of closing, and the buyer returns to the seller any prepaid taxes that extend beyond closing.

22. Oil in tank. There is usually an agreement on who owns the fuel at closing. If the seller owns the fuel, the buyer may have to pay for what is there. This can be quite a substantial item.

23. Leases. The seller should provide an accurate statement about the nature, terms, and conditions of each lease. Try to have this statement in the form of a warranty. Also, find out if the leases have been assigned to other tenants.

24. Utilities. The seller can be asked to warrant that there is adequate water, sewer, and/or electric service available to the property.

25. Inability to convey title. If the seller cannot convey perfect title, the buyer may be able to walk away from the contract or else achieve a reduction in the purchase price.

26. Date, time, and place of closing. These should all be established at the contract stage.

27. Breach remedies. If one or the other party breaches the contract, there remain expenses for attorneys, surveys, title reports, and other items. These costs can be assigned to either party or the seller can be entitled to keep the deposit as liquidated damages to pay for them.

28. Notice. The method and timing of notice between the parties should be clearly agreed upon. For example, if one party must secure a zoning change, notice of success or failure is important. That party should be required to mail or deliver notice to a specified place in a set time period.

29. Personal liability. The buyer or seller may want personal guarantees on specific parts of the contract.

There is a significant difference between a firm contract of sale with an unconditional obligation to close at a specified date and a contract of sale with negotiated conditions. The seller must be certain that any conditional item is reasonable before he removes the property from the marketplace. A purchaser, on the other hand, will want to include as many conditions as possible to be absolutely certain the real estate investment is safe and suitable. In all cases, conditions should be clear enough that, by objective standards, they can be met. If this is done, a purchaser or seller who knowingly fails to meet a condition within his control will still be under contractual obligations.

Source: *How to Make Money in Real Estate*, Steven James Lee, Boardroom Books, Springfield, NJ 07081.

Your Real Estate Taxes Can Be Much Lower

Many people pay too much in property taxes year after year without ever realizing it or questioning the system. Yet it is fairly easy to get property taxes reduced.

Statistics show that more than 60% of home owners who challenge assessments succeed. Our own firm's success rate on behalf of clients varies from 70% up to 100% in some counties.

No lawyer is needed to challenge an assessment, and there's no fee. All you have to do is put in the effort.

The savings you reap can become huge over time. Not only do you cut your tax bill every year, but your savings grow each year as property taxes go up on a percentage basis in line with inflation. And, by lowering your tax rate, you increase your home's resale value.

The Big Trap

The key to cutting your tax bill is understanding how the system works. The big trap is that many people believe their homes are assessed at bargain rates. That's because assessed value is typically only a percentage of market value. Thus, a house with a $200,000 market value may be assessed at only $100,000, and the owner may think he's getting a bargain tax rate.

What most people don't know is that property tax is computed by multiplying assessed value by an "equalization ratio" which is determined by the state. If the ratio on a $200,000 house assessed at $100,000 is 2.5, the owner is being taxed on a house value of $250,000 without even knowing it.

Equalization ratios are determined by the state and are applied county-wide or throughout a tax district. The ratios are increased periodically to keep track with inflation and market transactions. But the fixed ratio often can easily be shown to be inappropriate for a particular property. If you can change your equalization ratio, you can cut your tax bill.

Steps To Take

■Analyze your current assessment. Call your local tax assessment office and ask what equalization ratio is used to make the adjustment. Your tax bill may show an assessment at $100,000 but if the multiplier used is 2, then your assessment is really for $200,000. A challenge should be made if your home is actually worth less than $200,000.

■Justify your opinion of market value. Your opinion that the tax assessment is too high is probably right. Tax assessors usually base their assessment on the cost of replacing your home plus the land.

More accurate: A comparison of actual sales of similar homes in your area. This will produce a more realistic (and lower) valuation of your home. Sales prices and information about houses sold are a matter of public record at your local deed recording office.

Write all the information down in an organized format to be presented to the tax assessor. Don't forget to include adjustments for differences between your home's value and a recent local sale due to conditions, location, date of sale, amount of living space, etc.

■Research other assessments. Your property should be assessed at about the same rate as comparable homes in your neighborhood. If yours is higher, you are entitled to a reduction. Get information about other assessments at the assessor's office. (Your neighbors will never know.) All you need to find is three or four homes that are very similar to yours that are assessed at a lower value.

■Challenge the opinion of the tax assessor. Tax assessments are based on the market value of your land and the buildings on that land, in the opinion of the tax assessor. Yet tax assessors rarely have any kind of professional training in this area. Even professionals in the real estate business reach different opinions when valuing property.

■Compare any recent professional appraisals of your home with the assessor's. If you recently purchased your home, you paid your bank to perform an appraisal before it lent you the money. Call your lending officer and ask for a copy of that appraisal. If it's lower than the tax assessor's opinion, use it to show that you are overassessed.

■Hire your own appraiser. Tell the appraiser that you need it for a real estate reduction appeal. Shop around and get quotes from several appraisers. The cost is usually small compared to the amount of tax you will save, especially since a reduced assessment will stay in effect for several years.

■Look for the lowest value. Use anything you can to explain why your property's value is lower than what the tax assessor determined it to be. Put yourself in the place of a buyer who is trying to justify why you should lower the selling price of your home.

Examples: Water in the basement, radon or general deterioration in the condition of your home since the last assessment was made.

Look at the assessor's worksheet. Go to the tax assessment office and ask to see the worksheet that the assessor used for valuing your property. You have the right to see this document. Check to see if the assessor properly describes your home, land, zoning and public services. Check that the numbers of bathrooms and garages are correctly listed.

■Review property descriptions for mechanical errors. Check that the dimensions of the house were measured correctly and that the correct mathematics were used in calculating the number of square feet.

■Look for clerical errors. The amount of the assessment on the worksheet should be the same as the amount on your tax bill.

■Check that personal property wasn't included. Personal property is anything that is easily movable and is not fixed to land. Example: A shed that is not permanently affixed to your real estate. Items that can be removed relatively easily are considered personal property and are not subject to real estate taxation.

■Calmly present your facts. Go the assessor's office and tell the assessor what reduction you want and why. The assessor will probably make an adjustment if you have a good case. If the tax assessor doesn't agree to reduce your assessment, ask for a hearing with the local board of review. These boards have been established to give an impartial opinion. If the board decides against you, you can take your case to a court of law.

Source: Howard J. Udell is president of Property Tax Reduction Services, Inc., 2647 Russell St., Allentown, PA 18104.

Real Estate Income—Tax Free

Substitute for municipal bonds loophole. To get muni-like tax-free income from rental real estate, buy the property with a low enough mortgage so that your deduction for depreciation equals the income the property earns. The lower mortgage interest payments makes the cash flow, up to the depreciation amount, tax-free.

Opportunity: An arrangement of this kind is valuable for taxpayers with Adjusted Gross Income in excess of $150,000 who do not qualify for the $25,000 exception to the passive activity rules.

Reducing The Tax On Mutual Fund Gains

What has always been apparent to tax advisors seems to have escaped the attention of most taxpayers—that the way you keep your tax records can affect the amount of taxes you pay. An example can be found in bookkeeping for mutual fund purchases.

Mutual funds have always been a popular way to invest. Like many other investments, they can produce some nice gains, but when shares are sold it is possible to lose much of the profit through bad accounting. Lots of otherwise clever taxpayers have trouble figuring the tax cost basis of their shares in mutual funds for purposes of calculating gain or loss. That's because fund shares may have been bought regularly over a period of time and because taxable income and capital gains may have been used to buy additional shares. The problem gets worse when shares are switched from fund to fund within a family of funds.

Providentially, IRS regulations offer alternative methods of bookkeeping for those taxpayers who have better things to do than keep track of each separate transaction in each lot of fund shares.

The first averaging method prescribed is the "single category method" and it is quite simple. Every share the taxpayer owns in a particular fund is considered as being in the same pot. Each share's cost basis is the total adjusted cost of all the shares divided by the number of shares in the pot. The second system, the "double category method," divides all the shares in the fund into two pots, one for short-term holdings and the other for shares held six months or longer. Each category is averaged separately as in the single category method. The double category method slides along with the calendar, obviously, and is thus a bit more bothersome. As you can imagine, this method was particularly useful when long-term gains were taxed at favored rates.

To use either of the two cost-averaging methods sanctioned by the regulations, fund shares must be left in an appropriate custody account maintained by an agent.

Then there is the "first-in, first-out," or FIFO, method of accounting. It assumes simply that the earliest shares acquired that are still on hand are the first ones sold.

Even better is to sell the highest priced rather than the oldest shares first in order to reduce that taxable gain on the sale. To accomplish that, you must specifically identify each lot of fund shares by price or date acquired. That way the highest cost shares can be identified and the recognized gain reduced. Equally important, reinvested dividends will not be inadvertently taxed twice, first when they are distributed and immediately reinvested and again when the reinvestment shares are sold along with others with no indication that they cost anything in the first place. It's not easy to maintain all those records, but it is likely to produce lower taxes.

Source: *New Tax Loopholes for Investors*, Robert Garber, Boardroom Special Reports, Springfield, NJ 07081.

How To Get Money Out Of A Mutual Fund...Quickly

Most mutual fund investors don't think about getting their money out of a fund when they put it in. Too often, when financial markets dip and they want to redeem their shares, they find that getting their money back is time consuming, frustrating and sometimes costly.

Reasons:

■The phones are tied up. Mutual fund offices can be so inundated with orders to buy and sell shares that their switchboards may be busy at critical times. When you call requesting information about how to redeem shares, you may have to let the telephone ring for a few minutes before someone answers.

■The procedures for redeeming shares are bureaucratic. With most funds you must not only write a redemption letter requesting a check for the value of your investment, but you must also have your signature guaranteed by a commercial bank or by your broker. That can be time consuming, especially if you bought your shares directly from the fund instead of through a broker, and you don't happen to have an account with a commercial bank. Notarized signatures aren't acceptable and most funds will refuse to accept guarantees from savings and loan institutions. If your personal bank is an S&L, you'll have to go to a commercial bank that your bank has established a relationship with to have your signature guaranteed.

Preventive Measures

To avoid these obstacles:

■Make a copy of the section of the fund prospectus that refers to redemption procedures—and keep it handy. That way you won't have to make a phone call to get information on redemption procedures.

■Prepare a redemption letter in advance. Have your signature guaranteed by your broker or commercial bank so you can simply date the letter whenever you decide to pull out of the fund. Follow prospectus instructions for writing a redemption letter (Usually, all you need to do is request that a check be sent to your home address, and give the number of shares owned and your account number).

■Consider buying shares only in stock or bond funds managed by firms that also have money market funds to which you can switch part of or all of your account by telephone. That way you have access to the money via money market account checks, usually within two days. Caution: It's always a good idea to call in a switch as early in the day as possible, because after 3 p.m. on heavy-volume days, many fund offices can be especially busy.

■When you fill out the forms to purchase fund shares, complete the section for authorizing wire transfers of redemptions to your bank. That service allows you to have shares redeemed and the proceeds deposited directly in your checking or savings account, usually on the same day you make the request. If you need the money fast and you have trouble getting through by phone, you can request a bank transfer in a redemption letter sent by overnight mail.

Source: Sheldon Jacobs, publisher, *The No-Load Fund Investor*, Box 283, Hastings-on-Hudson, NY 10706.

Bond-Fund Traps

Check mutual funds' performance over a period of years, including both up and down markets. Be wary of bond funds' figures. Since there's no standard method of calculating yields, each fund uses whatever system makes it look best. Also be wary of government-securities-fund advertising, which suggests the government "guarantees" the fund's yield. Bonds themselves may be guaranteed, but prices fluctuate with the interest rate.

Source: *U.S. News & World Report.*

Buying Bonds Anonymously

Bearer bonds, although a perfectly legitimate form of debt security, have become a favorite investment for the underground economy. Why: They are a convenient way to stash cash, earn interest on it, and (illegally) hide that income from the IRS. This is possible because bearer bonds are not registered in the purchaser's name. They belong to anyone who possesses (bears) them.

Types of bonds that are bought in bearer form:

■Corporate issues predating the late 1960s. (After that, the Department of the Treasury required corporate bonds to be registered when sold.)

■Treasury notes and bonds (but not Treasury bills).

■Most federal government agency securities (such as GNMAs).

■Virtually all state and municipal issues.

Dangers: If lost or stolen, bearer-bond certificates are, for all practical purposes, impossible to trace and recover. Because there is no name on them, investors risk having someone else (perhaps a family member) cash them in without permission. And if the interest is not declared as income, and the IRS discovers the concealment, the bondholder faces criminal as well as civil penalties.

Scandalous Wall Street "Specials"

One of the more insidious stockbroker-dealer practices is the use of "specials" to dispose of inventory. When a brokerage firm wants to dump an over-the-counter (unlisted) security which it has in its own inventory, it substantially increases the commission it pays to its account executives if they sell it promptly.

Since the security comes out of the firm's inventory, the transaction is called a principal transaction. These are generally done on a net basis. On the confirmation slip that the customer receives, there is no breakdown between the actual price of the security and the commission charged. Result: The customer doesn't really know the exact commission or the stock's precise price. This obfuscation allows the broker to charge a higher price for the security than may be dictated by supply and demand. As a result of this ploy, the firm can afford to give its account executives the higher commissions.

Why is the account executive so eager to sell you a particular security? Does it really fit into your investment program? Does he have a research report recommending it?

There are two main reasons why brokers want to unload stocks in their inventory. They have become disenchanted with the stock's prospects, or the carrying (interest) charges have become excessive. Some firms announce "specials" to the account executives on an almost daily basis.

Safeguard: One of the most important safeguards any investor should employ is to ask his account executive for a research report on any recommendation that is made, even if it is only a brief one.

Confirmation slips should indicate when a brokerage firm is selling stock out of its own inventory by stating that it is a principal transaction. Some brokers, however, merely indicate that the transaction was done on a net basis and that the firm is a "market maker." An investor who sees these terms may have been an unwitting purchaser of a "special" which was sold to him only because his account executive was eager to get a higher commission. In order to mislead clients, some brokerage firms merely put a small code number on the front of the confirmation slip. On the back of that slip, in tiny print, one can find that the code number means that, in fact, a principal transaction was done.

Bottom line: Instruct your broker to always inform you beforehand whether the transaction is likely to be a principal or an agency transaction, which means that the broker is acting as a middleman or on behalf of another investor. Confirmation slips for agency transactions should state separate price and commission charges.

Smart Investments—U.S. Savings Bonds

U.S. Savings Bonds are smart investments for individuals—from both tax and economic points of view. They are exempt from state and local tax. And, they save your children under age 14 from paying the Kiddie Tax if the bond purchases are planned right.

There are two types of savings bonds:

■Series HH Bonds. The purchase price of an HH Bond is equal to its face value and the interest is paid twice a year. This interest is taxable each year.

■Series EE Bonds. The purchase price of an EE Bond is a discount price from its face value. When the bond matures, you can cash it in and receive that face value. You pay tax on the difference between the discount and face value.

Tax opportunity: You decide when to pay the tax on an EE Bond. Choices:

■Year of redemption. You can put off paying any tax until the year you cash in the bond. In that year, you can pay tax on the total appreciation since the year you purchased the bond.

Strategy: Use this method when you intend to hold the bond until a year when you will be in a lower tax bracket, such as after you retire.

■Year by year. You can elect to pay tax on the increased value as it occurs each year, even though you haven't received it yet.

Strategy: Use this method to prevent taxation on a large lump sum in the future. Children who have no other income may benefit by reporting the interest every year.

■After maturity. The original maturity period of U.S. Savings Bonds can usually be extended. If you decide to hold the bond beyond the original maturity period, just continue reporting the interest.

Series EE Bonds can help you escape the Kiddie Tax. By purchasing bonds that mature after the child turns age 14, all the income from the bond will be taxed at the child's tax rate when he/she cashes the bond in and pays the tax after age 14, regardless of the amount of his/her investment income.

Caution: Don't make the mistake of thinking that by purchasing a bond in your name and your child's name as co-owners you will shift income to your child. Interest on the bond is taxable to you if you bought it, even if you let your child cash it in and keep the total value.

Similarly, don't make the mistake of thinking that by transferring a co-owned bond into your child's name alone you will shift income successfully. You will have to report and pay tax on all the interest earned up until the date of the transfer on your tax return.

Instead of cashing in an EE Bond at maturity, you can convert it into an HH Bond. Advantage: The appreciation of the bond while it was still an EE Bond remains tax deferred until you cash in the HH Bond. However, since HH Bonds pay you interest every year, you will have to pay tax on this interest every year.

Source: Richard J. Shapiro, national director of taxes, Spicer & Oppenheim, CPAs, 7 World Trade Center, New York 10048.

Personal Bankruptcy Advantage

Tax considerations are hardly ever the main reason an individual files for bankruptcy. But the tax aspects of personal bankruptcy can be very favorable, especially for taxpayers who are heavily in debt to their employers or to their own closely held corporations. Main benefit:

■Cancellation of indebtedness. As a general rule, when a debt is forgiven, the debtor must report the amount forgiven as income. But a debt cancelled in bankruptcy is not treated as income.

Example: An individual had credit card charges of $10,000 last year. This year the credit card debt is discharged in bankruptcy. If any of the credit card charges were previously deducted (e.g., a business entertainment deduction) they would have to be reported as income. But the other part of the discharged debt wouldn't have to be reported.

Example: Five years ago, an individual borrowed heavily from his closely held corporation. For other reasons business is now so bad that the corporation must file for bankruptcy. If the individual also declares bankruptcy and the loan is discharged, he has a big tax windfall. He will not have to pick up the money he borrowed from the company as income.

Source: Edward Mendlowitz, Siegel, Mendlowitz & Rich, CPAs, New York 10017.

How To Beat The Banks Before They Beat You

Since deregulation, banks vary widely in their services and in the costs of those services. In order to turn the best profit, banks depend on the fact that customers don't know what to ask for. How you can get the most for your banking dollar:

Deal with the smallest bank you can find. After deregulation, most large banks decided to get rid of smaller depositors. They find it cheaper to serve one corporate account than 10 individual accounts. Smaller banks, on the other hand, are more responsive to individual depositors because they need this business.

Ask about checking accounts.

■What is the minimum-balance requirement? How does the bank calculate it? Watch out for a minimum-balance calculation that uses the lowest balance for the month. A figure based on the average daily balance is best.

■Does the balance on other accounts count toward the checking-account minimum balance?

■What is the clearing policy for deposits? This is especially important if you have a NOW account. Most banks hold checks 10 to 14 days, which means you lose interest and may be stuck with overdrafts.

■What is the overdraft charge? Often it is outrageous. In parts of the Midwest, for example, most banks charge $20.

Source: Edward F. Mrkvicka Jr., president, Reliance Enterprises, Inc., Marengo, IL 60152.

THE GREAT BOOK
OF BUSINESS SECRETS

Index